CLINICAL ANATOMY

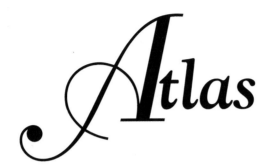
Atlas

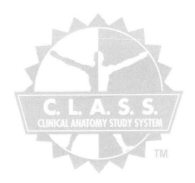
C.L.A.S.S.
CLINICAL ANATOMY STUDY SYSTEM
TM

OTHER PRODUCTS IN THE
CLINICAL ANATOMY STUDY SYSTEM

Clinical Anatomy Principles
Clinical Anatomy Dissections
Clinical Anatomy Interactive Lesson
Clinical Anatomy Interactive Lab Practical

CLINICAL ANATOMY

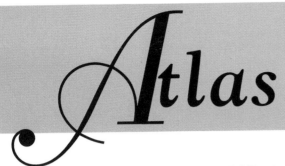

Atlas

ROBERT A. CHASE, M.D.
Emile Holman Professor Emeritus
Department of Surgery
Division of Human Anatomy
Stanford University School of Medicine
Stanford, California

JOHN A. GOSLING, M.D.
Professor, Division of Human Anatomy
Stanford University School of Medicine
Stanford, California
Professor and Chairman
Department of Anatomy
The Chinese University of Hong Kong
Hong Kong, China

JOHN DOLPH, M.A.
Lecturer, Division of Human Anatomy
Stanford University School of Medicine
Stanford, California

ERIC F. GLASGOW, M.D.
Professor, Division of Human Anatomy
Stanford University School of Medicine
Stanford, California
Honorary Professorial Fellow
Department of Anatomy
Monash University
Melbourne, Australia

LAWRENCE H. MATHERS, JR., M.D., PH.D.
Chief, Division of Human Anatomy
Associate Professor of Pediatrics and Surgery (Human Anatomy)
Stanford University School of Medicine
Stanford, California

with 603 illustrations

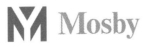 Mosby

St. Louis Baltimore Boston Carlsbad Chicago Naples New York Philadelphia Portland
London Madrid Mexico City Singapore Sydney Tokyo Toronto Wiesbaden

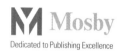
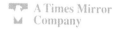

Editor: Emma D. Underdown
Editorial Assistant: Alicia E. Moten
Project Manager: John Rogers
Senior Production Editors: Helen Hudlin, Kathleen Teal
Designer: Dave Zielinski
Design Coordinator: Renée Duenow
Manufacturing Manager: Theresa Fuchs
Photography for cover image and section openers: John Phelan

Printed in the United States of America
Composition by Black Dot
Printing/binding by W. C. Brown Communications, Inc.

Mosby–Year Book, Inc.
11830 Westline Industrial Drive
St. Louis, Missouri 63146

ISBN 08151-4012-6

95 96 97 98 99 / 9 8 7 6 5 4 3 2 1

To students of medicine
who through many years have contributed to mutual learning
and strategies for acquiring and remembering
the critically important details of human anatomy.
It is their desire to understand human structure and function
that kindles our spirit both to teach and to learn.

Preface

Dissection in the laboratory offers students an opportunity to explore the human body in a way they have never before been able to do. While this opportunity is a privilege, it is also a very daunting task. The purpose of the *Clinical Anatomy Atlas* is to assist students who are learning anatomy to better understand what they are searching for in their laboratory quest.

The dissection photographs in this text have been carefully chosen to present the important structures from surface anatomy to deeper layers and tissues. Labels directly on the photographs help the student to quickly identify structures. We firmly believe that the lessons acquired from laboratory experience are best learned in the context of how they relate to the living person. Thus, throughout the *Atlas,* we have included clinical highlights to reinforce the relationships of normal anatomy to medical practice.

This atlas can be used alone as a laboratory aid or can accompany a textbook of anatomy in a curriculum that does not include a dissection laboratory. However, its most efficient use is as an integral part of the Clinical Anatomy Study System (C.L.A.S.S.). The *Clinical Anatomy Atlas* is cross-referenced to the *Clinical Anatomy Dissections* and vice versa; thus students in a laboratory can very quickly relate their dissection to a professionally completed one. The *Clinical Anatomy Atlas* is also closely correlated to the *Clinical Anatomy Principles* and offers color photographs to accompany the color drawings in that text. The *Clinical Anatomy Interactive Lab Practical* is another component in the study system that the student will find particularly useful in preparing for laboratory and class examinations. Finally, the individual foci of each of the texts are brought together in the *Clinical Anatomy Interactive Lesson,* a CD-ROM tutorial complete with text, illustrations, and animations.

ACKNOWLEDGEMENTS

We are deeply indebted to the team of anatomists responsible for producing *Human Anatomy: Text and Colour Atlas,* edition 2, by J.A. Gosling, P.F. Harris, J.R. Humpherson, I. Whitmore, and P.L.T. Willan. Many of the images in this text were photographed from their dissections by A.L. Bentley and J.L. Hargreaves. We are also grateful to the late Dr. David Bassett, author of the *Stereoscopic Atlas of Human Anatomy.* The Bassett stereo views were produced by the renowned Viewmaster inventor and stereo photographer, William B. Gruber.

Our profound thanks go to Emma Underdown, our Editor; to Helen Hudlin and Kathleen Teal, our Production Editors; and to their dedicated staff at Mosby.

Robert A. Chase, M.D.
John A. Gosling, M.D.
John Dolph, M.A.
Eric F. Glasgow, M.D.
Lawrence H. Mathers, Jr., M.D., Ph.D.

Stanford, California

Contents

Pelvis and Perineum

Lower Limb

CLINICAL ANATOMY

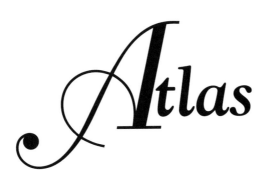

Atlas

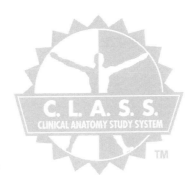

SECTION ONE

Thorax

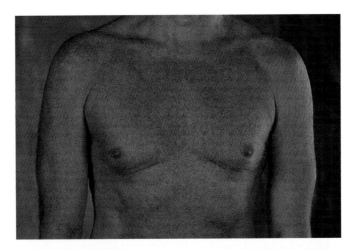

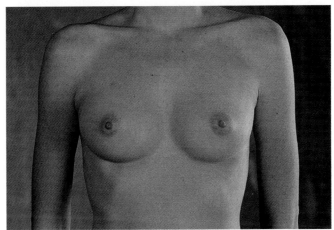

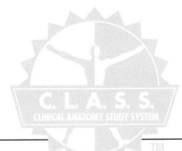

SEE **PRINCIPLES**, FIG. 1-1

1st rib   1st & 2nd   1st thoracic   Thoracic   Manubriosternal
            costal cartilages vertebra   inlet   Manubrium   joint

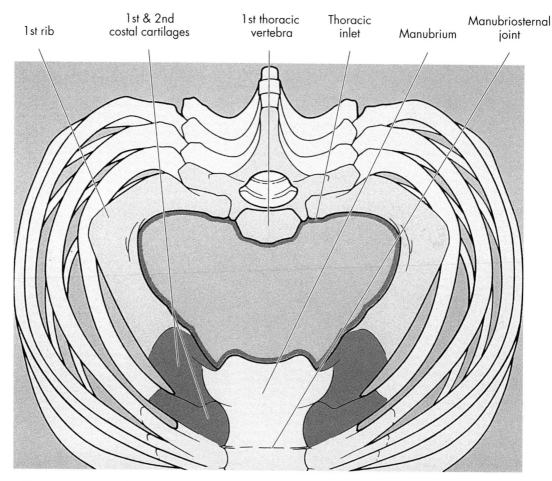

Figure 1-1   Boundaries of the thoracic inlet. *Structures passing from the thoracic outlet and cervical area to the upper limb may be compressed at the site of attachment of the scalenus anterior muscle to the first rib, in the interval between the first rib and clavicle, or where the pectoralis minor lies superficial to these structures. Sometimes a vestigial rib and its continuation as a fibrous cord originates at the C7 vertebrae. It may be asymptomatic and discovered by chance on routine chest x-ray. Alternately, it may cause angulation of vessels and nerves from the thoracic outlet to the upper limb (thoracic outlet syndrome).*

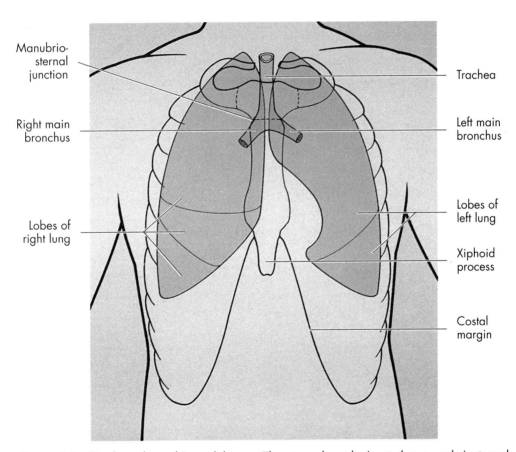

Figure 1-2 Trachea, bronchi, and lungs. The sternal angle is at the manubriosternal junction, the surface landmark used to identify the second rib cartilage and the T4-T5 vertebral level.

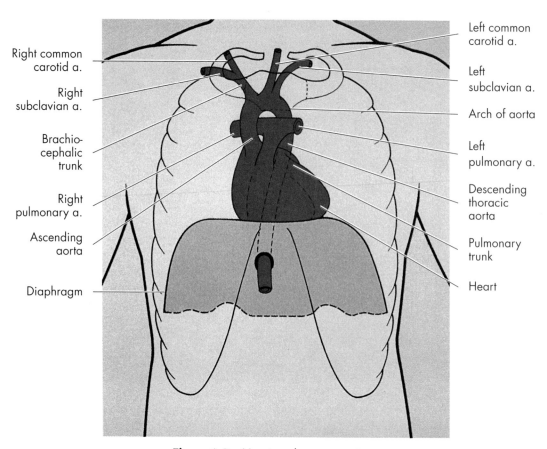

Right common
carotid a.

Right
subclavian a.

Brachio-
cephalic
trunk

Right
pulmonary a.

Ascending
aorta

Diaphragm

Left common
carotid a.

Left
subclavian a.

Arch of aorta

Left
pulmonary a.

Descending
thoracic
aorta

Pulmonary
trunk

Heart

Figure 1-3   Heart and great arteries.

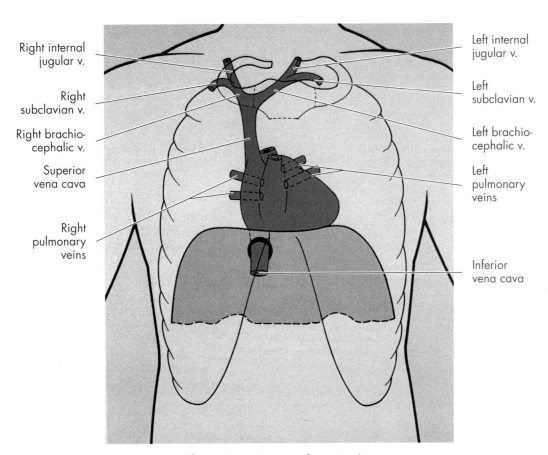

Right internal
jugular v.

Right
subclavian v.

Right brachio-
cephalic v.

Superior
vena cava

Right
pulmonary
veins

Left internal
jugular v.

Left
subclavian v.

Left brachio-
cephalic v.

Left
pulmonary
veins

Inferior
vena cava

Figure 1-4   Heart and great veins.

SEE PRINCIPLES, FIG. 1-1

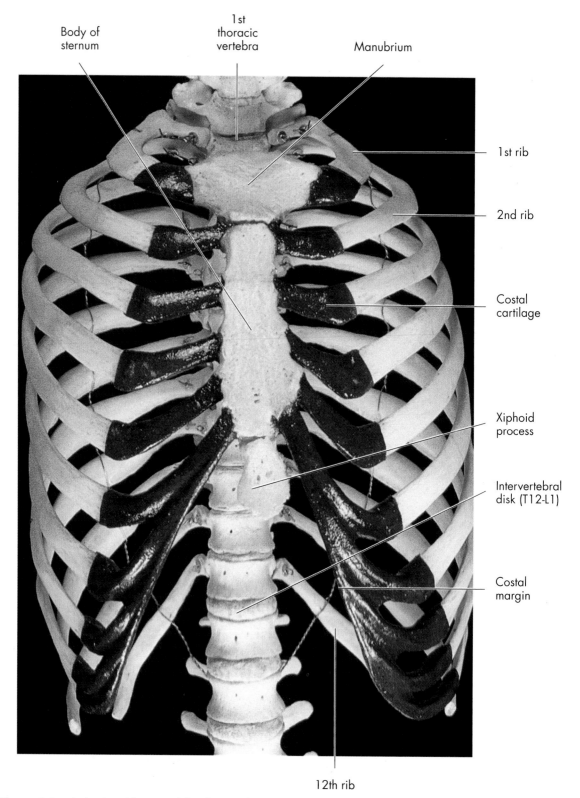

Figure 1-5　Articulated bones of the thorax showing the relationships between the vertebral column, ribs, costal cartilages, and sternum.

SEE PRINCIPLES, FIGS. 1-12, 1-14

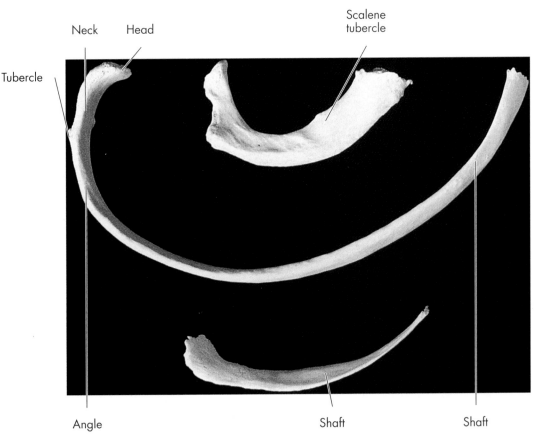

Figure 1-6   First, seventh, and twelfth ribs showing their surface features and relative sizes.

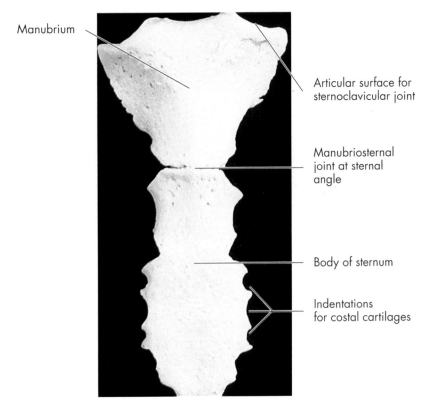

Figure 1-7   Manubrium and body of the sternum. The xiphoid process is absent.

SEE PRINCIPLES, FIG. 1-6

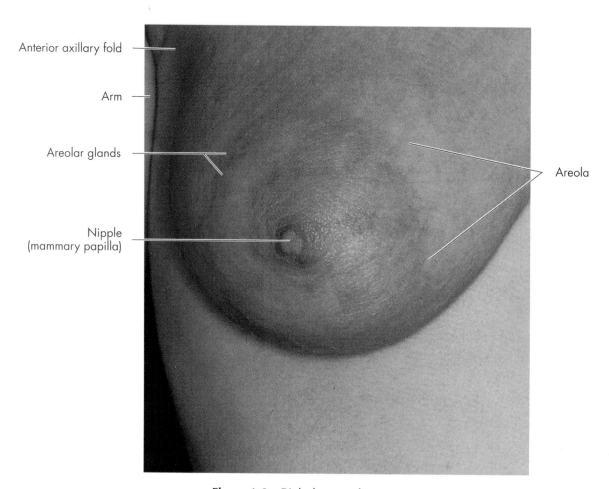

Anterior axillary fold

Arm

Areolar glands

Nipple
(mammary papilla)

Areola

Figure 1-8   Right breast of a young woman.

See **DISSECTIONS**, Section 1, p. 2
See **PRINCIPLES**, Fig. 1-6

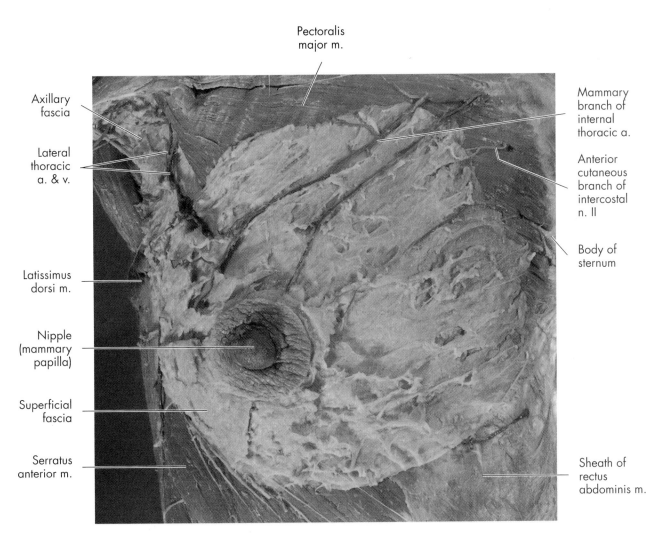

Pectoralis
major m.

Axillary
fascia

Lateral
thoracic
a. & v.

Latissimus
dorsi m.

Nipple
(mammary
papilla)

Superficial
fascia

Serratus
anterior m.

Mammary
branch of
internal
thoracic a.

Anterior
cutaneous
branch of
intercostal
n. II

Body of
sternum

Sheath of
rectus
abdominis m.

Figure 1-9   Right female breast dissected in situ.

SEE PRINCIPLES, FIG. 1-25

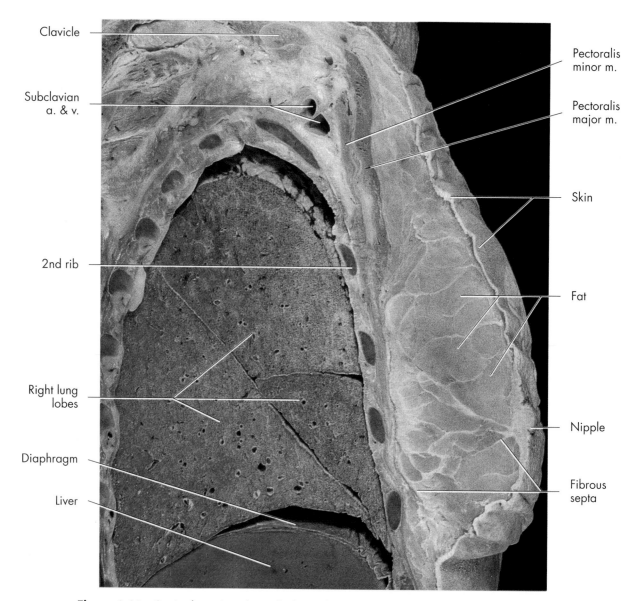

Clavicle

Subclavian
a. & v.

2nd rib

Right lung
lobes

Diaphragm

Liver

Pectoralis
minor m.

Pectoralis
major m.

Skin

Fat

Nipple

Fibrous
septa

Figure 1-10   Sagittal section through the right breast and underlying chest wall. In this dissection, the glandular structure of the breast cannot be distinguished. *About one in ten women will develop cancer of the breast during her lifetime. Such tumors most commonly spread via lymphatics in the axilla and clavicular area. Cancer in the medial half of the breast may spread to the internal mammary (internal thoracic) chain of nodes found adjacent to the internal thoracic blood vessels. Surgery for removal of the breast (mastectomy) requires the surgeon to know the anatomy of blood vessels to the breast. Branches from intercostal vessels, lateral thoracic branches of the axillary artery and vein, and perforating branches from the internal thoracic vessels are primary sources of blood supply to the breast.*

See DISSECTIONS, Section 1, p. 2
See PRINCIPLES, Fig. 1-17

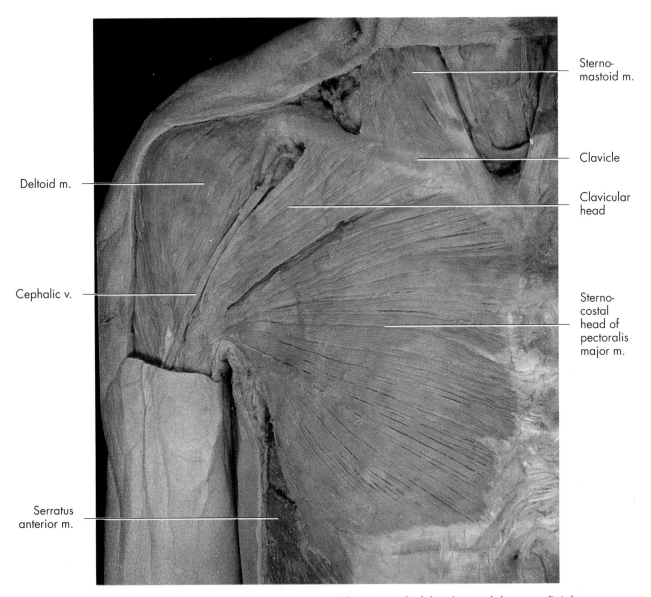

Figure 1-11   Pectoralis major muscle revealed by removal of the skin and the superficial and deep fascia.

See DISSECTIONS, Section 1, p. 2
See PRINCIPLES, Fig. 1-17

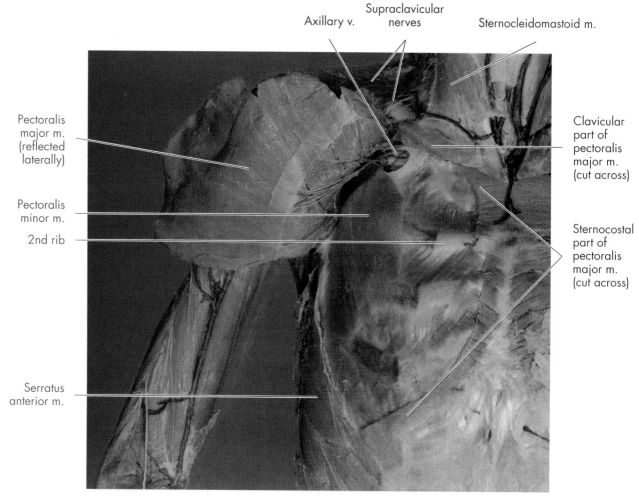

Axillary v.   Supraclavicular nerves   Sternocleidomastoid m.

Pectoralis major m. (reflected laterally)

Clavicular part of pectoralis major m. (cut across)

Pectoralis minor m.

2nd rib

Sternocostal part of pectoralis major m. (cut across)

Serratus anterior m.

Figure 1-12   Left pectoralis major muscle has been reflected. Its clavicular, sternocostal and abdominal origins have been preserved. The pectoralis minor is covered by a layer of the clavipectoral fascia.

SEE DISSECTIONS, SECTION 1, P. 3
SEE PRINCIPLES, FIG. 1-15, TABLE 1-2

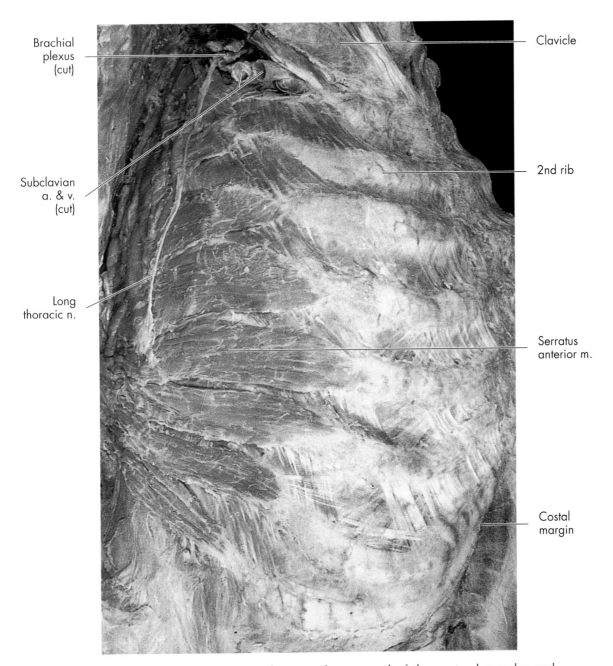

Brachial
plexus
(cut)

Clavicle

Subclavian
a. & v.
(cut)

2nd rib

Long
thoracic n.

Serratus
anterior m.

Costal
margin

Figure 1-13 Serratus anterior muscle seen after removal of the pectoral muscles and displacement of the scapula backwards.

14   **Clinical Anatomy Atlas**

SEE DISSECTIONS, SECTION 1, P. 3
SEE PRINCIPLES, FIG. 1-15, TABLE 1-2

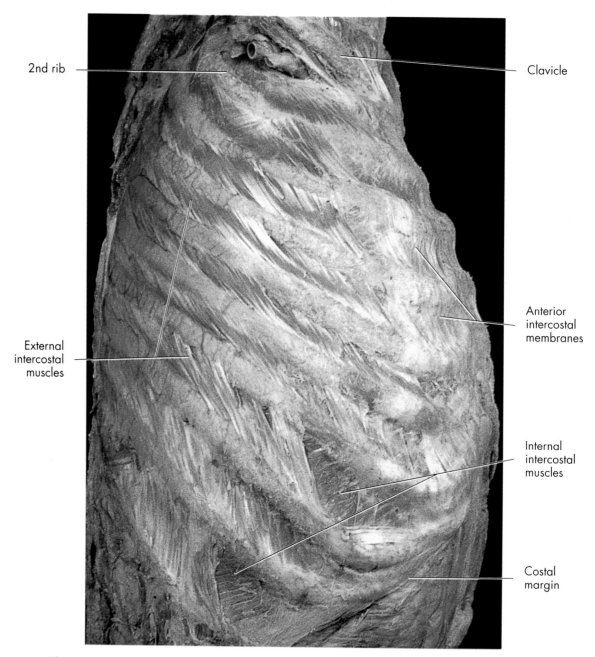

2nd rib

Clavicle

External
intercostal
muscles

Anterior
intercostal
membranes

Internal
intercostal
muscles

Costal
margin

Figure 1-14   External intercostal muscles exposed by removal of the upper limb and the serratus anterior.

See **DISSECTIONS, Section 1, p. 3**
See **PRINCIPLES, Fig. 1-15, Table 1-2**

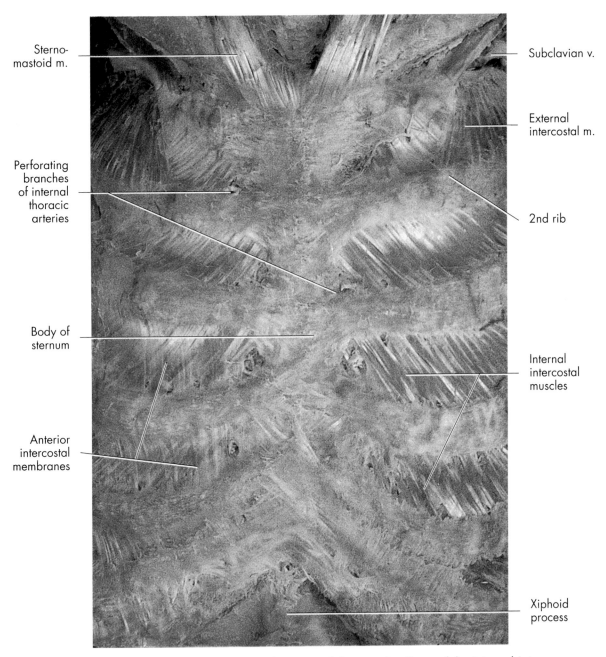

Sterno-
mastoid m.

Subclavian v.

External
intercostal m.

Perforating
branches
of internal
thoracic
arteries

2nd rib

Body of
sternum

Internal
intercostal
muscles

Anterior
intercostal
membranes

Xiphoid
process

Figure 1-15   Anterior intercostal membranes and the anterior fibers of the internal intercostal muscles.

SEE DISSECTIONS, SECTION 1, P. 3
SEE PRINCIPLES, FIG. 1-15, TABLE 1-2

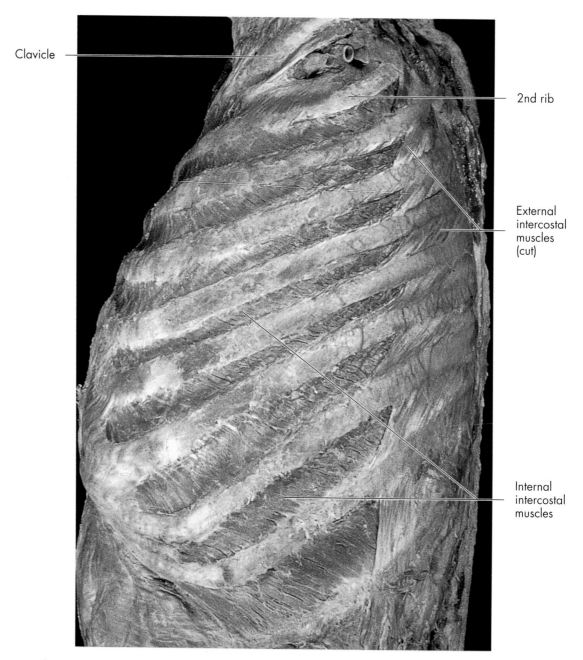

Clavicle

2nd rib

External
intercostal
muscles
(cut)

Internal
intercostal
muscles

Figure 1-16   Internal intercostal muscles exposed by removal of the anterior parts of the external intercostal muscles.

See DISSECTIONS, Section 1, p. 3
See PRINCIPLES, Fig. 1-15, Table 1-2

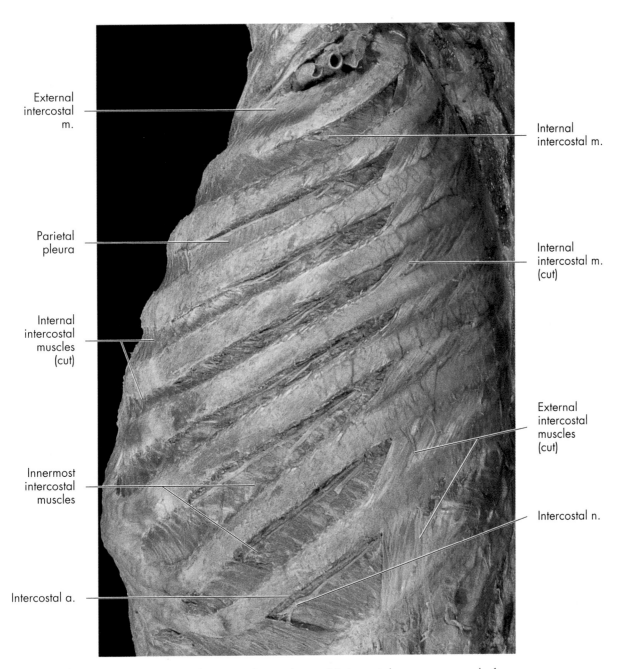

External
intercostal
m.

Parietal
pleura

Internal
intercostal
muscles
(cut)

Innermost
intercostal
muscles

Intercostal a.

Internal
intercostal m.

Internal
intercostal m.
(cut)

External
intercostal
muscles
(cut)

Intercostal n.

Figure 1-17 Innermost intercostal muscles and intercostal nerves exposed after removing parts of the internal intercostal muscles. In the third intercostal space, the innermost intercostal muscle has been removed to expose the parietal pleura.

See **DISSECTIONS**, Section 1, p. 3

See **PRINCIPLES**, Fig. 1-22

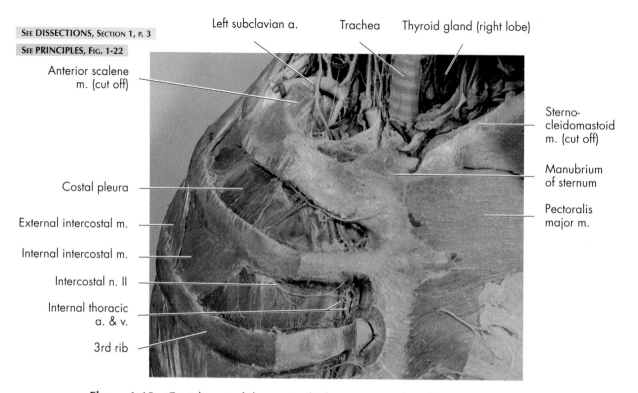

Left subclavian a.   Trachea   Thyroid gland (right lobe)

Anterior scalene m. (cut off)

Sterno-cleidomastoid m. (cut off)

Manubrium of sternum

Pectoralis major m.

Costal pleura

External intercostal m.

Internal intercostal m.

Intercostal n. II

Internal thoracic a. & v.

3rd rib

Figure 1-18 Costal part of the parietal pleura exposed in the anterior portions of the first and second intercostal spaces. Some structures related to the thoracic inlet are visible.

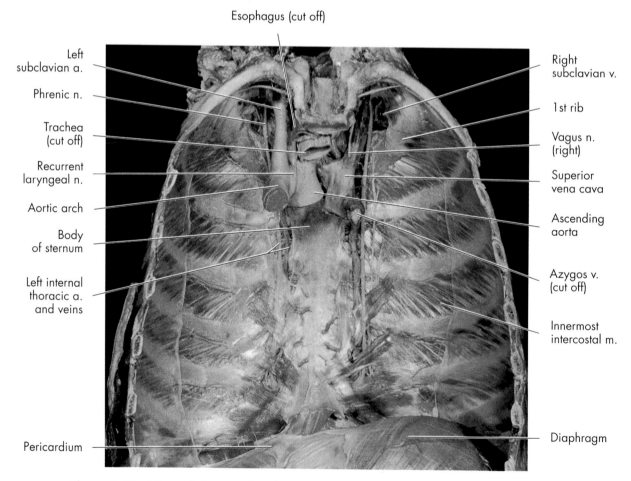

Esophagus (cut off)

Left subclavian a.

Phrenic n.

Trachea (cut off)

Recurrent laryngeal n.

Aortic arch

Body of sternum

Left internal thoracic a. and veins

Pericardium

Right subclavian v.

1st rib

Vagus n. (right)

Superior vena cava

Ascending aorta

Azygos v. (cut off)

Innermost intercostal m.

Diaphragm

Figure 1-19 View of the anterior thoracic wall from within. All the thoracic viscera have been removed except those structures that pass through the superior thoracic aperture (thoracic inlet). The pleura and endothoracic fascia have been excised.

See DISSECTIONS, Section 1, p. 4
See PRINCIPLES, Fig. 1-21

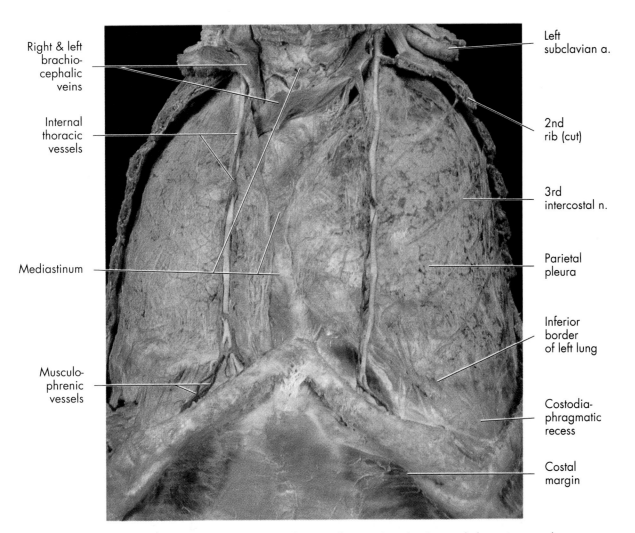

Right & left brachio-cephalic veins

Internal thoracic vessels

Mediastinum

Musculo-phrenic vessels

Left subclavian a.

2nd rib (cut)

3rd intercostal n.

Parietal pleura

Inferior border of left lung

Costodia-phragmatic recess

Costal margin

Figure 1-20   Removal of the anterior chest wall exposing the internal thoracic vessels and costal part of the parietal pleura, through which the lungs are visible.

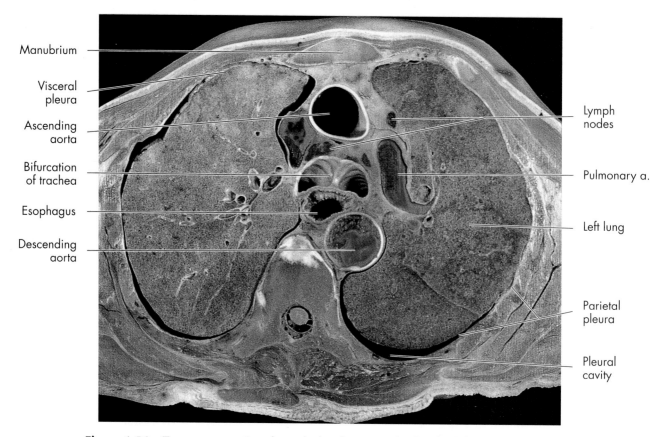

Manubrium

Visceral
pleura

Ascending
aorta

Bifurcation
of trachea

Esophagus

Descending
aorta

Lymph
nodes

Pulmonary a.

Left lung

Parietal
pleura

Pleural
cavity

Figure 1-21   Transverse section through the thorax at the level of the tracheal bifurcation and the fourth thoracic vertebra, viewed from inferior to superior.

See DISSECTIONS, Section 1, p. 4
See PRINCIPLES, Fig. 1-24

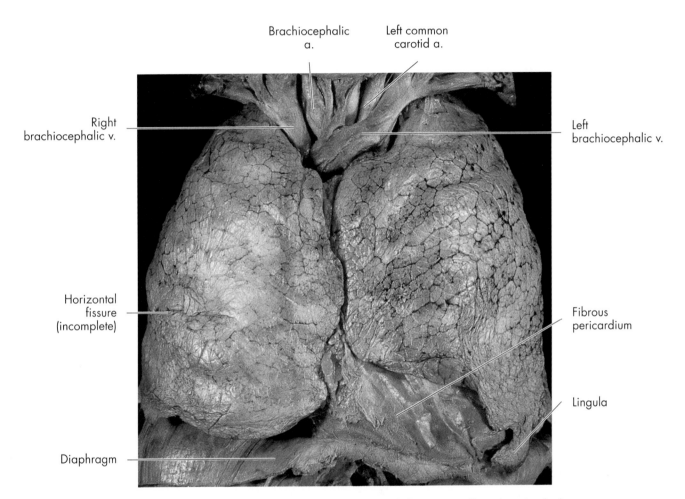

Brachiocephalic a.

Left common carotid a.

Right brachiocephalic v.

Left brachiocephalic v.

Horizontal fissure (incomplete)

Fibrous pericardium

Lingula

Diaphragm

Figure 1-22 Lungs after removal of the anterolateral thoracic wall and parietal pleura. In this specimen the lungs overlie more of the mediastinum than is usual.

SEE **DISSECTIONS**, SECTION 1, P. 4

SEE **PRINCIPLES**, FIG. 1-25

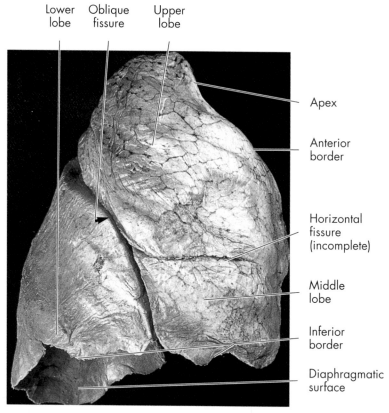

Figure 1-23   Costal surface of the right lung showing oblique and horizontal fissures and the upper, middle, and lower lobes.

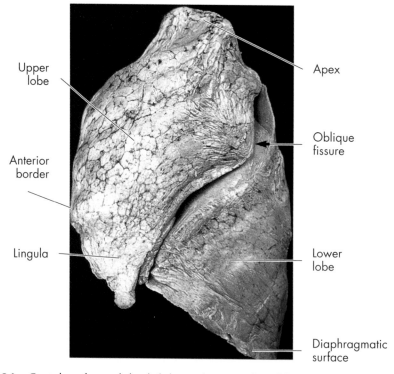

Figure 1-24   Costal surface of the left lung showing the oblique fissure and upper and lower lobes.

See **DISSECTIONS, Section 1, p. 4**
See **PRINCIPLES, Fig. 1-25**

Horizontal fissure
(incomplete)

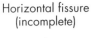

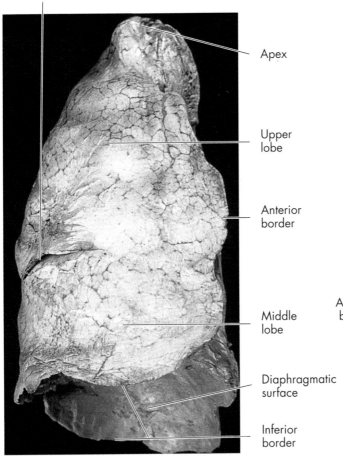

Apex

Upper
lobe

Anterior
border

Middle
lobe

Diaphragmatic
surface

Inferior
border

Figure 1-25   Right lung showing its concave inferior
surface and sharp anterior and inferior borders.

Anterior
border

Apex

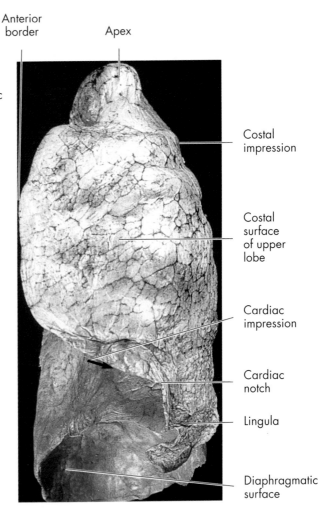

Costal
impression

Costal
surface
of upper
lobe

Cardiac
impression

Cardiac
notch

Lingula

Diaphragmatic
surface

Figure 1-26   Left lung showing the cardiac notch and
lingula, both of which are particularly prominent in
this specimen.

See DISSECTIONS, Section 1, p. 4
See PRINCIPLES, Fig. 1-25

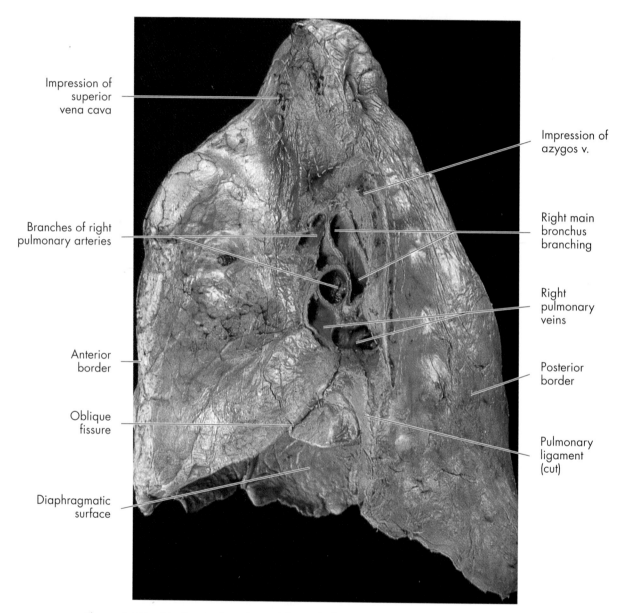

Impression of
superior
vena cava

Impression of
azygos v.

Branches of right
pulmonary arteries

Right main
bronchus
branching

Right
pulmonary
veins

Anterior
border

Posterior
border

Oblique
fissure

Pulmonary
ligament
(cut)

Diaphragmatic
surface

Figure 1-27   Mediastinal surface of the right lung, showing the hilum lying close to the rounded posterior border.

See **DISSECTIONS**, Section 1, p. 4

See **PRINCIPLES**, Fig. 1-25

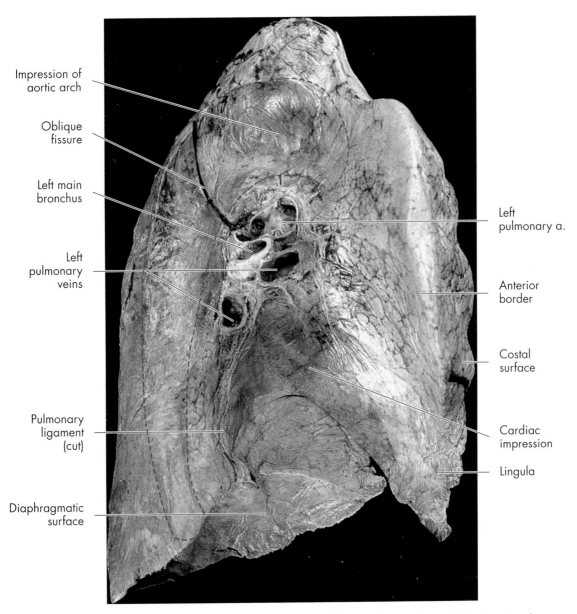

Impression of
aortic arch

Oblique
fissure

Left main
bronchus

Left
pulmonary
veins

Pulmonary
ligament
(cut)

Diaphragmatic
surface

Left
pulmonary a.

Anterior
border

Costal
surface

Cardiac
impression

Lingula

Figure 1-28   Mediastinal surface of the left lung, showing impressions of the heart and aorta.

SEE PRINCIPLES, FIG. 1-27

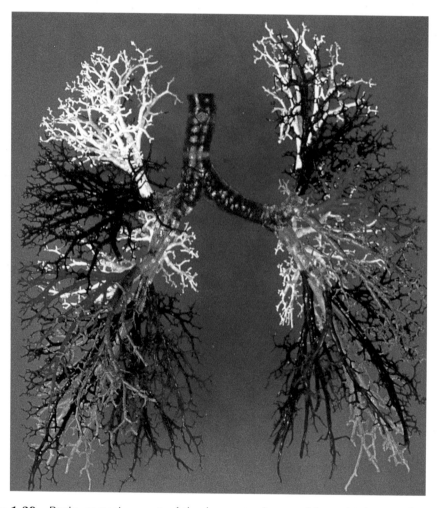

Figure 1-29   Resin corrosion cast of the lower trachea and bronchial tree. The amber portions of the specimen relate to the trachea, the main (primary) bronchi, and the lobar (secondary) bronchi, while the colored portions are the segmental (tertiary) bronchi and their branches. *Removal of a whole lung (pneumonectomy), a single lobe (lobectomy), or a single segment (segmental resection) at surgery requires an intimate knowledge of the relationships of bronchi, arteries, veins, and lymphatics. In addition, a knowledge of associated mediastinal structures, such as the phrenic nerves, the pulmonary arteries and veins, and the pericardium, is very important.*

SEE PRINCIPLES, FIG. 1-54

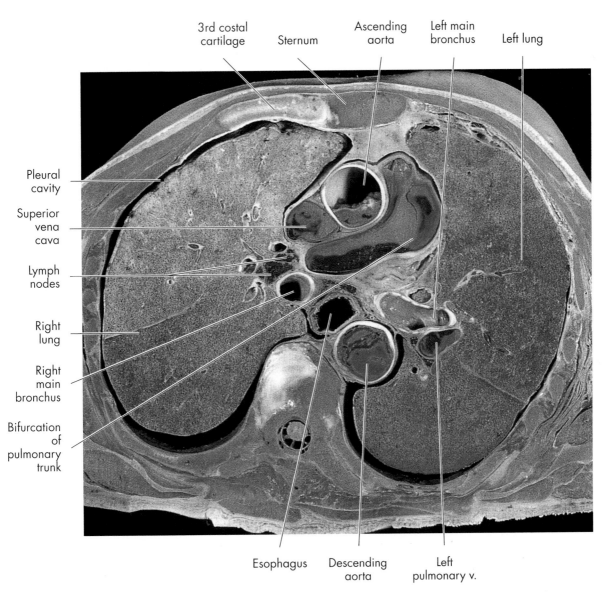

Figure 1-30 Transverse section through the thorax at the level of the fifth thoracic vertebra looking from inferior to superior.

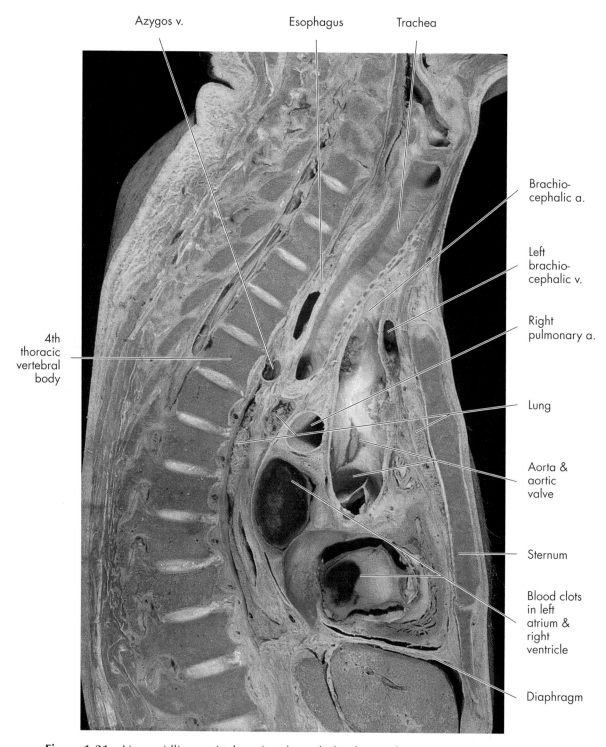

Azygos v.   Esophagus   Trachea

Brachio-
cephalic a.

Left
brachio-
cephalic v.

Right
pulmonary a.

4th
thoracic
vertebral
body

Lung

Aorta &
aortic
valve

Sternum

Blood clots
in left
atrium &
right
ventricle

Diaphragm

Figure 1-31   Near-midline sagittal section through the thorax showing some mediastinal structures.

See **DISSECTIONS**, **Section 1**, p. 5
See **PRINCIPLES**, Fig. 1-37

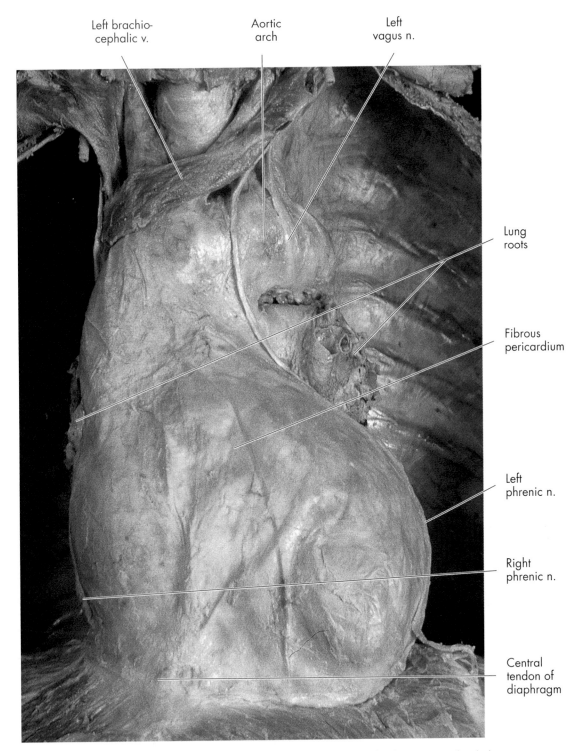

Figure 1-32 Fibrous pericardium and phrenic nerves revealed after removal of the lungs.

See DISSECTIONS, Section 1, p. 5

See PRINCIPLES, Fig. 1-33

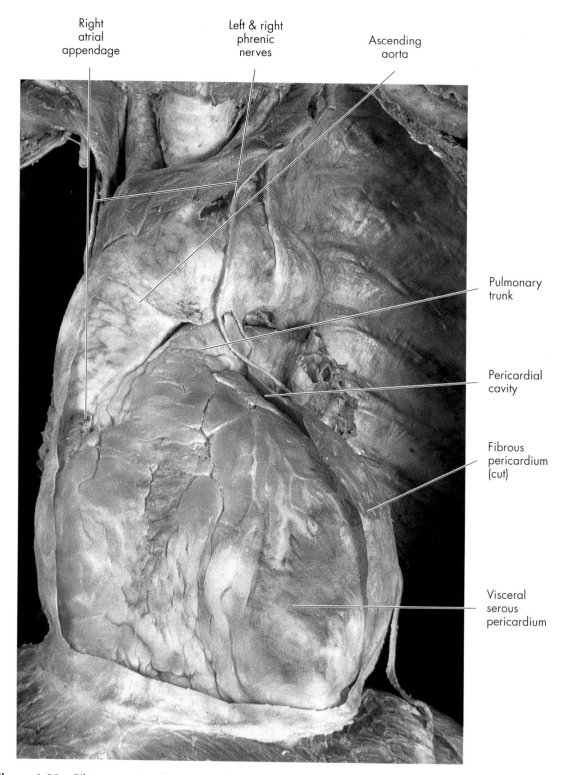

Right atrial appendage

Left & right phrenic nerves

Ascending aorta

Pulmonary trunk

Pericardial cavity

Fibrous pericardium (cut)

Visceral serous pericardium

Figure 1-33   Fibrous pericardium opened to expose the visceral pericardium covering the anterior surface of the heart.

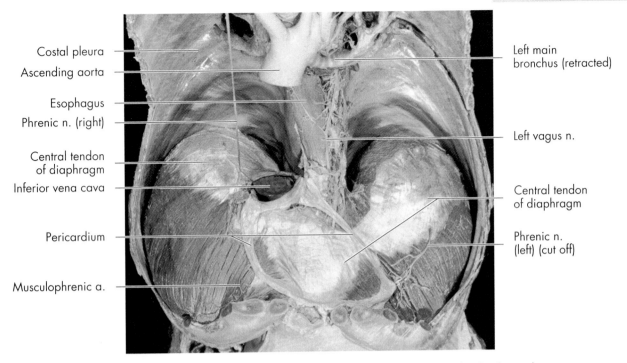

Costal pleura

Ascending aorta

Esophagus

Phrenic n. (right)

Central tendon
of diaphragm

Inferior vena cava

Pericardium

Musculophrenic a.

Left main
bronchus (retracted)

Left vagus n.

Central tendon
of diaphragm

Phrenic n.
(left) (cut off)

Figure 1-34 Diaphragm viewed from above with the pleura removed. The lungs have been removed and the tracheobronchial tree has been displaced posteriorly to provide an unobstructed view of the diaphragm. A narrow band of pericardium has been preserved along the margin of its diaphragmatic attachment. *Congenital herniation of abdominal contents into the thoracic cavity is a result of incomplete development of the diaphragm. Most commonly it occurs posteriorly on the left. In adults, most diaphragmatic hernias occur at the esophageal hiatus. The cardiac part of the stomach may slip upward through the hiatus (sliding hiatus hernia). Acid gastric contents may be regurgitated or inflammation and ulceration may occur resulting in pain (heartburn), bleeding, or obstruction. Surgical repair of the hernia may be required if simple measures such as antacids, weight loss, and changed sleeping posture fail.*

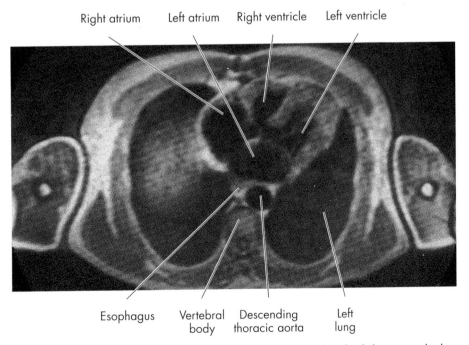

Right atrium   Left atrium   Right ventricle   Left ventricle

Esophagus   Vertebral
body   Descending
thoracic aorta   Left
lung

Figure 1-35 Transverse magnetic resonance image at the level of the seventh thoracic vertebra (viewed from below up).

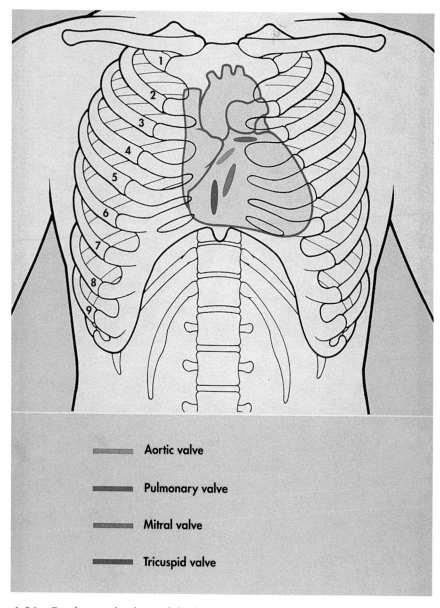

Figure 1-36   Borders and valves of the heart and their relationships to the anterior chest wall.

See **DISSECTIONS**, Section 1, p. 6
See **PRINCIPLES**, Fig. 1-35

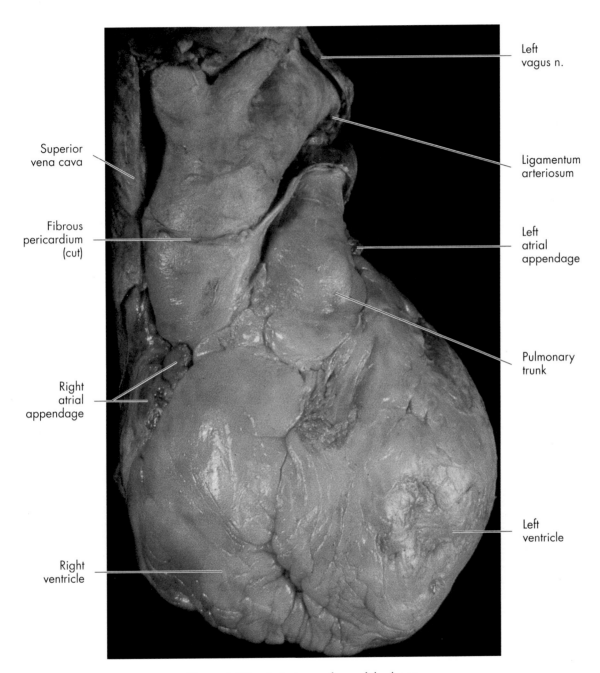

Left
vagus n.

Ligamentum
arteriosum

Left
atrial
appendage

Pulmonary
trunk

Left
ventricle

Superior
vena cava

Fibrous
pericardium
(cut)

Right
atrial
appendage

Right
ventricle

Figure 1-37   Anterior surface of the heart.

See **DISSECTIONS**, Section 1, p. 6

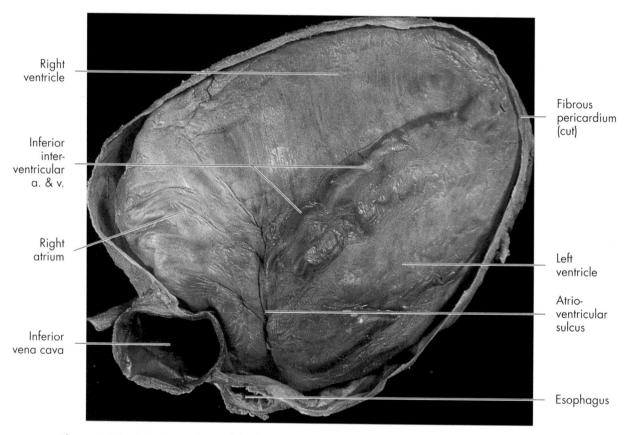

Right
ventricle

Inferior
inter-
ventricular
a. & v.

Right
atrium

Inferior
vena cava

Fibrous
pericardium
(cut)

Left
ventricle

Atrio-
ventricular
sulcus

Esophagus

Figure 1-38   Inferior surface of the heart. The inferior part of the fibrous pericardium has been removed with the diaphragm.

See **DISSECTIONS**, Section 1, p. 6
See **PRINCIPLES**, Fig. 1-39

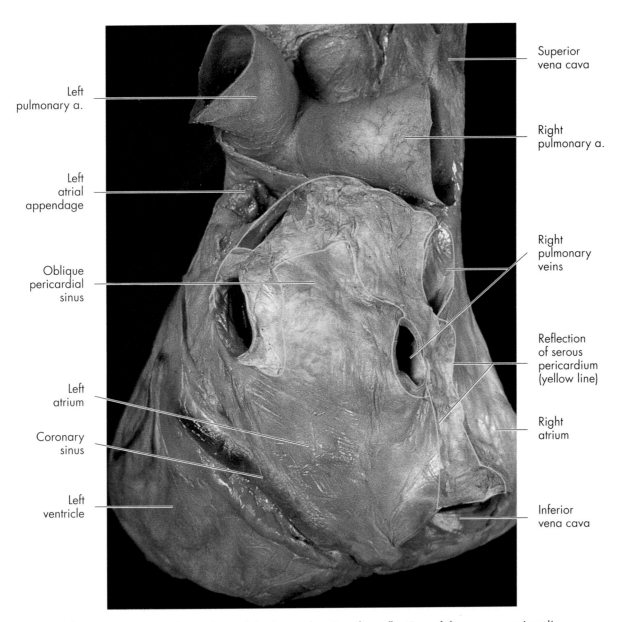

Figure 1-39 Posterior surface of the heart showing the reflection of the serous pericardium (see yellow line) and the site of the oblique pericardial sinus.

See DISSECTIONS, Section 1, p. 7
See PRINCIPLES, Fig. 1-41

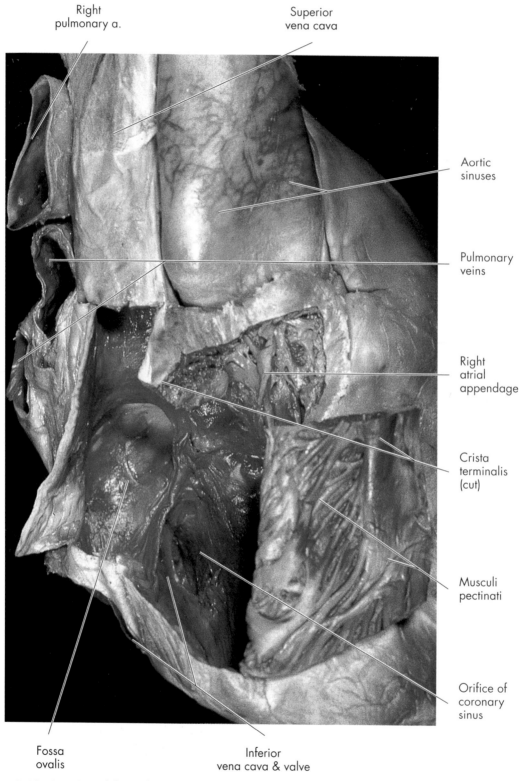

Right
pulmonary a.

Superior
vena cava

Aortic
sinuses

Pulmonary
veins

Right
atrial
appendage

Crista
terminalis
(cut)

Musculi
pectinati

Orifice of
coronary
sinus

Fossa
ovalis

Inferior
vena cava & valve

Figure 1-40 Interior of the right atrium and atrial appendage exposed by reflection and excision of part of the anterior atrial wall. Note the fossa ovalis site of the fetal foramen ovale. *Failure of closure of the foramen ovale at birth results in a patent foramen ovale, allowing flow between the right atrium and left atrium.*

SEE DISSECTIONS, SECTION 1, P. 7

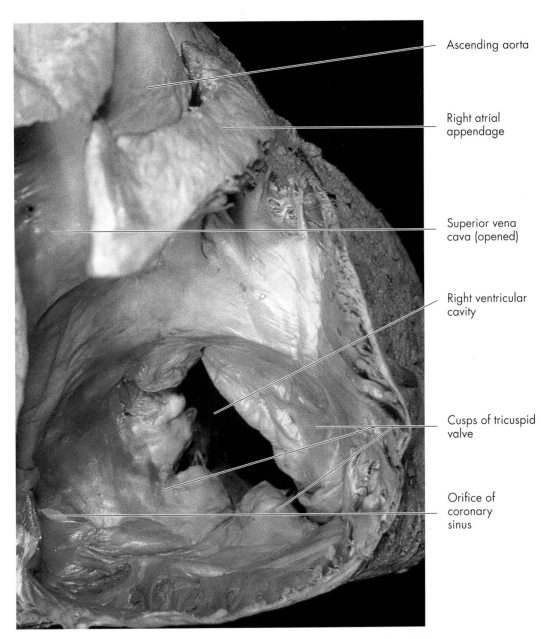

Ascending aorta

Right atrial
appendage

Superior vena
cava (opened)

Right ventricular
cavity

Cusps of tricuspid
valve

Orifice of
coronary
sinus

Figure 1-41   Tricuspid valve revealed after removal of the lateral wall of the right atrium.

SEE DISSECTIONS, SECTION 1, P. 7

SEE PRINCIPLES, FIG. 1-43

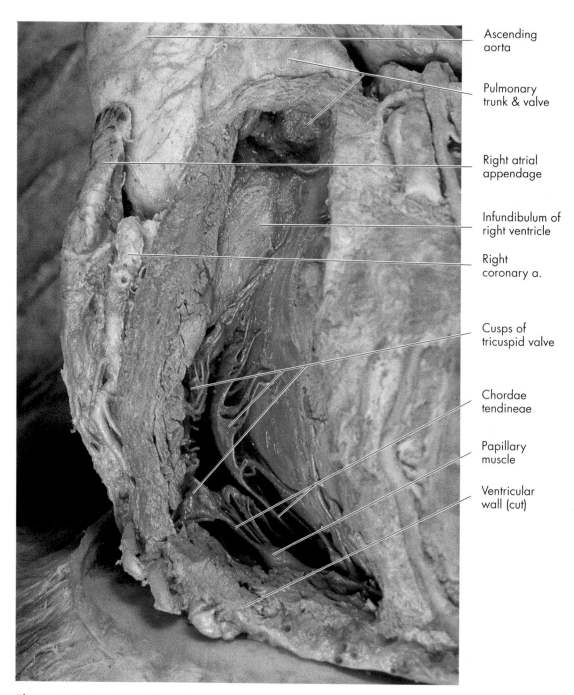

Ascending
aorta

Pulmonary
trunk & valve

Right atrial
appendage

Infundibulum of
right ventricle

Right
coronary a.

Cusps of
tricuspid valve

Chordae
tendineae

Papillary
muscle

Ventricular
wall (cut)

Figure 1-42   Interior of the right ventricle seen after removal of its anterior wall.

SEE DISSECTIONS, SECTION 1, P. 7

SEE PRINCIPLES, FIG. 1-43

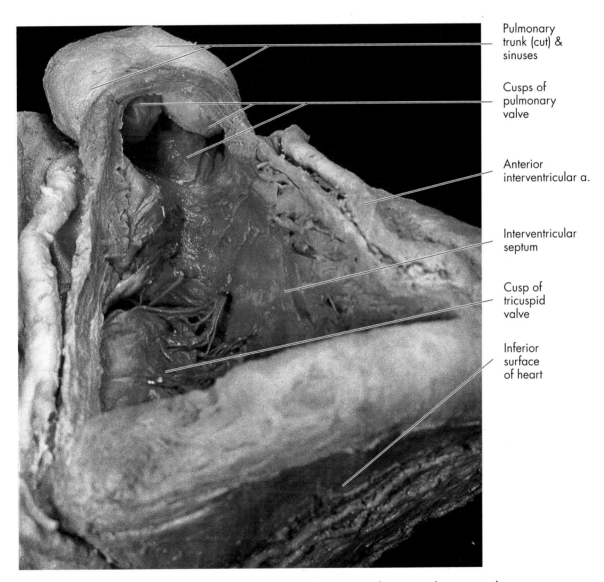

Pulmonary
trunk (cut) &
sinuses

Cusps of
pulmonary
valve

Anterior
interventricular a.

Interventricular
septum

Cusp of
tricuspid
valve

Inferior
surface
of heart

Figure 1-43   Ventricular surfaces of the cusps of the pulmonary valve seen after removal
of part of the anterior wall of the right ventricle.

See DISSECTIONS, Section 1, pp. 6, 7
See PRINCIPLES, Fig. 1-42

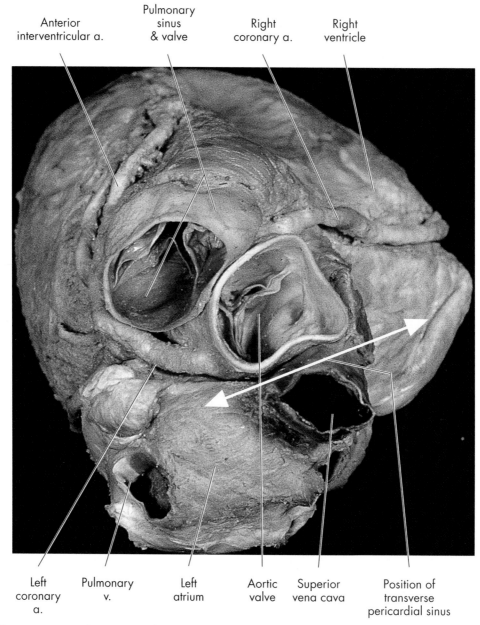

Anterior
interventricular a.

Pulmonary
sinus
& valve

Right
coronary a.

Right
ventricle

Left
coronary
a.

Pulmonary
v.

Left
atrium

Aortic
valve

Superior
vena cava

Position of
transverse
pericardial sinus

Figure 1-44   Pulmonary and aortic valves seen from above with a view of the transverse pericardial sinus. (*white arrow*).

SEE DISSECTIONS, SECTION 1, P. 7
SEE PRINCIPLES, FIG. 1-44

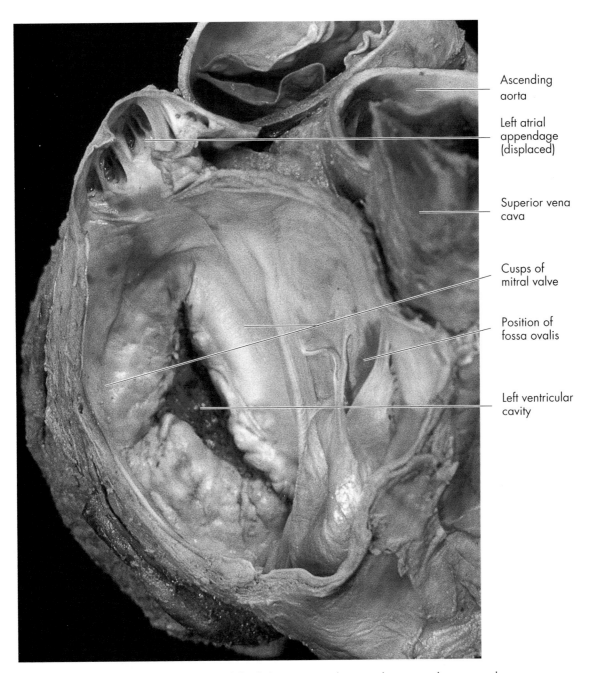

Ascending
aorta

Left atrial
appendage
(displaced)

Superior vena
cava

Cusps of
mitral valve

Position of
fossa ovalis

Left ventricular
cavity

Figure 1-45   Mitral valve and interior of the left atrium and appendage seen by removal of the posterior wall of the chamber.

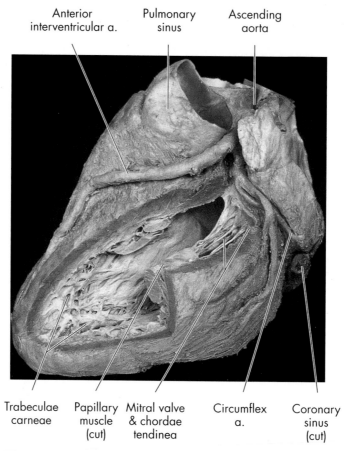

Anterior interventricular a. Pulmonary sinus Ascending aorta

Trabeculae carneae Papillary muscle (cut) Mitral valve & chordae tendinea Circumflex a. Coronary sinus (cut)

Figure 1-46   Interior of the left ventricle seen after removal of part of its wall.

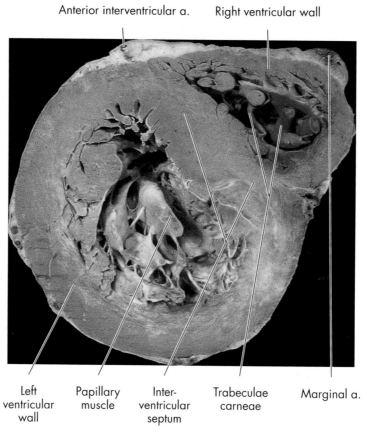

Anterior interventricular a. Right ventricular wall

Left ventricular wall Papillary muscle Inter-ventricular septum Trabeculae carneae Marginal a.

Figure 1-47   Section through the heart showing apical portions of the left and right ventricles.

SEE DISSECTIONS, SECTION 1, P. 7

SEE PRINCIPLES, FIG. 1-48

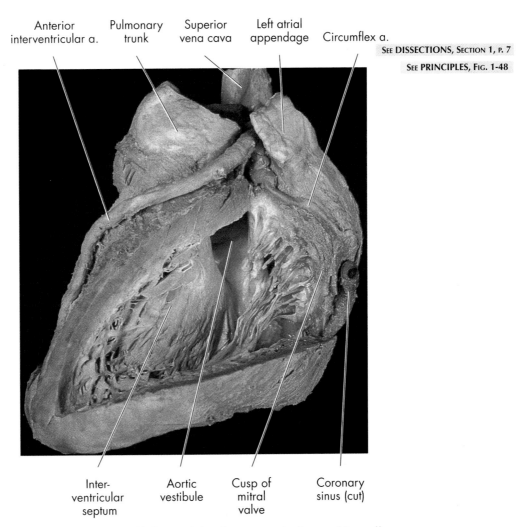

Anterior
interventricular a.   Pulmonary
trunk   Superior
vena cava   Left atrial
appendage   Circumflex a.

Inter-
ventricular
septum   Aortic
vestibule   Cusp of
mitral
valve   Coronary
sinus (cut)

Figure 1-48   Interior of left ventricle after removal of part of its wall.

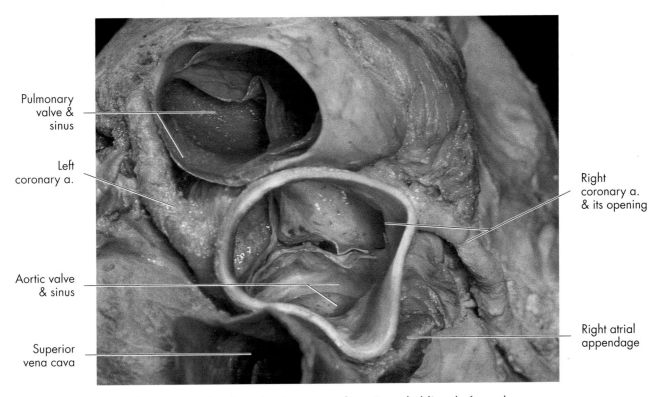

Pulmonary
valve &
sinus

Left
coronary a.

Aortic valve
& sinus

Superior
vena cava

Right
coronary a.
& its opening

Right atrial
appendage

Figure 1-49   Aortic and pulmonary valves viewed obliquely from above.

See DISSECTIONS, Section 1, p. 7
See PRINCIPLES, Figs. 1-44, 1-50

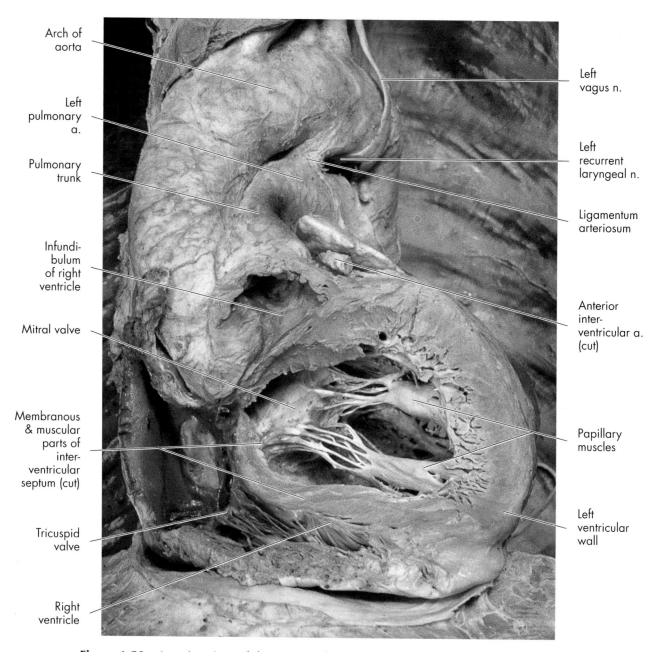

Arch of aorta

Left pulmonary a.

Pulmonary trunk

Infundi- bulum of right ventricle

Mitral valve

Membranous & muscular parts of inter- ventricular septum (cut)

Tricuspid valve

Right ventricle

Left vagus n.

Left recurrent laryngeal n.

Ligamentum arteriosum

Anterior inter- ventricular a. (cut)

Papillary muscles

Left ventricular wall

Figure 1-50   Anterior view of the aorta, pulmonary trunk, and ligamentum arteriosum. Most of the muscular part of the interventricular septum has been removed to show the interior of the left ventricle.

SEE DISSECTIONS, SECTION 1, P. 7

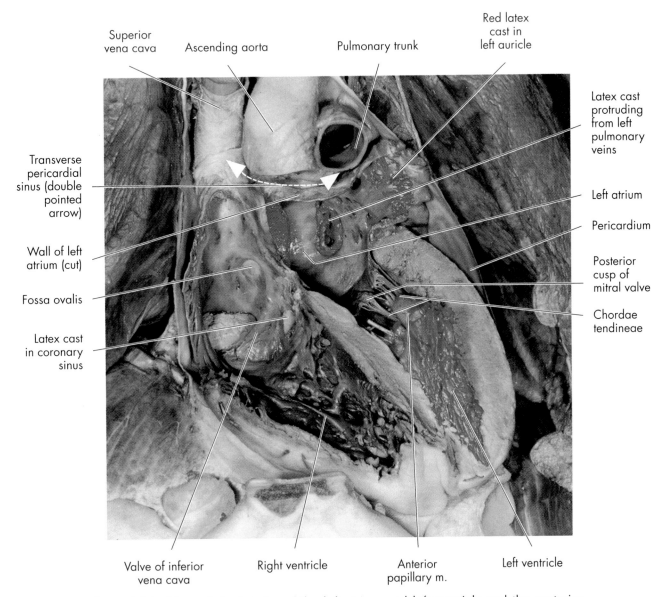

Superior vena cava · Ascending aorta · Pulmonary trunk · Red latex cast in left auricle

Latex cast protruding from left pulmonary veins

Transverse pericardial sinus (double pointed arrow)

Left atrium

Pericardium

Wall of left atrium (cut)

Posterior cusp of mitral valve

Fossa ovalis

Chordae tendineae

Latex cast in coronary sinus

Valve of inferior vena cava · Right ventricle · Anterior papillary m. · Left ventricle

Figure 1-51   View of the interior of the left atrium and left ventricle and the posterior cusp of the mitral valve. *Diseases of the heart valves resulting from such systemic causes as rheumatic fever and metabolic disorders may result in scar tissue constriction or stenosis of a valve or destruction of leaflets, producing insufficiency. Sometimes the chordae tendinae, which tether the edges of the mitral and tricuspid valves, rupture resulting in valvular insufficiency or even prolapse. Defective valves may be effectively replaced by open heart surgery.*

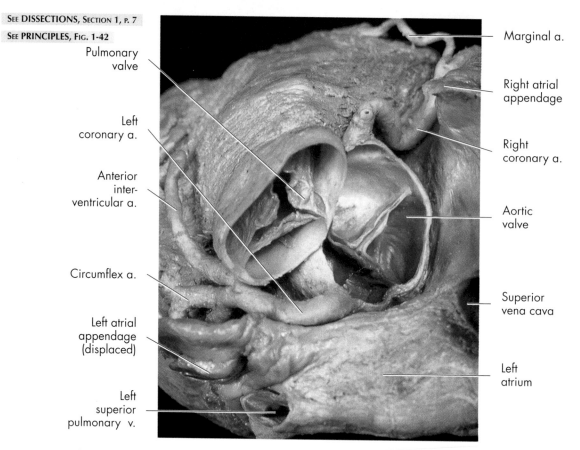

Pulmonary valve

Left coronary a.

Anterior inter-ventricular a.

Circumflex a.

Left atrial appendage (displaced)

Left superior pulmonary v.

Marginal a.

Right atrial appendage

Right coronary a.

Aortic valve

Superior vena cava

Left atrium

Figure 1-52 Origins of the right and left coronary arteries from the root of the ascending aorta seen from above.

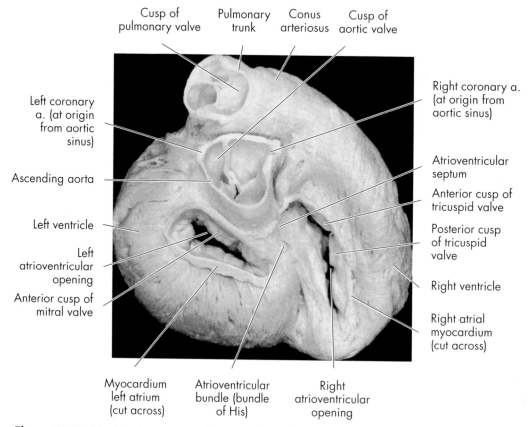

Cusp of pulmonary valve

Pulmonary trunk

Conus arteriosus

Cusp of aortic valve

Left coronary a. (at origin from aortic sinus)

Ascending aorta

Left ventricle

Left atrioventricular opening

Anterior cusp of mitral valve

Right coronary a. (at origin from aortic sinus)

Atrioventricular septum

Anterior cusp of tricuspid valve

Posterior cusp of tricuspid valve

Right ventricle

Right atrial myocardium (cut across)

Myocardium left atrium (cut across)

Atrioventricular bundle (bundle of His)

Right atrioventricular opening

Figure 1-53 Ventricular myocardium, cardiac valves, and ostia seen from above. The atria have been removed close to their attachments to the atrioventricular valve rings.

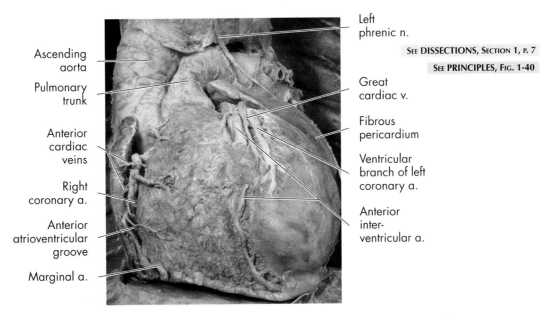

Ascending aorta

Pulmonary trunk

Anterior cardiac veins

Right coronary a.

Anterior atrioventricular groove

Marginal a.

Left phrenic n.

SEE DISSECTIONS, SECTION 1, P. 7

SEE PRINCIPLES, FIG. 1-40

Great cardiac v.

Fibrous pericardium

Ventricular branch of left coronary a.

Anterior inter-ventricular a.

Figure 1-54 Right and left coronary arteries and their branches on the anterior surface of the heart.

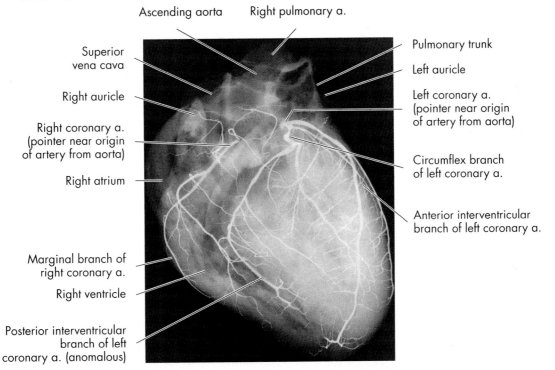

Ascending aorta

Right pulmonary a.

Superior vena cava

Right auricle

Right coronary a. (pointer near origin of artery from aorta)

Right atrium

Marginal branch of right coronary a.

Right ventricle

Posterior interventricular branch of left coronary a. (anomalous)

Pulmonary trunk

Left auricle

Left coronary a. (pointer near origin of artery from aorta)

Circumflex branch of left coronary a.

Anterior interventricular branch of left coronary a.

Figure 1-55 Coronary angiogram. The heart is viewed from the front. Contrast medium has been injected into the right and left coronary arteries; an anomalous arrangement is present in this specimen. The right coronary artery terminates by descending along the right margin of the heart. The left coronary artery gives rise to the posterior interventricular branch, which is normally the terminal branch of the right coronary artery. *Insufficient blood flow through the coronary arteries, particularly during exercise and tachycardia (rapid heart beat), results in cardiac muscle ischemia (inadequate oxygenation). This causes pain (angina pectoris) in the chest and often in the referred areas of the axilla and medial aspect of the upper arm. Visceral afferent sympathetic fibers from the heart enter upper thoracic spinal level—the same region in which somatic sensory nerves from the arm and axilla enter. Visceral heart pain is misinterpreted as pain from this area (referred pain). Complete occlusion without adequate collateral blood supply from other coronary arteries results in an area of muscle death (infarct). Coronary arteries have little or no collateral communication with one another and thus they are known as end arteries. When proximal parts of coronary arteries become seriously and symptomatically occluded, procedures such as dilitation of the arteries from within under imaging control may be effective. Alternately, bypass grafts using segments of veins to connect the aorta to the coronary arteries beyond the site of obstruction may be indicated.*

Marginal a.   Right   Inferior
                     ventricle   interventricular a.

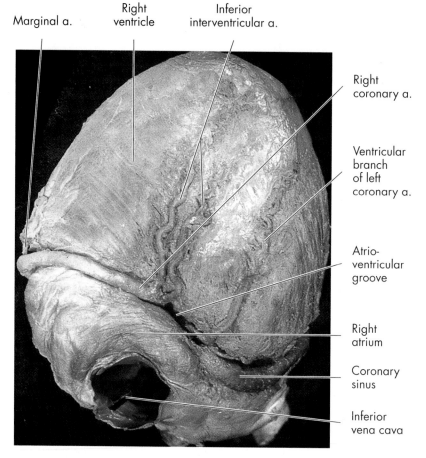

Right
coronary a.

Ventricular
branch
of left
coronary a.

Atrio-
ventricular
groove

Right
atrium

Coronary
sinus

Inferior
vena cava

Figure 1-56 Right and left coronary arteries and their branches on the inferior surface of the heart. The inferior interventricular artery is duplicated in this specimen.

Pulmonary   Anterior   Ascending   Superior
trunk   interventricular a.   aorta   vena cava

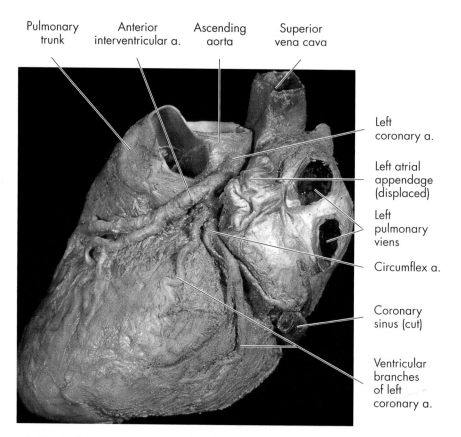

Left
coronary a.

Left atrial
appendage
(displaced)

Left
pulmonary
viens

Circumflex a.

Coronary
sinus (cut)

Ventricular
branches
of left
coronary a.

Figure 1-57 Left coronary artery and its branches viewed from the left.

SEE **DISSECTIONS**, SECTION 1, P. 7
SEE **PRINCIPLES**, FIG. 1-39

Posterior v.
of left
ventricle

Great
cardiac v.

Left
atrial
appendage

Left
pulmonary
veins

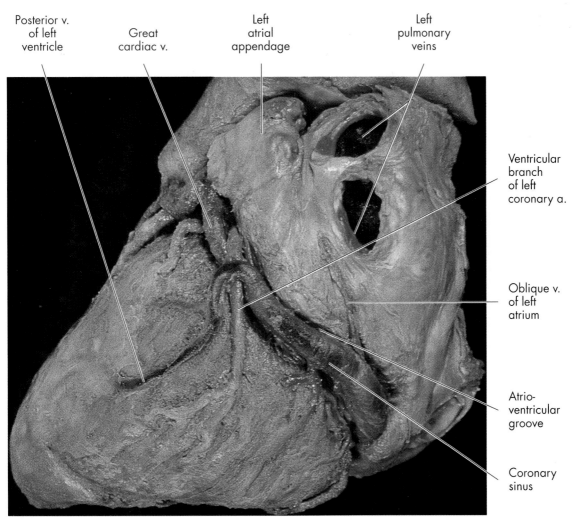

Ventricular
branch
of left
coronary a.

Oblique v.
of left
atrium

Atrio-
ventricular
groove

Coronary
sinus

Figure 1-58 Oblique view of the coronary sinus lying in the atrioventricular groove.

See **DISSECTIONS**, Section 1, p. 7
See **PRINCIPLES**, Fig. 1-39

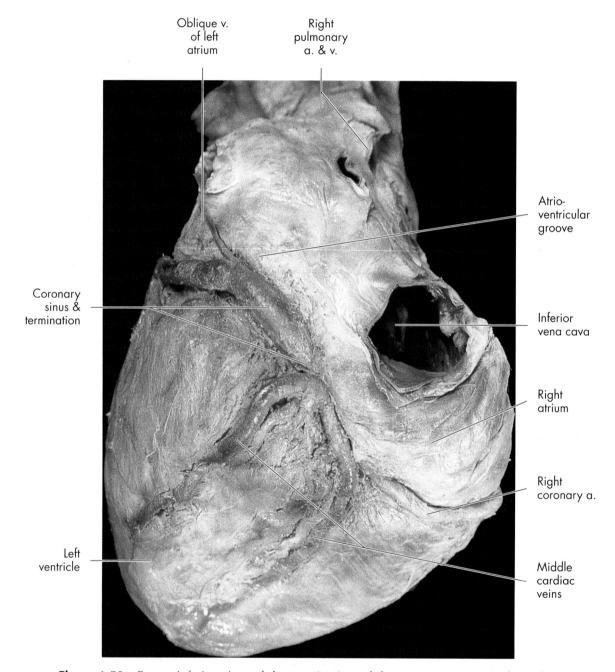

Oblique v. of left atrium

Right pulmonary a. & v.

Atrio-ventricular groove

Coronary sinus & termination

Inferior vena cava

Right atrium

Right coronary a.

Left ventricle

Middle cardiac veins

Figure 1-59   Posteroinferior view of the termination of the coronary sinus in the right atrium.

See PRINCIPLES, Fig. 1-48

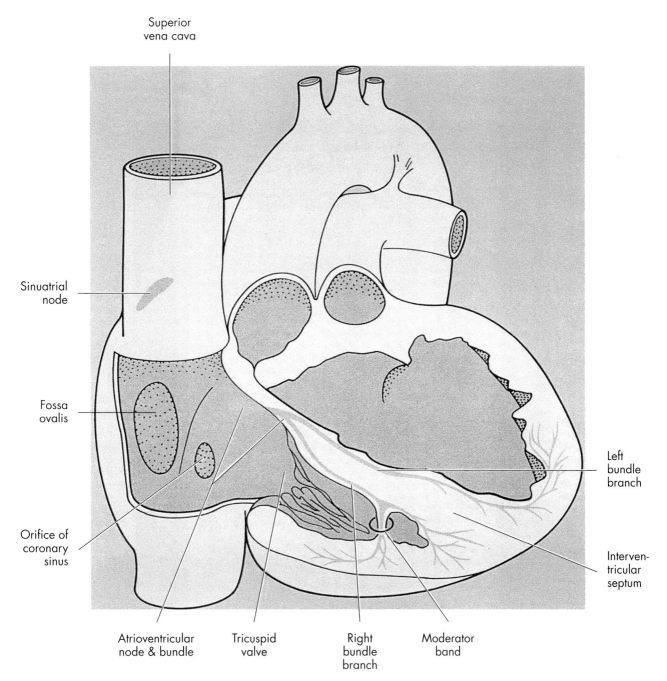

Superior
vena cava

Sinuatrial
node

Fossa
ovalis

Orifice of
coronary
sinus

Left
bundle
branch

Interven-
tricular
septum

Atrioventricular
node & bundle

Tricuspid
valve

Right
bundle
branch

Moderator
band

Figure 1-60 Location of the conducting tissues.

See PRINCIPLES, Fig. 1-36

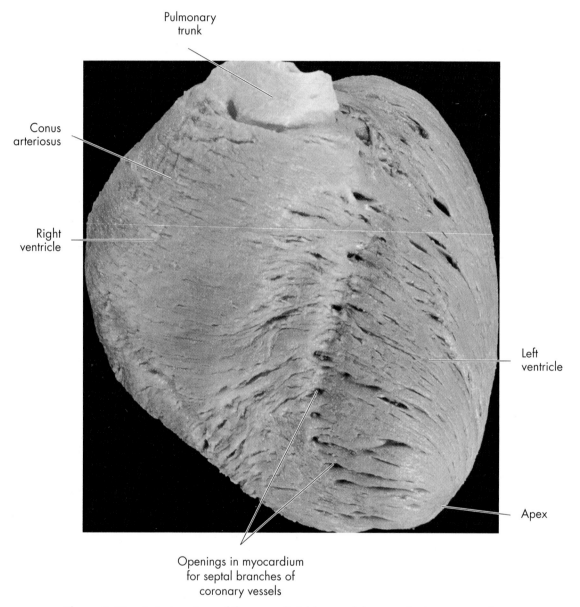

Pulmonary
trunk

Conus
arteriosus

Right
ventricle

Left
ventricle

Apex

Openings in myocardium
for septal branches of
coronary vessels

Figure 1-61   Anterior view of the superficial layer of the ventricular myocardium.

See **PRINCIPLES**, Fig. 1-36

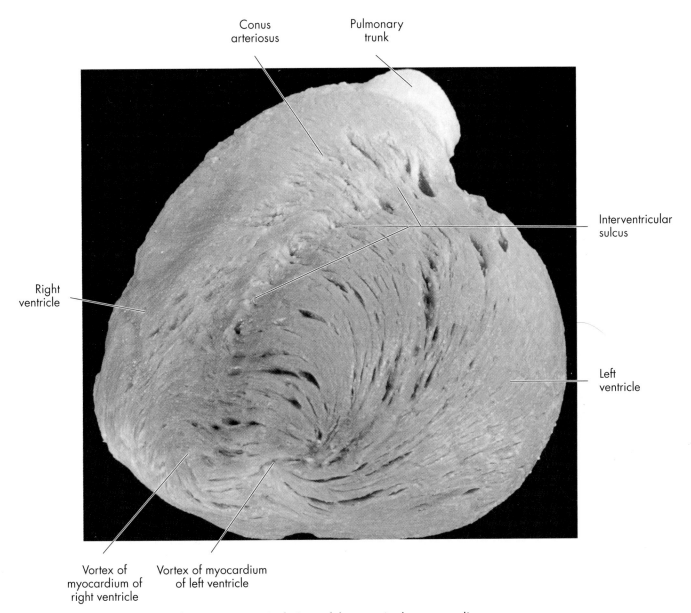

Conus
arteriosus

Pulmonary
trunk

Interventricular
sulcus

Right
ventricle

Left
ventricle

Vortex of
myocardium of
right ventricle

Vortex of myocardium
of left ventricle

Figure 1-62   Apical view of the ventricular myocardium.

See DISSECTIONS, Section 1, p. 7

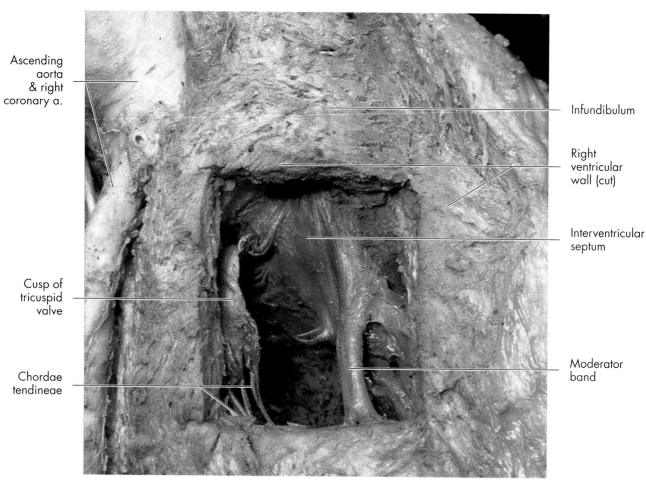

Ascending
aorta
& right
coronary a.

Infundibulum

Right
ventricular
wall (cut)

Interventricular
septum

Cusp of
tricuspid
valve

Chordae
tendineae

Moderator
band

Figure 1-63   Moderator band seen through a window cut in the anterior wall of the right ventricle.

See DISSECTIONS, Section 1, p. 10
See PRINCIPLES, Fig. 1-35

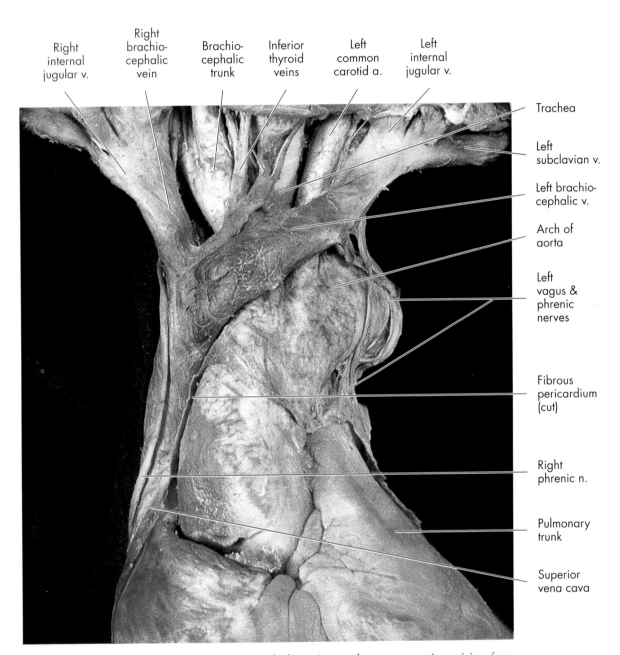

Right internal jugular v.

Right brachio-cephalic vein

Brachio-cephalic trunk

Inferior thyroid veins

Left common carotid a.

Left internal jugular v.

Trachea

Left subclavian v.

Left brachio-cephalic v.

Arch of aorta

Left vagus & phrenic nerves

Fibrous pericardium (cut)

Right phrenic n.

Pulmonary trunk

Superior vena cava

Figure 1-64 Relationship of the brachiocephalic veins to the great arteries arising from the aortic arch.

See DISSECTIONS, Section 1, pp. 10, 11
See PRINCIPLES, Fig. 1-55

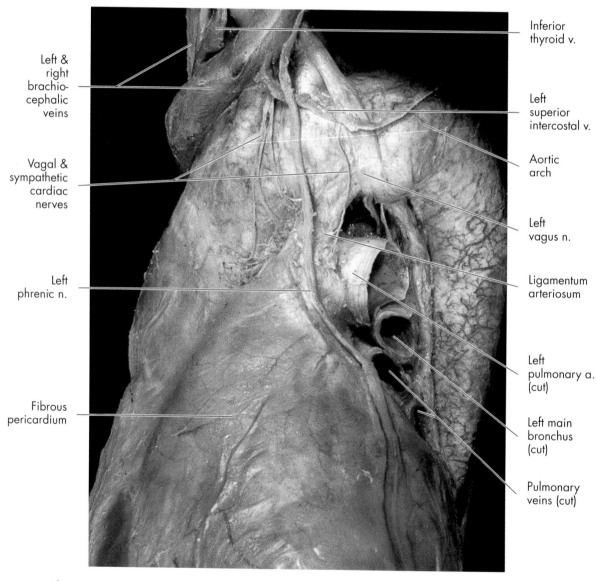

Left &
right
brachio-
cephalic
veins

Vagal &
sympathetic
cardiac
nerves

Left
phrenic n.

Fibrous
pericardium

Inferior
thyroid v.

Left
superior
intercostal v.

Aortic
arch

Left
vagus n.

Ligamentum
arteriosum

Left
pulmonary a.
(cut)

Left main
bronchus
(cut)

Pulmonary
veins (cut)

Figure 1-65   Oblique view of the arch of the aorta showing the course of the left vagus and phrenic nerves.

See **DISSECTIONS, Section 1, pp. 10, 11**

See **PRINCIPLES, Fig. 1-54**

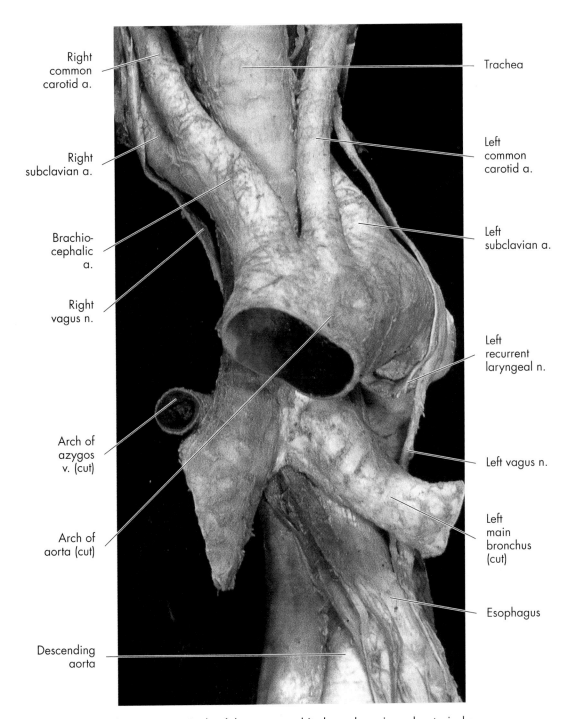

Right common carotid a.

Right subclavian a.

Brachiocephalic a.

Right vagus n.

Arch of azygos v. (cut)

Arch of aorta (cut)

Descending aorta

Trachea

Left common carotid a.

Left subclavian a.

Left recurrent laryngeal n.

Left vagus n.

Left main bronchus (cut)

Esophagus

Figure 1-66   Arch of the aorta and its branches viewed anteriorly.

See DISSECTIONS, Section 1, pp. 5, 10

See PRINCIPLES, Fig. 1-53

Right
internal
thoracic
a. (cut)

Right
brachio-
cephalic v.

Brachio-
cephalic
a.

Left
common
carotid a.

Trachea

Left
brachio-
cephalic v.

Fibrous
pericardium
(cut)

Left lung
root

Right
phrenic n.

Superior
vena cava

Right
lung root

Right
atrium

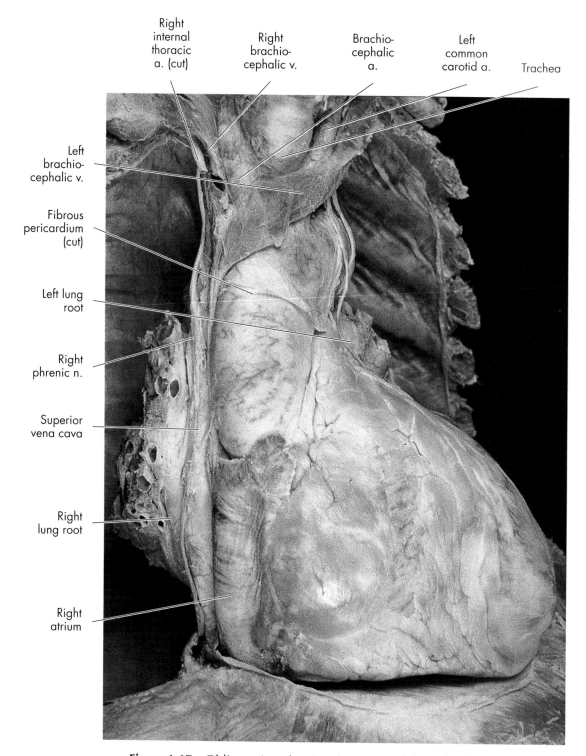

Figure 1-67   Oblique view showing the course of the right phrenic nerve.

SEE DISSECTIONS, SECTION 1, PP. 5, 10

SEE PRINCIPLES, FIG. 1-53

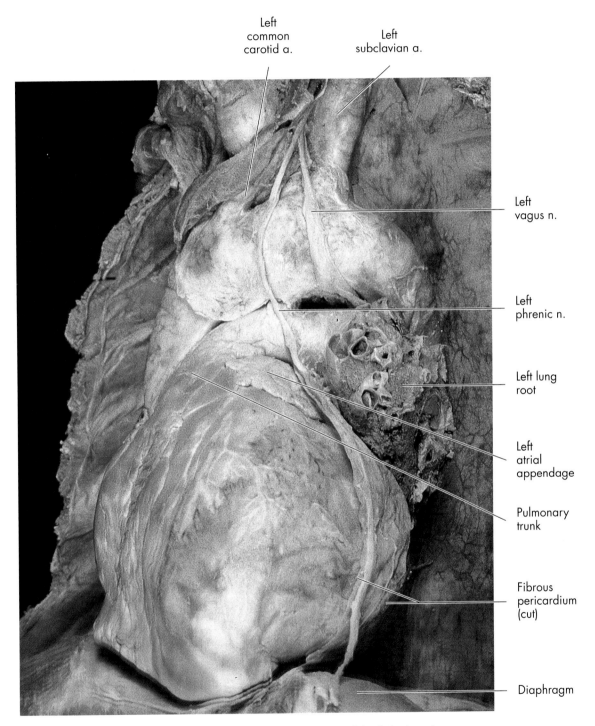

Left
common
carotid a.

Left
subclavian a.

Left
vagus n.

Left
phrenic n.

Left lung
root

Left
atrial
appendage

Pulmonary
trunk

Fibrous
pericardium
(cut)

Diaphragm

Figure 1-68   Oblique view of the intrathoracic course of the left phrenic nerve.

SEE **DISSECTIONS**, SECTION 1, PP. 5, 6

SEE **PRINCIPLES**, FIG. 1-34

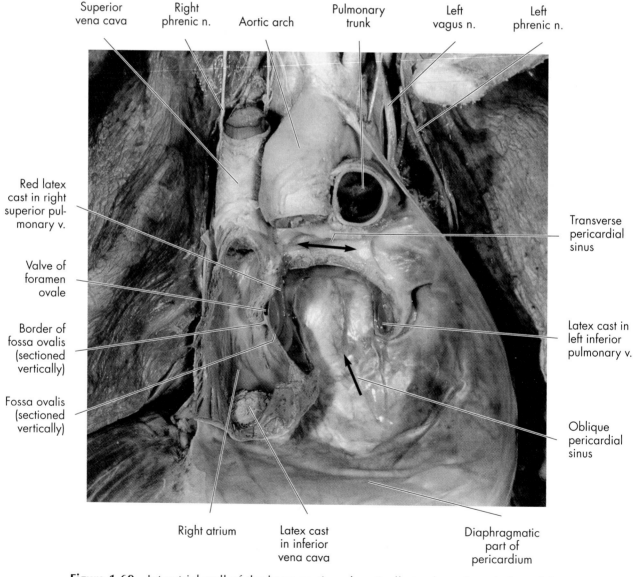

Superior
vena cava

Right
phrenic n.

Aortic arch

Pulmonary
trunk

Left
vagus n.

Left
phrenic n.

Red latex
cast in right
superior pul-
monary v.

Valve of
foramen
ovale

Border of
fossa ovalis
(sectioned
vertically)

Fossa ovalis
(sectioned
vertically)

Transverse
pericardial
sinus

Latex cast in
left inferior
pulmonary v.

Oblique
pericardial
sinus

Right atrium

Latex cast
in inferior
vena cava

Diaphragmatic
part of
pericardium

Figure 1-69   Interatrial wall of the heart sectioned vertically to show the relation of the fossa ovalis to the left atrium. The remains of both ventricles and part of the posterior wall of the left atrium are removed to show the oblique sinus.

See **DISSECTIONS**, Section 1, p. 8

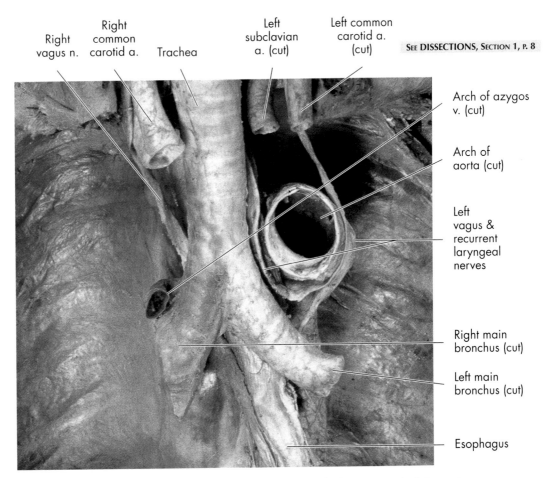

Right vagus n. — Right common carotid a. — Trachea — Left subclavian a. (cut) — Left common carotid a. (cut)

Arch of azygos v. (cut)

Arch of aorta (cut)

Left vagus & recurrent laryngeal nerves

Right main bronchus (cut)

Left main bronchus (cut)

Esophagus

Figure 1-70 Trachea and left and right main bronchi exposed after removal of the anterior part of the aortic arch.

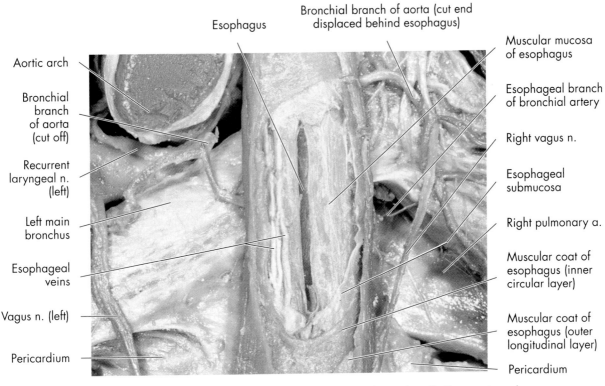

Esophagus — Bronchial branch of aorta (cut end displaced behind esophagus)

Muscular mucosa of esophagus

Aortic arch

Bronchial branch of aorta (cut off)

Esophageal branch of bronchial artery

Right vagus n.

Recurrent laryngeal n. (left)

Esophageal submucosa

Left main bronchus

Right pulmonary a.

Esophageal veins

Muscular coat of esophagus (inner circular layer)

Vagus n. (left)

Muscular coat of esophagus (outer longitudinal layer)

Pericardium

Pericardium

Figure 1-71 A nonstandard posterior view with the esophageal wall dissected to show its muscle layers and mid-thoracic relationships.

SEE **DISSECTIONS**, SECTION 1, PP. 8, 9, 10, 11

SEE **PRINCIPLES**, FIG. 1-56

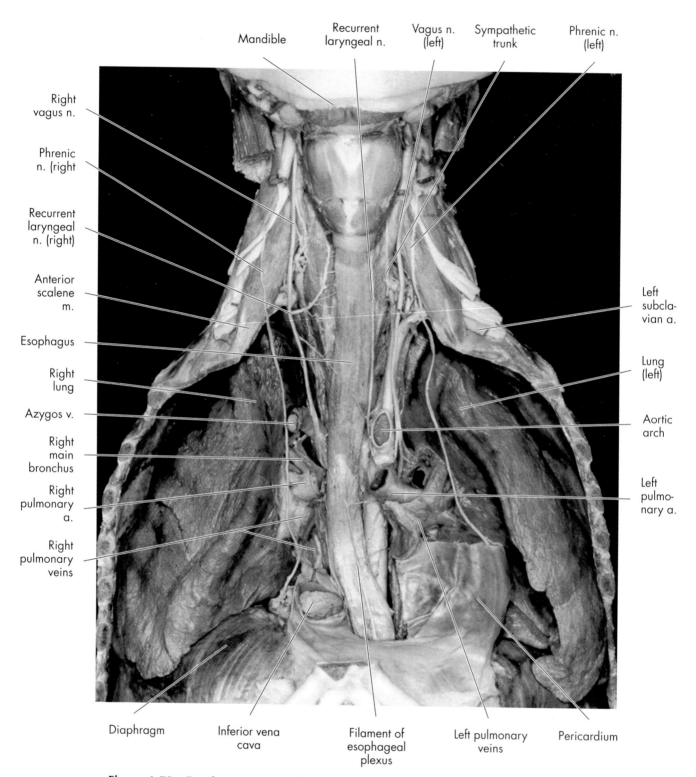

Figure 1-72 Esophagus exposed by removing the trachea, right pulmonary artery, and part of the pericardium from the specimen in Figure 1-71.

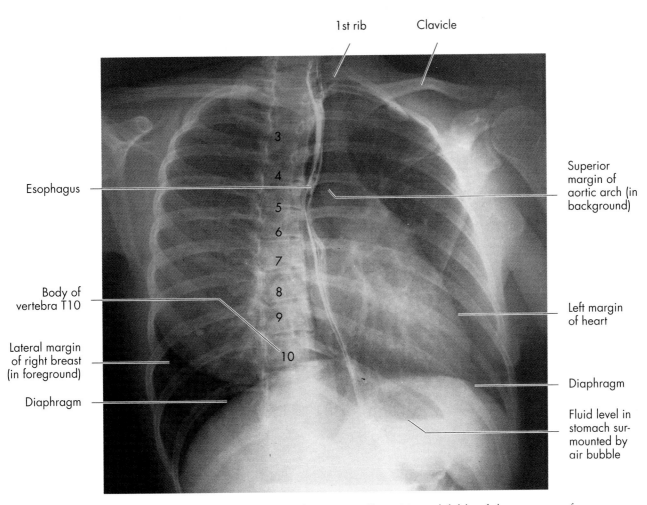

Figure 1-73   Esophagus outlined by a barium swallow. Normal folds of the mucosa of the esophagus are indicated in several areas by vertical striation of the barium mass. The upper margin of the aortic arch is faintly visible opposite the upper border of the fifth thoracic vertebral body. The esophagus is deflected posteriorly by the aortic arch and the right main bronchus.

SEE **DISSECTIONS,** SECTION 1, P. 8

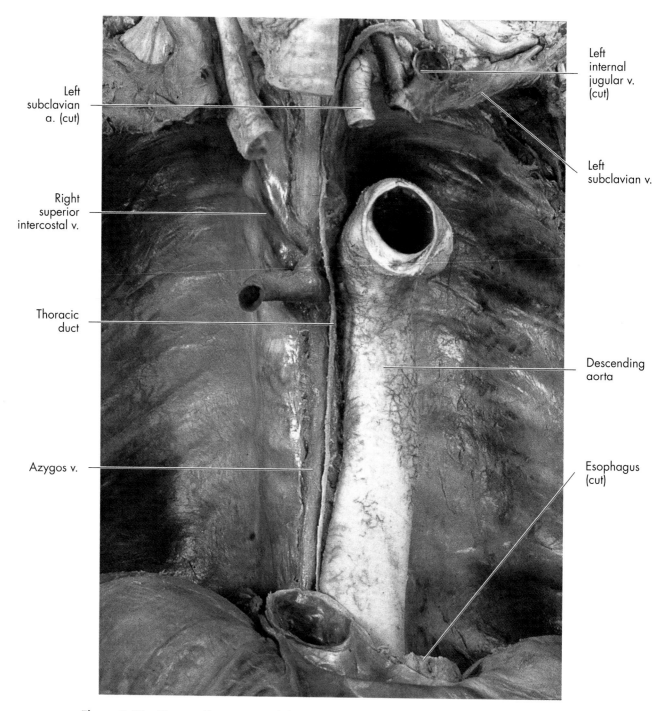

Left
subclavian
a. (cut)

Right
superior
intercostal v.

Thoracic
duct

Azygos v.

Left
internal
jugular v.
(cut)

Left
subclavian v.

Descending
aorta

Esophagus
(cut)

Figure 1-74   Descending aorta and thoracic duct exposed after removal of the thoracic
part of the esophagus.

See DISSECTIONS, Section 1, pp. 4, 8
See PRINCIPLES, Figs. 1-3, 1-55, A

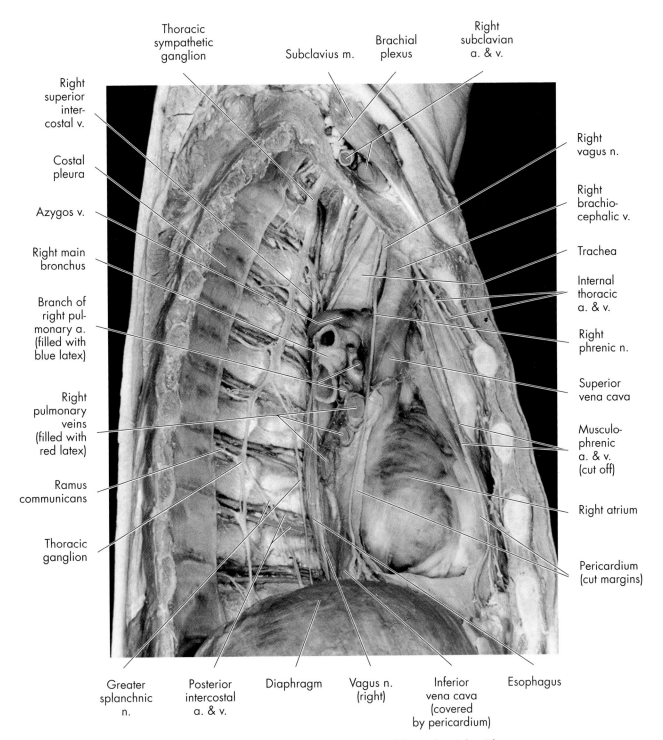

Thoracic sympathetic ganglion

Subclavius m.

Brachial plexus

Right subclavian a. & v.

Right superior intercostal v.

Costal pleura

Azygos v.

Right main bronchus

Branch of right pulmonary a. (filled with blue latex)

Right pulmonary veins (filled with red latex)

Ramus communicans

Thoracic ganglion

Right vagus n.

Right brachiocephalic v.

Trachea

Internal thoracic a. & v.

Right phrenic n.

Superior vena cava

Musculophrenic a. & v. (cut off)

Right atrium

Pericardium (cut margins)

Greater splanchnic n.

Posterior intercostal a. & v.

Diaphragm

Vagus n. (right)

Inferior vena cava (covered by pericardium)

Esophagus

Figure 1-75 Mediastinal contents viewed from the right side.

See **DISSECTIONS,** Section 1, pp. 4, 8

See **PRINCIPLES,** Fig. 1-55, *B*

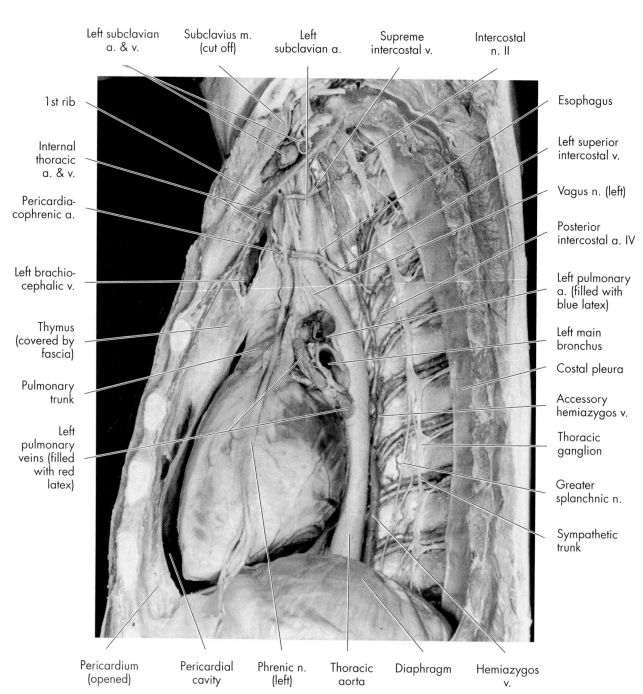

Left subclavian a. & v.

Subclavius m. (cut off)

Left subclavian a.

Supreme intercostal v.

Intercostal n. II

1st rib

Internal thoracic a. & v.

Pericardia-cophrenic a.

Left brachio-cephalic v.

Thymus (covered by fascia)

Pulmonary trunk

Left pulmonary veins (filled with red latex)

Esophagus

Left superior intercostal v.

Vagus n. (left)

Posterior intercostal a. IV

Left pulmonary a. (filled with blue latex)

Left main bronchus

Costal pleura

Accessory hemiazygos v.

Thoracic ganglion

Greater splanchnic n.

Sympathetic trunk

Pericardium (opened)

Pericardial cavity

Phrenic n. (left)

Thoracic aorta

Diaphragm

Hemiazygos v.

Figure 1-76   Mediastinal contents viewed from the left side with pleura removed in the paravertebral area.

SEE **DISSECTIONS, SECTION 1, PP. 4, 8**
SEE **PRINCIPLES, FIG. 1-55,** *A & B*

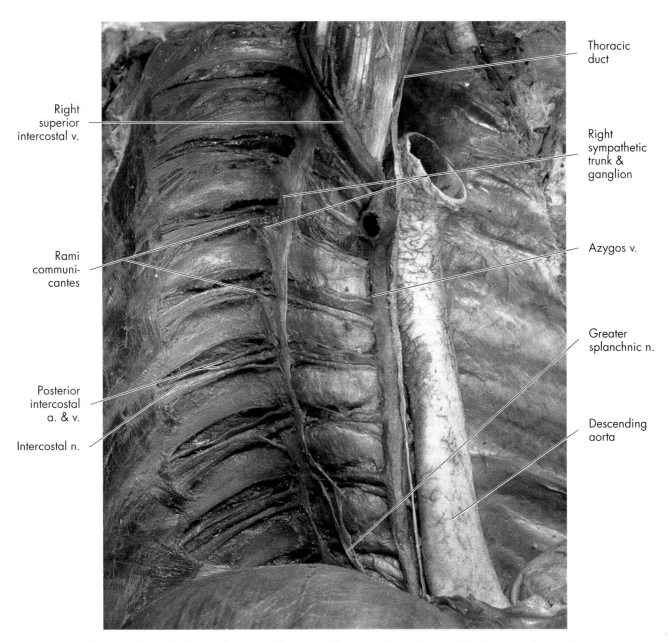

Thoracic
duct

Right
superior
intercostal v.

Right
sympathetic
trunk &
ganglion

Rami
communi-
cantes

Azygos v.

Posterior
intercostal
a. & v.

Greater
splanchnic n.

Intercostal n.

Descending
aorta

Figure 1-77   Oblique view of right sympathetic trunk and posterior intercostal vessels and intercostal nerves after removal of the parietal pleura.

SEE **DISSECTIONS**, SECTION 1, P. 1
SEE **PRINCIPLES**, FIG. 1-55, *B*

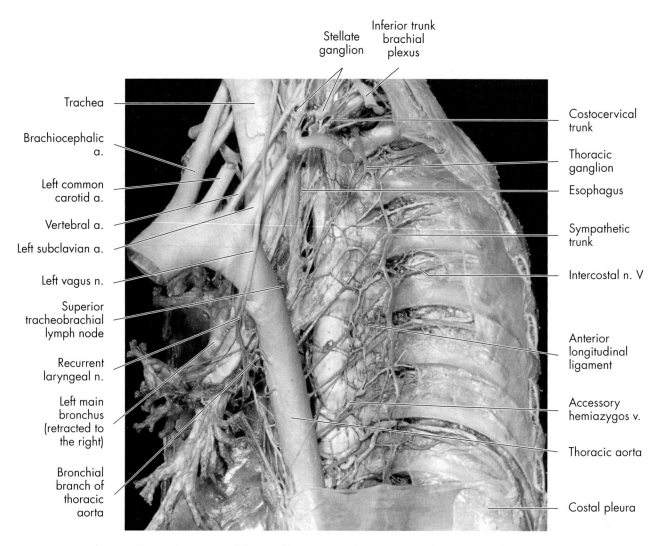

Stellate
ganglion

Inferior trunk
brachial
plexus

Trachea

Brachiocephalic
a.

Left common
carotid a.

Vertebral a.

Left subclavian a.

Left vagus n.

Superior
tracheobrachial
lymph node

Recurrent
laryngeal n.

Left main
bronchus
(retracted to
the right)

Bronchial
branch of
thoracic
aorta

Costocervical
trunk

Thoracic
ganglion

Esophagus

Sympathetic
trunk

Intercostal n. V

Anterior
longitudinal
ligament

Accessory
hemiazygos v.

Thoracic aorta

Costal pleura

Figure 1-78   Dissection of the mediastinum and paravertebral structures shown from the
lateral view.

SECTION TWO

Head and Neck

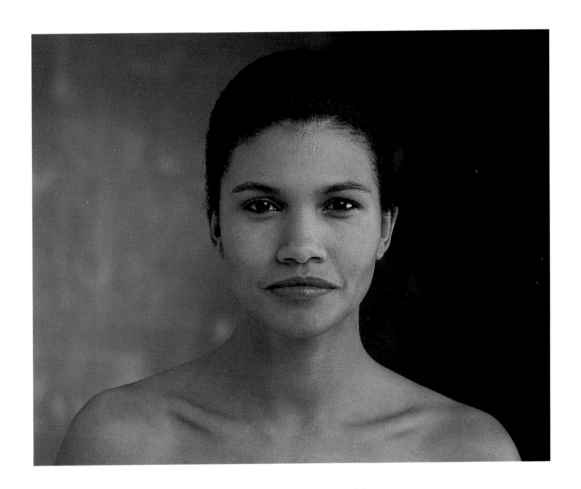

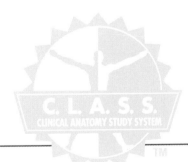

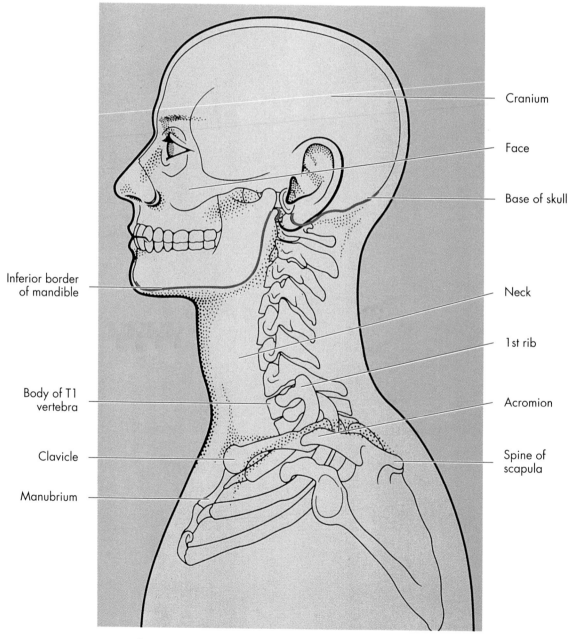

Cranium

Face

Base of skull

Inferior border
of mandible

Neck

1st rib

Body of T1
vertebra

Acromion

Clavicle

Spine of
scapula

Manubrium

Figure 2-1   Regions and skeleton of the head and neck.

See PRINCIPLES, Fig. 2-41

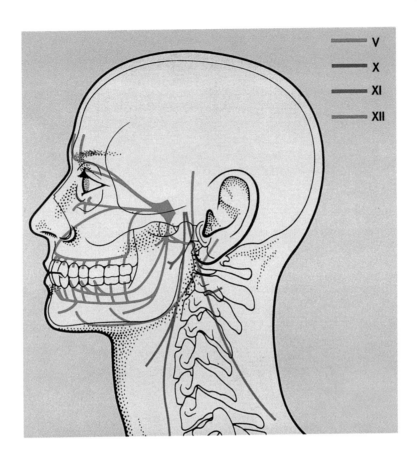

	V
	X
	XI
	XII

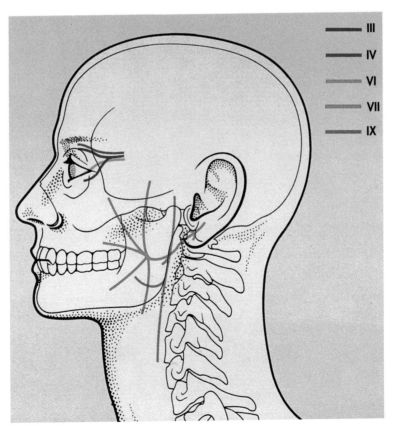

	III
	IV
	VI
	VII
	IX

Figure 2-2   Lateral projection of the extracranial parts of some cranial nerves.

SEE **PRINCIPLES**, FIG. 2-40

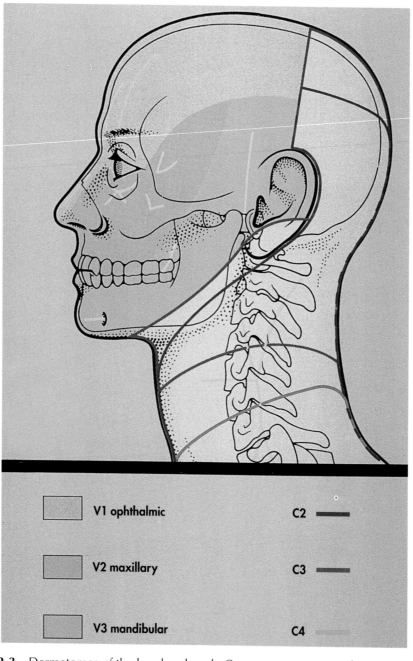

Figure 2-3   Dermatomes of the head and neck. Cutaneous nerves are shown in yellow.

See PRINCIPLES, Figs. 2-46, 2-47

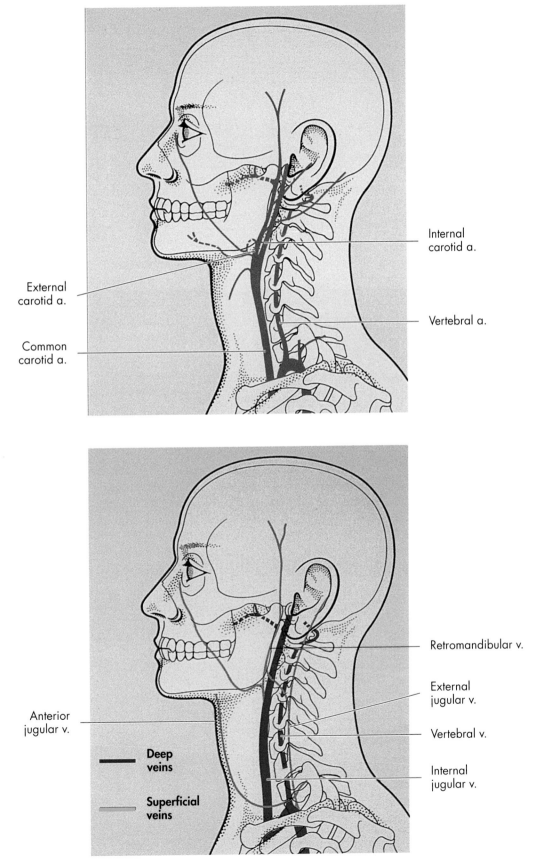

External
carotid a.

Common
carotid a.

Internal
carotid a.

Vertebral a.

Anterior
jugular v.

Deep
veins

Superficial
veins

Retromandibular v.

External
jugular v.

Vertebral v.

Internal
jugular v.

Figure 2-4 Main arteries and veins of the head and neck.

See PRINCIPLES, Fig. 2-60

Carotid
sheath   Cervical fascial layers   Investing fascia

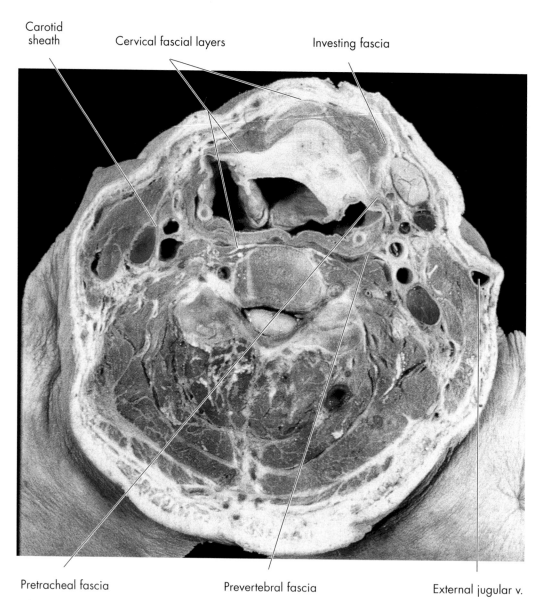

Pretracheal fascia   Prevertebral fascia   External jugular v.

Figure 2-5   Transverse section of the neck at the level of C4 showing the layers of cervical fascia.

See **DISSECTIONS**, **Section** 2, p. 15

See **PRINCIPLES**, Fig. 2-68

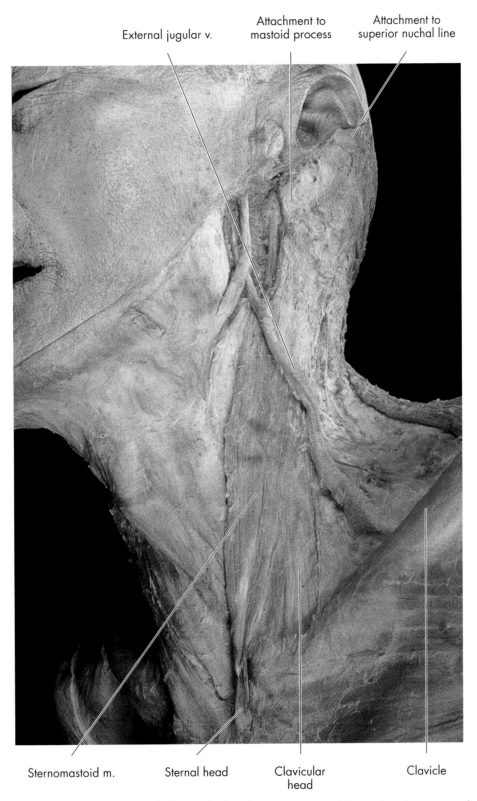

Sternomastoid m.   Sternal head   Clavicular   Clavicle
                                             head

External jugular v.   Attachment to   Attachment to
                           mastoid process   superior nuchal line

Figure 2-6 Oblique view of the neck showing sternomastoid muscle after removal of the investing fascia covering the sternomastoid and the trapezius.

See DISSECTIONS, Section 2, p. 15

See PRINCIPLES, Fig. 2-68

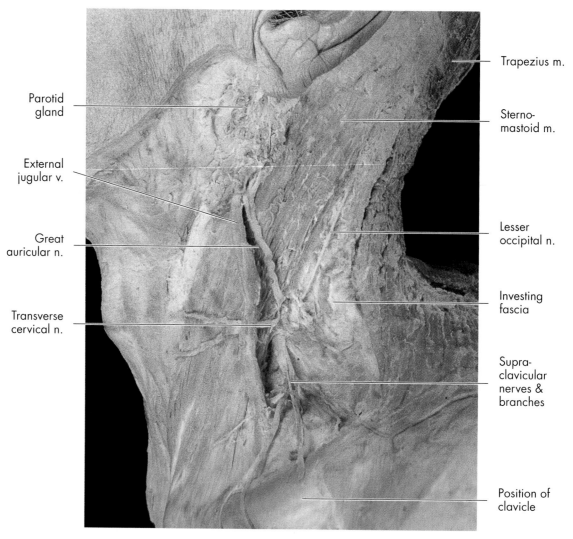

Parotid gland

External jugular v.

Great auricular n.

Transverse cervical n.

Trapezius m.

Sterno-mastoid m.

Lesser occipital n.

Investing fascia

Supra-clavicular nerves & branches

Position of clavicle

Figure 2-7   Boundaries and roof of the posterior triangle of the neck are the posterior border of the sternomastoid, the anterior border of the trapezius, and the mid one third of the clavicle. External jugular vein and cutaneous branches of the cervical plexus, lying superficial to the roof, are also visible.

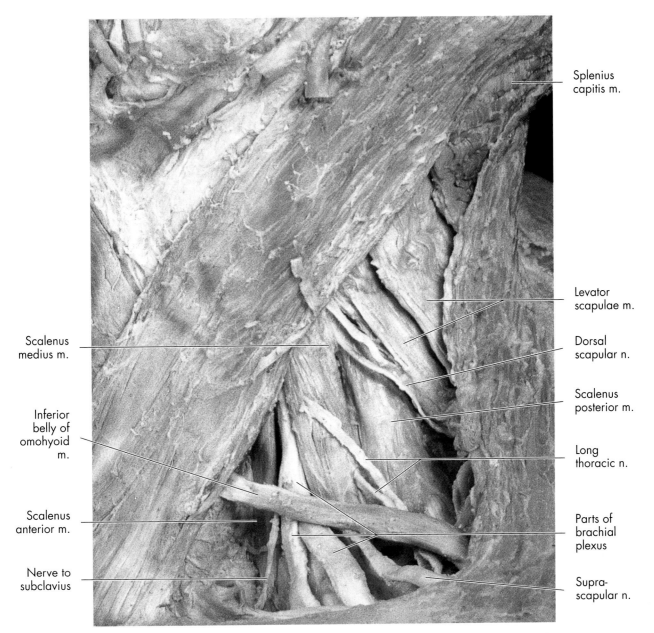

Figure 2-8 Floor of the posterior triangle from which the prevertebral fascia has been removed. The inferior belly of the omohyoid muscle, one of the contents of the triangle, is still present.

See **PRINCIPLES**, Figs. 2-31, *A*; 2-68

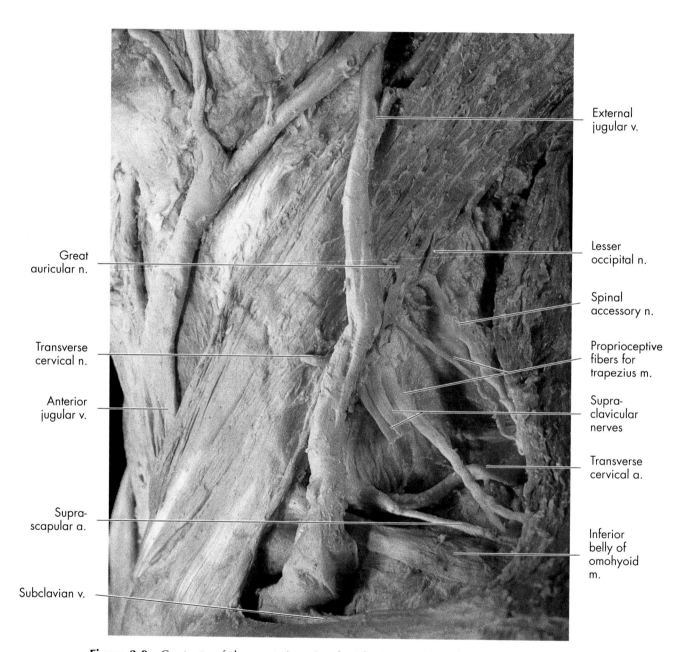

Great
auricular n.

Transverse
cervical n.

Anterior
jugular v.

Supra-
scapular a.

Subclavian v.

External
jugular v.

Lesser
occipital n.

Spinal
accessory n.

Proprioceptive
fibers for
trapezius m.

Supra-
clavicular
nerves

Transverse
cervical a.

Inferior
belly of
omohyoid
m.

Figure 2-9 Contents of the posterior triangle. The external jugular vein is continuous
with the anterior jugular system.

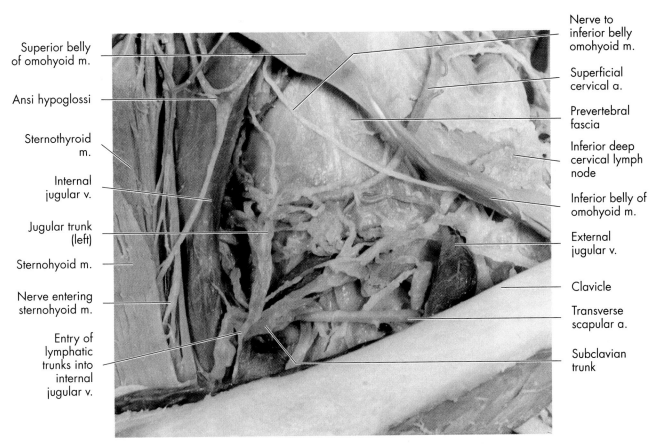

Superior belly of omohyoid m.

Ansi hypoglossi

Sternothyroid m.

Internal jugular v.

Jugular trunk (left)

Sternohyoid m.

Nerve entering sternohyoid m.

Entry of lymphatic trunks into internal jugular v.

Nerve to inferior belly omohyoid m.

Superficial cervical a.

Prevertebral fascia

Inferior deep cervical lymph node

Inferior belly of omohyoid m.

External jugular v.

Clavicle

Transverse scapular a.

Subclavian trunk

Figure 2-10 Middle layer of cervical fascia removed from the jugular/subclavian triangle with the omohyoid muscle retracted superiorly. The thoracic duct, although not visible, enters the subclavian/jugular angle with the lymphatic trunks visible in this dissection. *The thoracic duct enters the venous system at the junction of the left internal jugular and left subclavian veins. Sometimes cancer arising below the diaphragm (i.e., stomach) may spread to a left supraclavicular node (sentinel node) creating a palpable lump. Biopsy of lymph nodes in this area is performed with care to avoid injury to the thoracic duct, which might lead to a fistula draining lymph from the neck wound.*

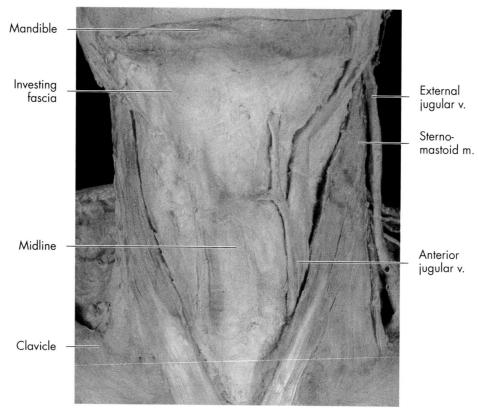

Mandible

Investing fascia

Midline

Clavicle

External jugular v.

Sterno-mastoid m.

Anterior jugular v.

Figure 2-11 Boundaries and roofs of both anterior triangles of the neck. Boundaries are anterior border of the sternomastoid muscle, margin of the mandible, and the midline of the neck. Midline is the division between the two triangles.

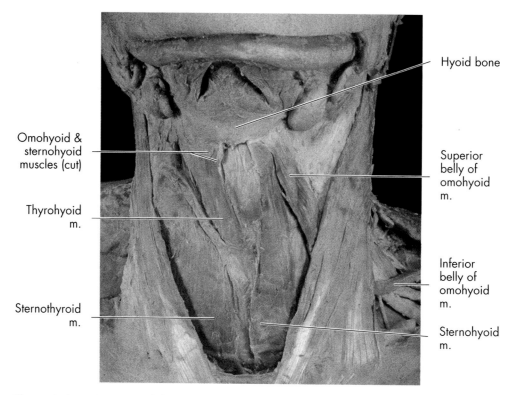

Omohyoid & sternohyoid muscles (cut)

Thyrohyoid m.

Sternothyroid m.

Hyoid bone

Superior belly of omohyoid m.

Inferior belly of omohyoid m.

Sternohyoid m.

Figure 2-12 Contents of the anterior triangle. The right omohyoid and sternohyoid muscles have been removed to show the deeper thyrohyoid and sternothyroid muscles.

See DISSECTIONS, Section 2, p. 15

See PRINCIPLES, Figs. 2-63, 2-74

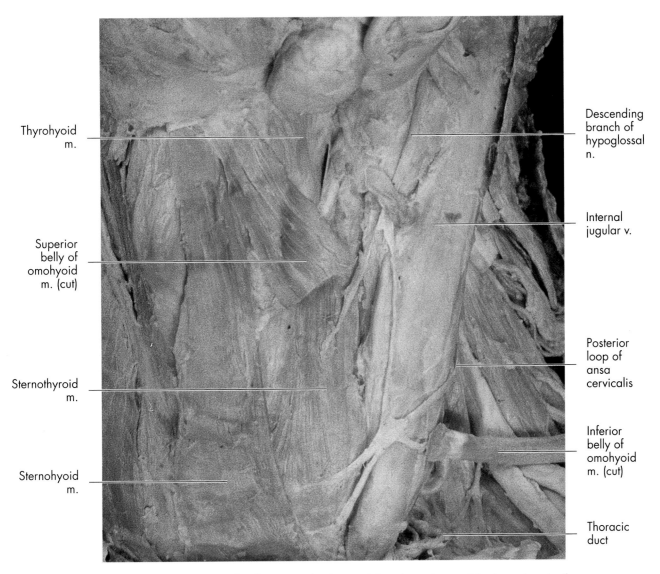

Thyrohyoid m.

Superior belly of omohyoid m. (cut)

Sternothyroid m.

Sternohyoid m.

Descending branch of hypoglossal n.

Internal jugular v.

Posterior loop of ansa cervicalis

Inferior belly of omohyoid m. (cut)

Thoracic duct

Figure 2-13 Ansa cervicalis, lying on the internal jugular vein, and its branches to the strap muscles on the left side of the neck.

SEE PRINCIPLES, FIG. 2-78

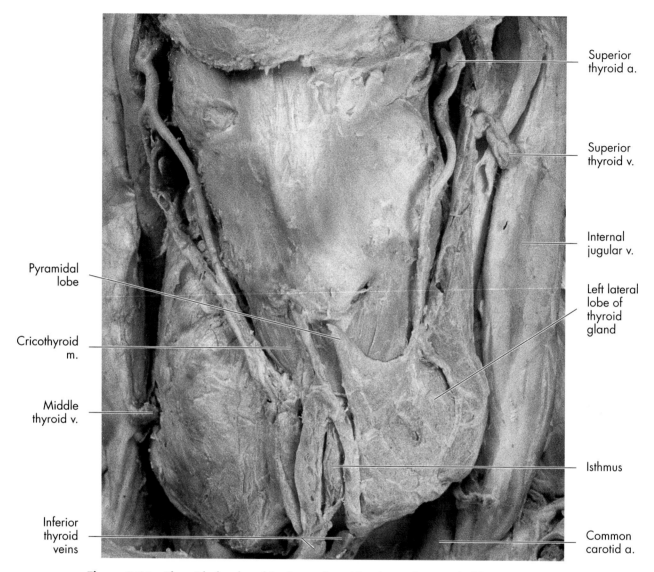

Superior thyroid a.

Superior thyroid v.

Internal jugular v.

Left lateral lobe of thyroid gland

Isthmus

Common carotid a.

Pyramidal lobe

Cricothyroid m.

Middle thyroid v.

Inferior thyroid veins

Figure 2-14   Thyroid gland and its immediate blood supply revealed by removal of the pretracheal fascia. *The thyroid gland is subject to hyper- and hypo-functional disorders and tumors that sometimes require surgical removal of all or part of the gland. A knowledge of arterial supply from the superior and inferior thyroid arteries and venous drainage via the superior middle and inferior thyroid veins and occasionally thyroidea ima vessels is essential. Even more crucial is an understanding of the relationship of the superior laryngeal nerves and superior thyroid vessels and the recurrent laryngeal nerve running just posterior to the gland in the groove between the trachea and esophagus. The parathyroid glands are subject to accidental removal with the thyroid since they lie on the posterior surface of the right and left thyroid lobes.*

SEE DISSECTIONS, SECTION 1, P. 9; SECTION 2, P. 15

SEE PRINCIPLES, FIG. 2-78

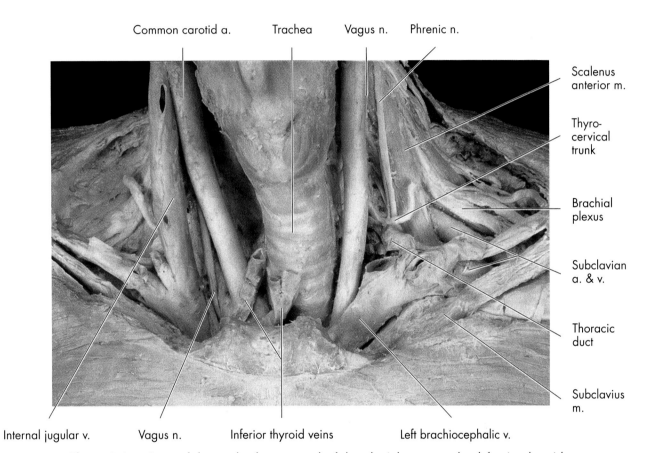

Figure 2-15 Root of the neck after removal of the clavicles, pretracheal fascia, thyroid gland, carotid sheath, and left internal jugular vein.

SEE DISSECTIONS, SECTION 1, P. 9; SECTION 2, P. 15

SEE PRINCIPLES, FIG. 3-17

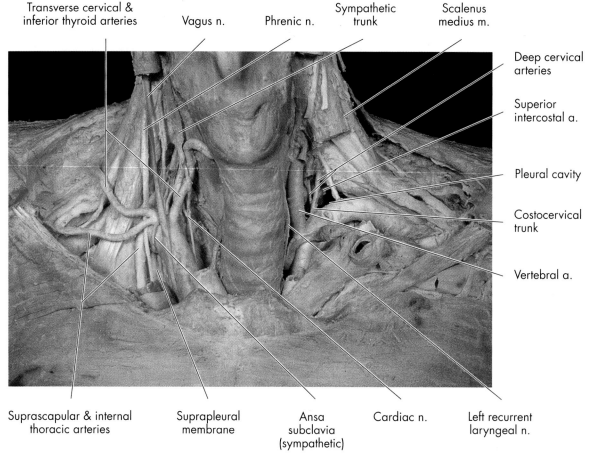

Transverse cervical &
inferior thyroid arteries

Vagus n.

Phrenic n.

Sympathetic
trunk

Scalenus
medius m.

Deep cervical
arteries

Superior
intercostal a.

Pleural cavity

Costocervical
trunk

Vertebral a.

Suprascapular & internal
thoracic arteries

Suprapleural
membrane

Ansa
subclavia
(sympathetic)

Cardiac n.

Left recurrent
laryngeal n.

Figure 2-16   Deeper structures of the root of neck revealed by removal of most of the left vagus and phrenic nerves, the left scalenus anterior, both common carotid arteries, and the large veins. *The phrenic nerve is readily accessible to the surgeon as it passes across the anterior surface of the scalenus anterior muscle obliquely from superolateral to infraomedial. The nerve may be blocked temporarily with local anesthetic injected in the region or the nerve may be exposed and crushed to paralyze the hemidiaphragm for many weeks or it may be cut to secure permanent paralysis. Temporary interruption may be used for singultus (hiccups). Prolonged paralysis may be used to rest the lung in pulmonary disease such as tuberculosis, and permanent paralysis may help obliterate dead space left after a pneumonectomy.*

See DISSECTIONS, Section 2, p. 16

See PRINCIPLES, Fig. 2-81

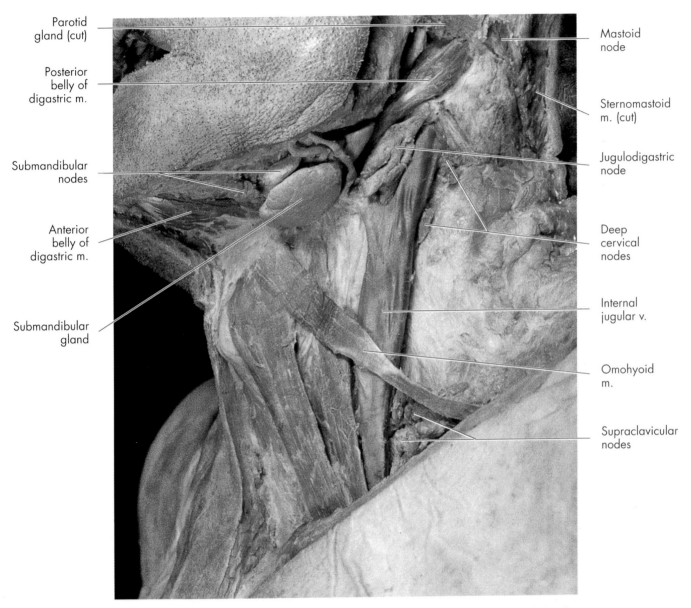

Parotid gland (cut)

Posterior belly of digastric m.

Submandibular nodes

Anterior belly of digastric m.

Submandibular gland

Mastoid node

Sternomastoid m. (cut)

Jugulodigastric node

Deep cervical nodes

Internal jugular v.

Omohyoid m.

Supraclavicular nodes

Figure 2-17   Internal jugular vein and some cervical lymph nodes, revealed after removal of sternomastoid and part of the parotid gland.

See DISSECTIONS, Section 2, p. 16

See PRINCIPLES, Fig. 2-68

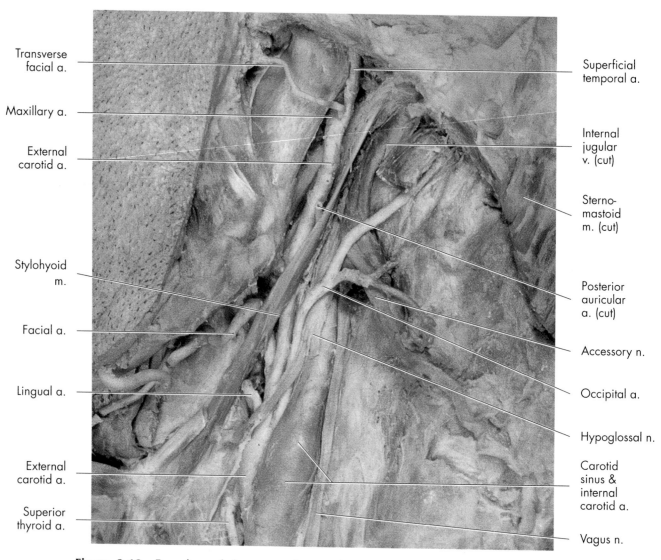

Transverse facial a.

Maxillary a.

External carotid a.

Stylohyoid m.

Facial a.

Lingual a.

External carotid a.

Superior thyroid a.

Superficial temporal a.

Internal jugular v. (cut)

Sterno-mastoid m. (cut)

Posterior auricular a. (cut)

Accessory n.

Occipital a.

Hypoglossal n.

Carotid sinus & internal carotid a.

Vagus n.

Figure 2-18 Branches of the external carotid artery and the vagus, accessory, and hypoglossal nerves after removal of part of the internal jugular vein, carotid sheath, and the posterior belly of the digastric muscle.

See **PRINCIPLES, FIG. 2-1,** *A*

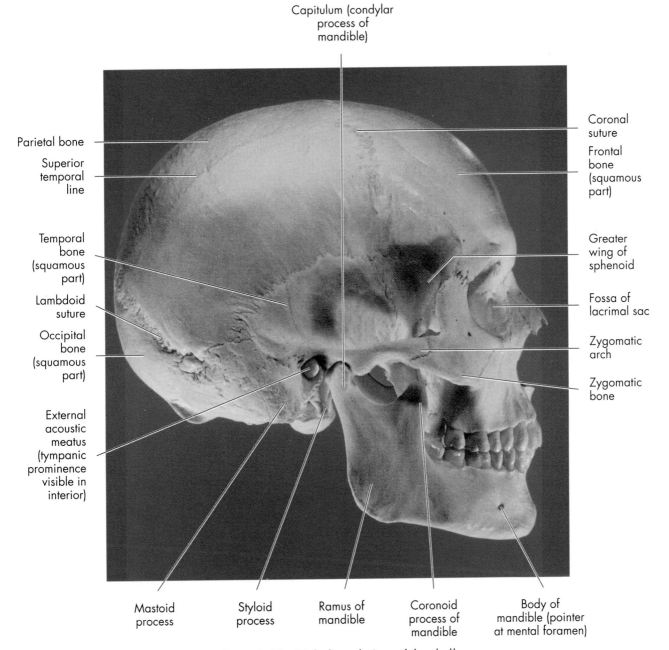

Capitulum (condylar process of mandible)

Parietal bone

Superior temporal line

Temporal bone (squamous part)

Lambdoid suture

Occipital bone (squamous part)

External acoustic meatus (tympanic prominence visible in interior)

Coronal suture

Frontal bone (squamous part)

Greater wing of sphenoid

Fossa of lacrimal sac

Zygomatic arch

Zygomatic bone

Mastoid process

Styloid process

Ramus of mandible

Coronoid process of mandible

Body of mandible (pointer at mental foramen)

Figure 2-19   Right lateral view of the skull.

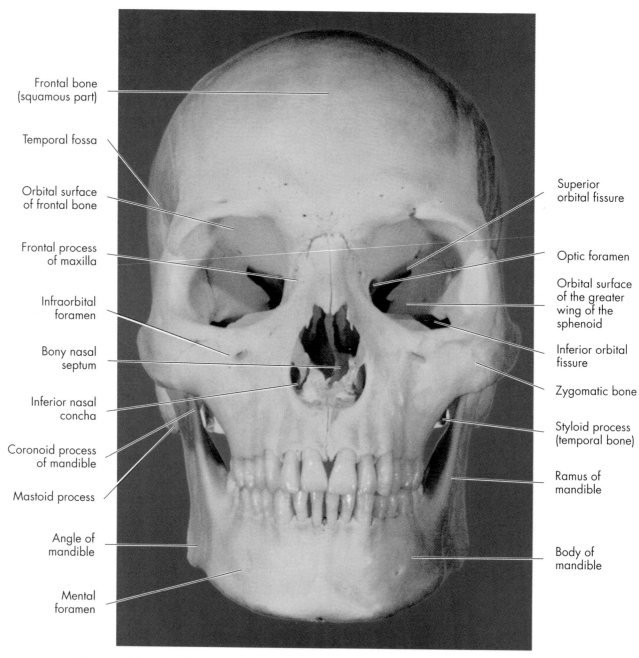

Frontal bone
(squamous part)

Temporal fossa

Orbital surface
of frontal bone

Frontal process
of maxilla

Infraorbital
foramen

Bony nasal
septum

Inferior nasal
concha

Coronoid process
of mandible

Mastoid process

Angle of
mandible

Mental
foramen

Superior
orbital fissure

Optic foramen

Orbital surface
of the greater
wing of the
sphenoid

Inferior orbital
fissure

Zygomatic bone

Styloid process
(temporal bone)

Ramus of
mandible

Body of
mandible

Figure 2-20   Anterior view of the skull. There is a supraorbital foramen on the right and a supraorbital notch on the left. Note the deviation of the bony nasal septum.

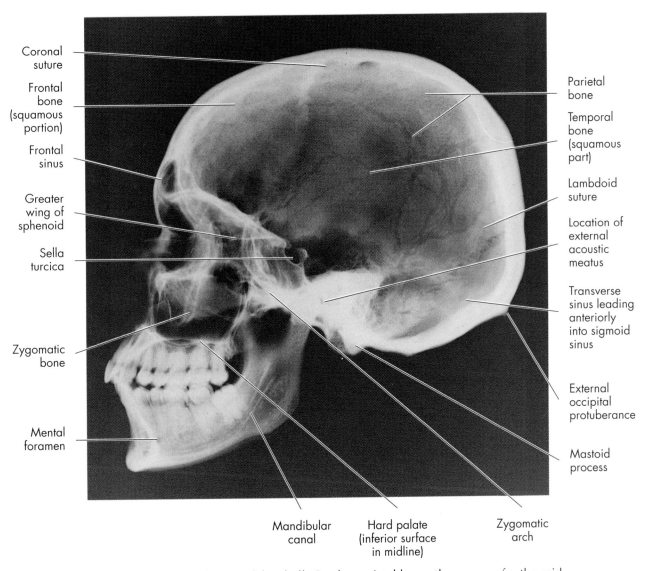

Figure 2-21 Left lateral x-ray of the skull. On the parietal bone, the grooves for the middle meningeal artery are visible anteriorly, and channels for the temporal posterior diploic vein are visible posteriorly. Occipital condyles of the mastoid process are visible slightly anteriorly.

SEE PRINCIPLES, FIG. 2-2

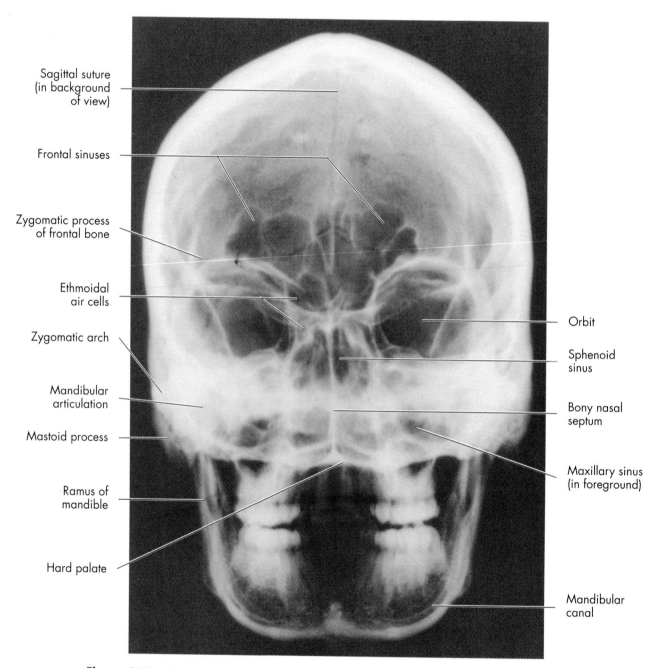

Sagittal suture
(in background
of view)

Frontal sinuses

Zygomatic process
of frontal bone

Ethmoidal
air cells

Zygomatic arch

Mandibular
articulation

Mastoid process

Ramus of
mandible

Hard palate

Orbit

Sphenoid
sinus

Bony nasal
septum

Maxillary sinus
(in foreground)

Mandibular
canal

Figure 2-22 Anteroposterior x-ray of the skull. The sella turcica and the clinoid processes lie posterior to the ethymoidal cells.

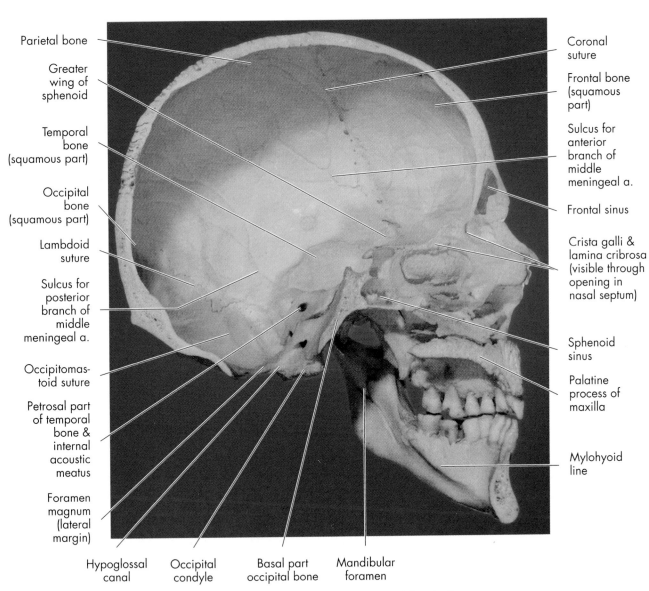

Parietal bone

Greater
wing of
sphenoid

Temporal
bone
(squamous part)

Occipital
bone
(squamous part)

Lambdoid
suture

Sulcus for
posterior
branch of
middle
meningeal a.

Occipitomas-
toid suture

Petrosal part
of temporal
bone &
internal
acoustic
meatus

Foramen
magnum
(lateral
margin)

Hypoglossal
canal

Occipital
condyle

Basal part
occipital bone

Mandibular
foramen

Coronal
suture

Frontal bone
(squamous
part)

Sulcus for
anterior
branch of
middle
meningeal a.

Frontal sinus

Crista galli &
lamina cribrosa
(visible through
opening in
nasal septum)

Sphenoid
sinus

Palatine
process of
maxilla

Mylohyoid
line

Figure 2-23   Midsagittal section of the skull.

SEE DISSECTIONS, SECTION 2, P. 10

SEE PRINCIPLES, FIG. 2-42

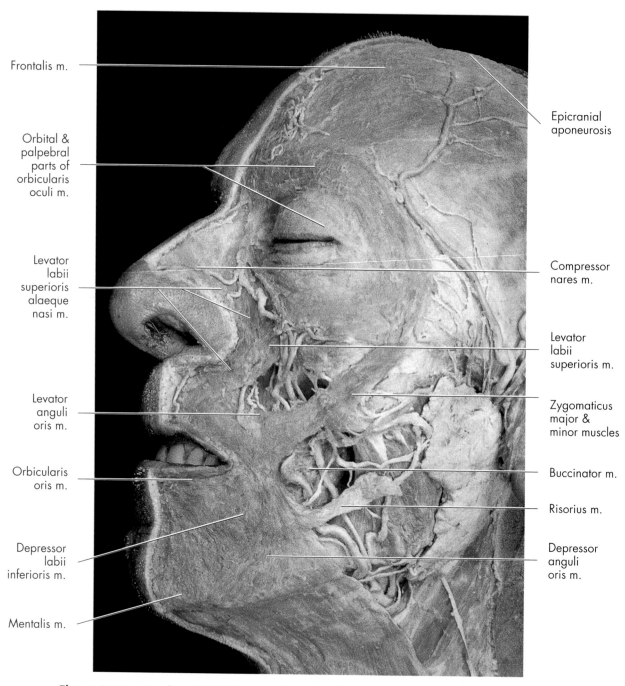

Frontalis m.

Orbital &
palpebral
parts of
orbicularis
oculi m.

Levator
labii
superioris
alaeque
nasi m.

Levator
anguli
oris m.

Orbicularis
oris m.

Depressor
labii
inferioris m.

Mentalis m.

Epicranial
aponeurosis

Compressor
nares m.

Levator
labii
superioris m.

Zygomaticus
major &
minor muscles

Buccinator m.

Risorius m.

Depressor
anguli
oris m.

Figure 2-24 Muscles of facial expression. The skin and subcutaneous fat have been removed.

SEE DISSECTIONS, SECTION 2, P. 10
SEE PRINCIPLES, FIG. 2-42

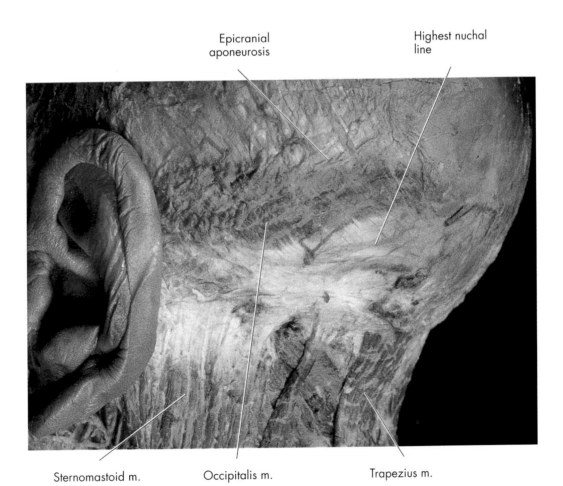

Epicranial
aponeurosis

Highest nuchal
line

Sternomastoid m.   Occipitalis m.   Trapezius m.

Figure 2-25   Posterior view showing the occipitalis muscle and part of the epicranial aponeurosis.

SEE DISSECTIONS, SECTION 2, P. 10

SEE PRINCIPLES, FIG. 2-42

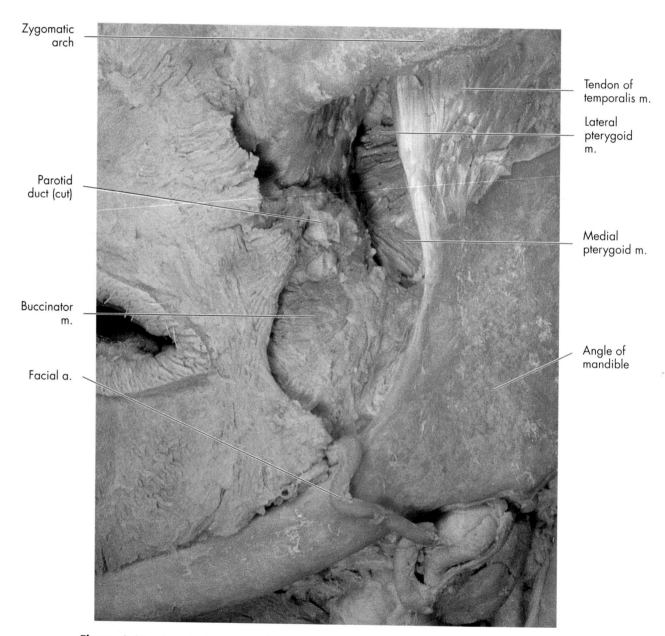

Zygomatic arch

Tendon of temporalis m.

Lateral pterygoid m.

Parotid duct (cut)

Medial pterygoid m.

Buccinator m.

Angle of mandible

Facial a.

Figure 2-26 Buccinator seen after removal of some superficial facial muscles, the parotid gland and most of its duct, and the masseter muscle.

See DISSECTIONS, SECTION 2, p. 10
See PRINCIPLES, FIG. 2-42

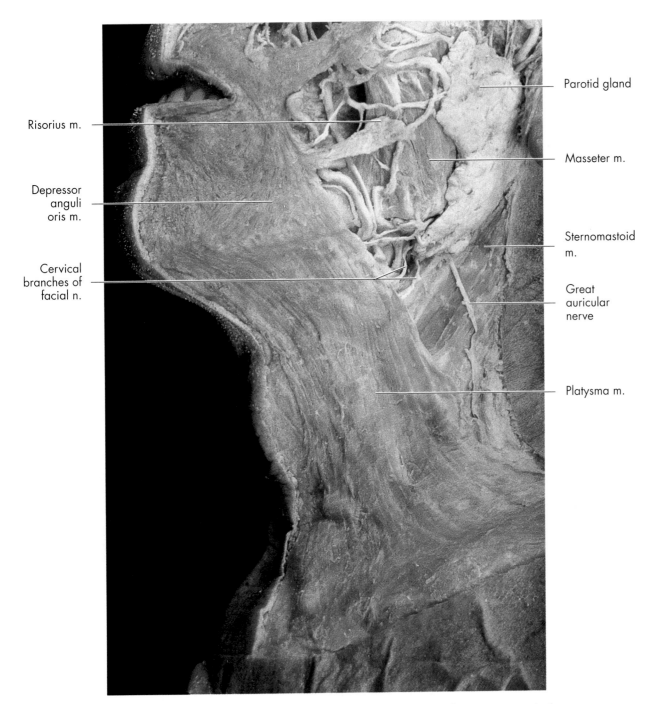

Risorius m.

Depressor anguli oris m.

Cervical branches of facial n.

Parotid gland

Masseter m.

Sternomastoid m.

Great auricular nerve

Platysma m.

Figure 2-27 Platysma, the largest muscle of facial expression, and its nerve supply from the cervical branches of the facial nerve.

See DISSECTIONS, Section 2, p. 10
See PRINCIPLES, Figs. 2-44, 2-48, *A*

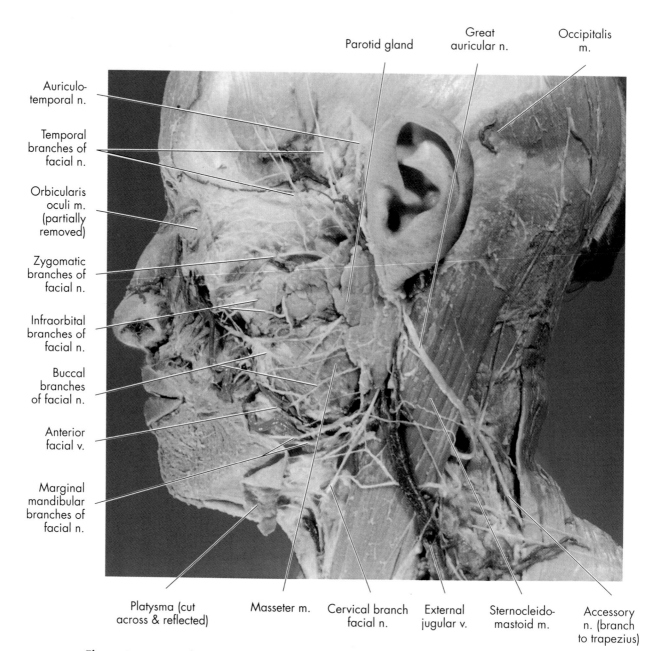

Parotid gland   Great auricular n.   Occipitalis m.

Auriculo-temporal n.

Temporal branches of facial n.

Orbicularis oculi m. (partially removed)

Zygomatic branches of facial n.

Infraorbital branches of facial n.

Buccal branches of facial n.

Anterior facial v.

Marginal mandibular branches of facial n.

Platysma (cut across & reflected)   Masseter m.   Cervical branch facial n.   External jugular v.   Sternocleido-mastoid m.   Accessory n. (branch to trapezius)

Figure 2-28   Overlying fascia removed to reveal the parotid gland and various branches of the facial nerve. The course of the external carotid artery and anterior facial vein is displayed. In the neck, the platysma has been extensively cut away and the external layer of deep cervical fascia removed. *Parotid removal (parotidectomy) requires meticulous attention to anatomic detail to avoid injury to the important facial nerve whose branches course between the superficial and deep lobes of the gland. Facial paralysis may occur with malignant parotid tumors and even with severe inflammation of the parotid gland. Facial paralysis may also occur with several systemic disorders that result in inflammatory swelling around the nerve within the facial canal just before the nerve exits from the stylomastoid foramen (Bell's palsy). Such paralysis often subsides spontaneously but sometimes requires steroid therapy and even surgical decompression of the tunnel.*

See PRINCIPLES, Fig. 2-40

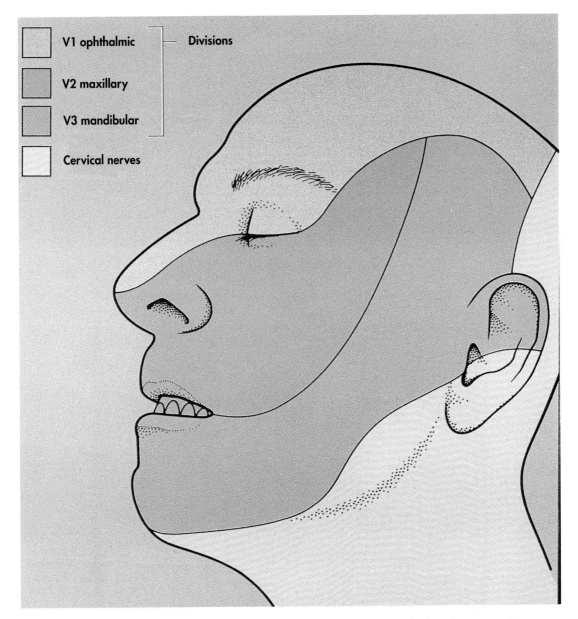

Figure 2-29 Dermatomes of the face. Areas of the face are supplied with sensory fibers from the different division of the trigeminal nerve.

SEE DISSECTIONS, SECTION 2, P. 10

SEE PRINCIPLES, FIGS. 2-37, 2-38, 2-45, 2-48, *B*

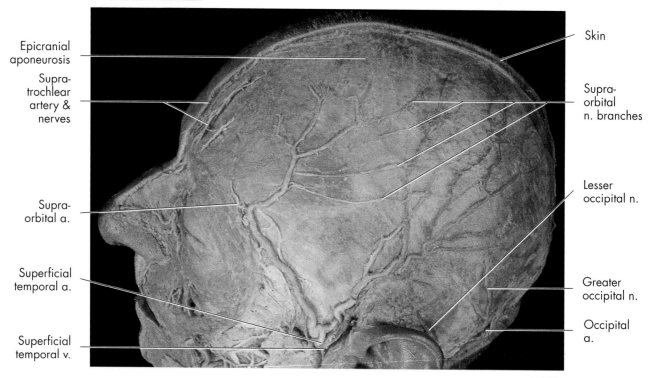

Epicranial aponeurosis

Supra-trochlear artery & nerves

Supra-orbital a.

Superficial temporal a.

Superficial temporal v.

Skin

Supra-orbital n. branches

Lesser occipital n.

Greater occipital n.

Occipital a.

Figure 2-30   Vessels and nerves of the scalp lying on the epicranial aponeurosis.

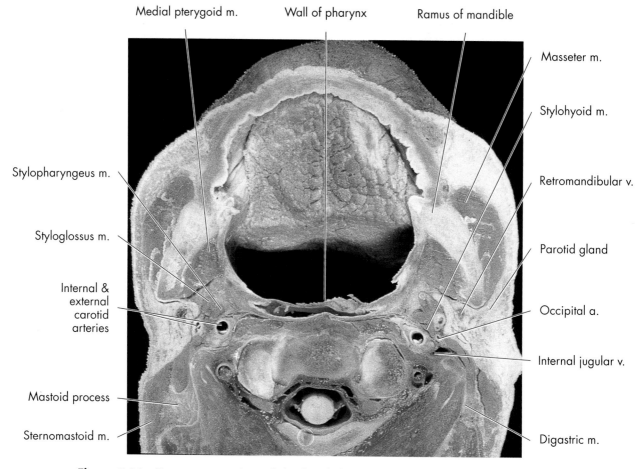

Medial pterygoid m.

Wall of pharynx

Ramus of mandible

Masseter m.

Stylohyoid m.

Retromandibular v.

Parotid gland

Occipital a.

Internal jugular v.

Digastric m.

Stylopharyngeus m.

Styloglossus m.

Internal & external carotid arteries

Mastoid process

Sternomastoid m.

Figure 2-31   Transverse section of the head through the parotid glands. They extend deeply as far as the styloid processes.

See DISSECTIONS, Section 2, p. 10

See PRINCIPLES, Fig. 2-48, A

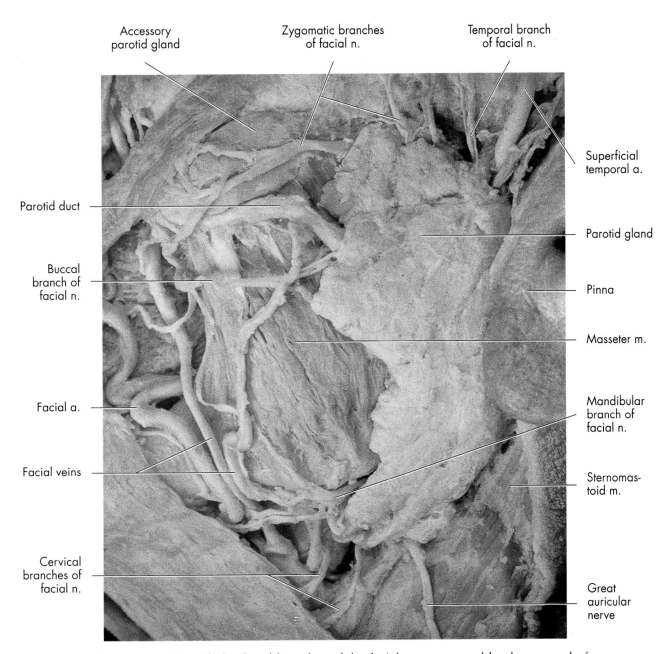

Figure 2-32   Parotid gland and branches of the facial nerve exposed by the removal of the superficial layer of the parotid fascia.

SEE DISSECTIONS, SECTION 2, P. 11
SEE PRINCIPLES, FIG. 2-47

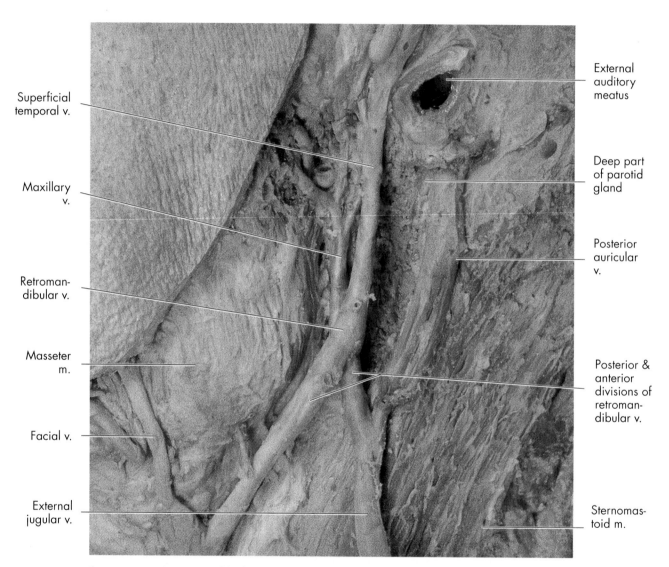

Superficial
temporal v.

Maxillary
v.

Retroman-
dibular v.

Masseter
m.

Facial v.

External
jugular v.

External
auditory
meatus

Deep part
of parotid
gland

Posterior
auricular
v.

Posterior &
anterior
divisions of
retroman-
dibular v.

Sternomas-
toid m.

Figure 2-33   Retromandibular vein and its communications seen after removal of the superficial portion of the parotid gland.

See DISSECTIONS, Section 2, p. 11
See PRINCIPLES, Figs. 2-46, *A;* 2-53

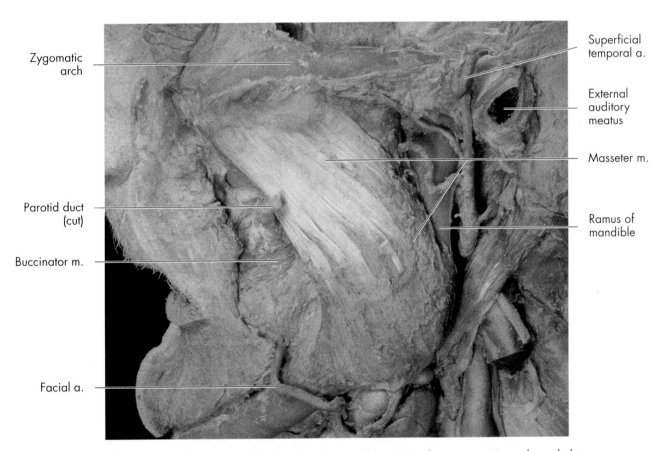

Zygomatic arch

Parotid duct (cut)

Buccinator m.

Facial a.

Superficial temporal a.

External auditory meatus

Masseter m.

Ramus of mandible

Figure 2-34   Masseter muscle showing its attachment to the zygomatic arch and the angle of the mandible, after removal of the parotid gland.

See DISSECTIONS, Section 2, p. 11

See PRINCIPLES, Figs. 2-46, *A* and *B;* 2-53

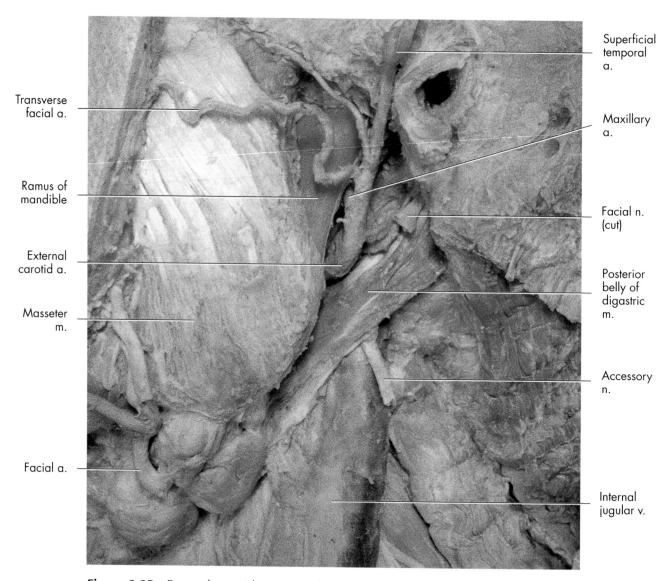

Transverse facial a.

Ramus of mandible

External carotid a.

Masseter m.

Facial a.

Superficial temporal a.

Maxillary a.

Facial n. (cut)

Posterior belly of digastric m.

Accessory n.

Internal jugular v.

Figure 2-35   External carotid artery and its terminal branches revealed by complete excision of the parotid gland.

SEE **DISSECTIONS**, SECTION 2, P. 12

SEE **PRINCIPLES**, FIGS. 2-46, *A;* 2-53

Temporalis m.   Zygomatic   Capsule of
                         arch (cut)   temporomandibular
                                                joint

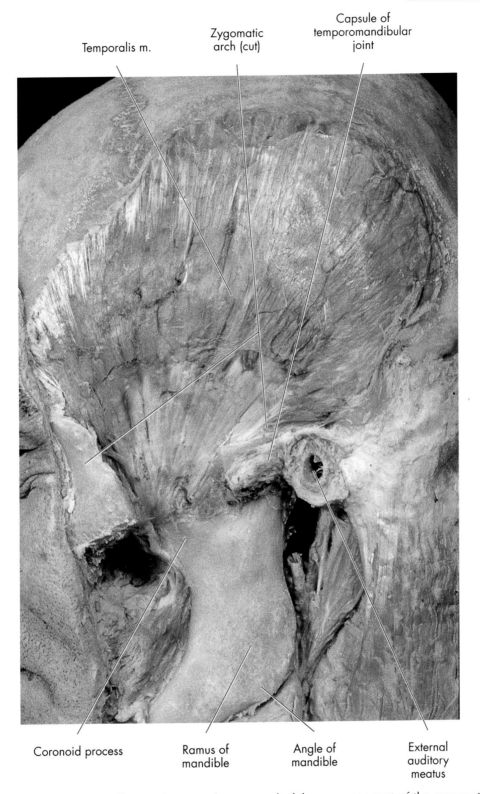

Coronoid process   Ramus of   Angle of   External
                    mandible   mandible   auditory
                                                meatus

Figure 2-36   Temporalis muscle seen after removal of the masseter, part of the zygomatic arch, and the temporal fascia.

SEE DISSECTIONS, SECTION 2, P. 12
SEE PRINCIPLES, FIG. 2-50

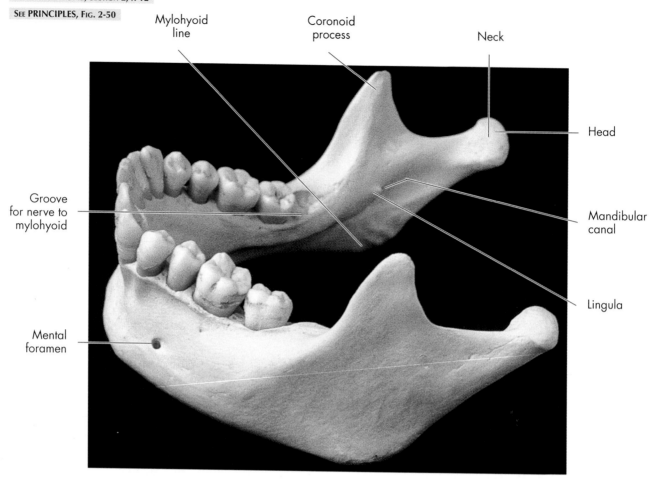

Mylohyoid line

Coronoid process

Neck

Head

Groove for nerve to mylohyoid

Mandibular canal

Lingula

Mental foramen

Figure 2-37   Mandible. The right wisdom tooth is partially erupted.

Coronoid process

Ramus of mandible

Body of mandible

Angle of mandible

Mandibular canal

Condyloid process of mandible

Figure 2-38   Posteroanterior oblique x-ray of the mandible.

See **PRINCIPLES**, Figs. 2-122, 2-123

Infraorbital
foramen

Maxillary sinus
(opened)

Molar II
(permanent)

Molar I
(permanent)

Molar II
(deciduous)

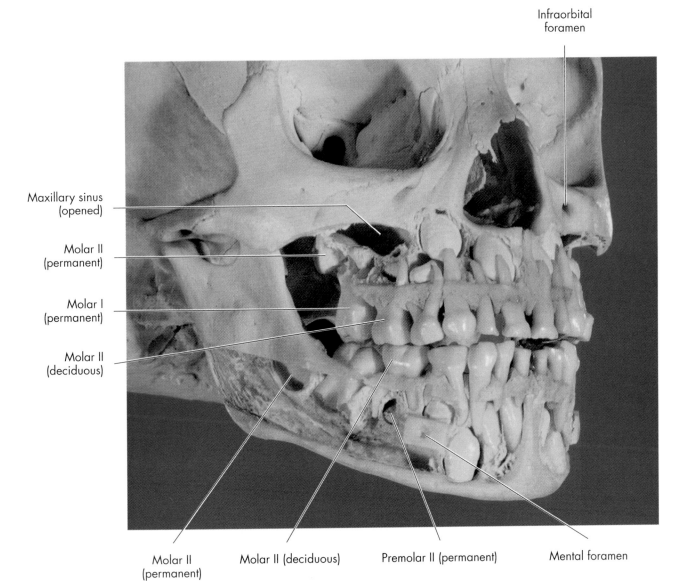

Molar II
(permanent)   Molar II (deciduous)   Premolar II (permanent)   Mental foramen

Figure 2-39   Deciduous and permanent teeth at 6 years of age. Parts of the maxilla and mandible have been cut away to reveal the roots of the deciduous teeth and the nonerupted permanent teeth in various stages of development. The maxillary sinus has been opened.

S ee DISSECTIONS, Section 2, p. 12
S ee PRINCIPLES, Fig. 2-51

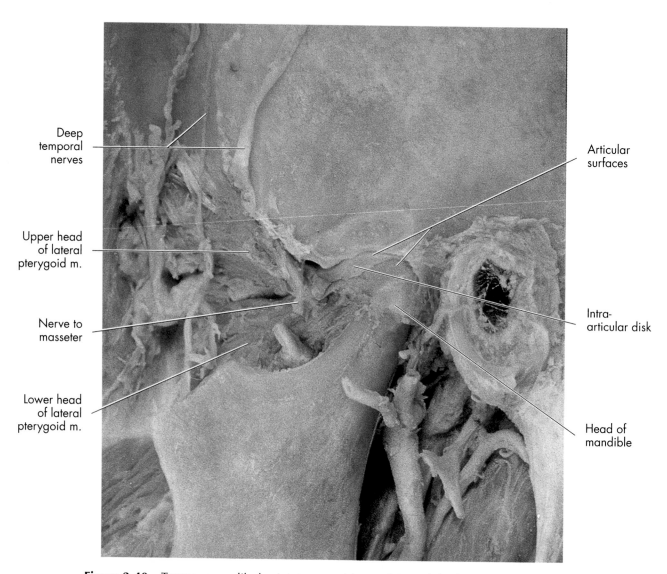

Deep
temporal
nerves

Upper head
of lateral
pterygoid m.

Nerve to
masseter

Lower head
of lateral
pterygoid m.

Articular
surfaces

Intra-
articular disk

Head of
mandible

Figure 2-40   Temporomandibular joint opened by excision of the lateral part of its capsule.

See DISSECTIONS, Section 2, p. 12

See PRINCIPLES, Fig. 2-53

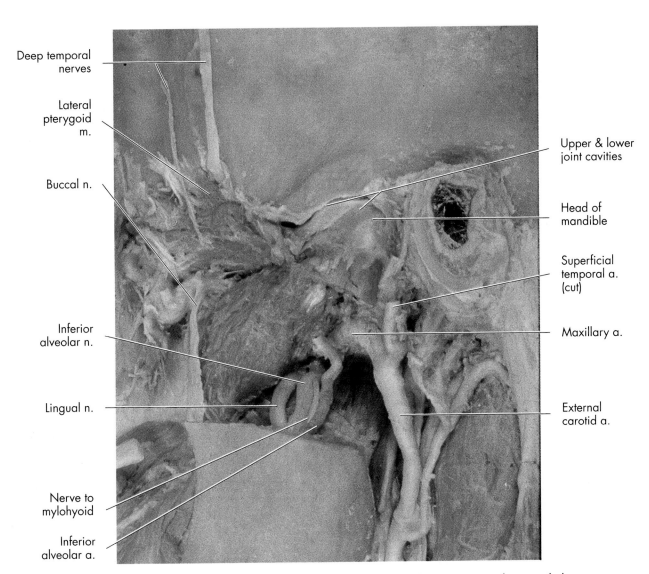

Deep temporal
nerves

Lateral
pterygoid
m.

Buccal n.

Inferior
alveolar n.

Lingual n.

Nerve to
mylohyoid

Inferior
alveolar a.

Upper & lower
joint cavities

Head of
mandible

Superficial
temporal a.
(cut)

Maxillary a.

External
carotid a.

Figure 2-41   Contents of the infratemporal fossa seen after excision of part of the mandible.

108   **Clinical Anatomy Atlas**

S<small>EE</small> **DISSECTIONS**, S<small>ECTION</small> 2, <small>P.</small> 13

S<small>EE</small> **PRINCIPLES**, F<small>IGS.</small> 2-55, 2-56

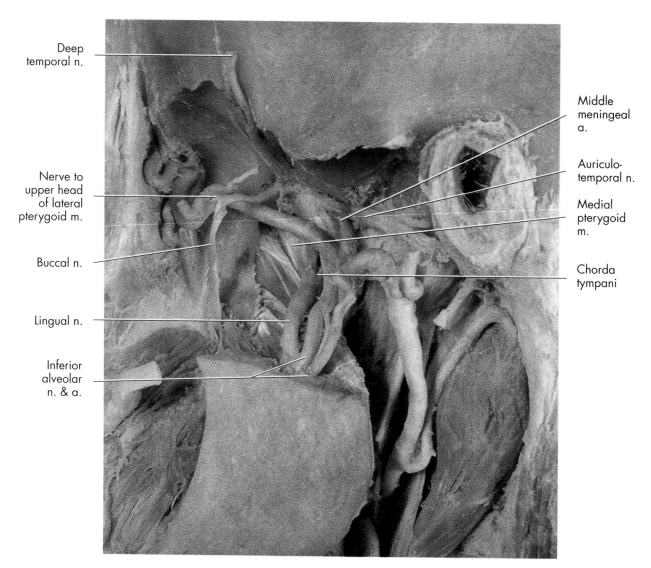

Deep temporal n.

Nerve to upper head of lateral pterygoid m.

Buccal n.

Lingual n.

Inferior alveolar n. & a.

Middle meningeal a.

Auriculo-temporal n.

Medial pterygoid m.

Chorda tympani

Figure 2-42   Branches of the mandibular division of the trigeminal nerve and the maxillary artery revealed by removal of the mandibular head and lateral pterygoid.

SEE DISSECTIONS, SECTION 2, PP. 13 AND 14

SEE PRINCIPLES, FIG. 2-56

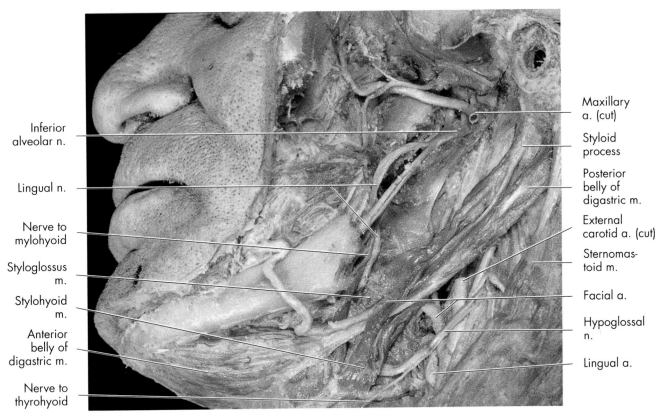

Inferior alveolar n.

Lingual n.

Nerve to mylohyoid

Styloglossus m.

Stylohyoid m.

Anterior belly of digastric m.

Nerve to thyrohyoid

Maxillary a. (cut)

Styloid process

Posterior belly of digastric m.

External carotid a. (cut)

Sternomas- toid m.

Facial a.

Hypoglossal n.

Lingual a.

Figure 2-43 Digastric and stylohyoid muscles seen after removal of part of the mandible. The superficial part of the submandibular gland has also been excised.

See DISSECTIONS, SECTION 2, PP. 13 AND 14

See PRINCIPLES, FIG. 2-56

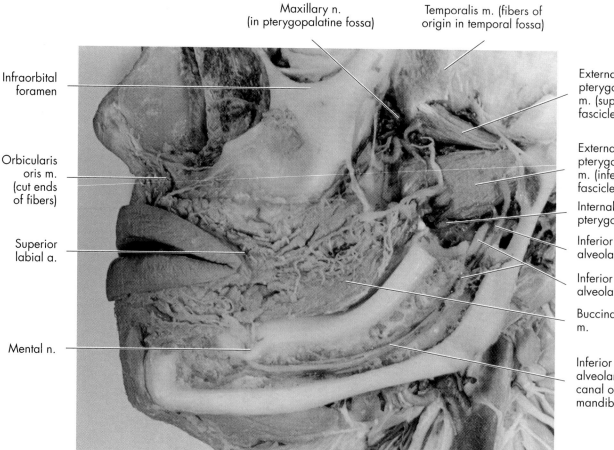

Maxillary n.
(in pterygopalatine fossa)

Temporalis m. (fibers of
origin in temporal fossa)

Infraorbital
foramen

Orbicularis
oris m.
(cut ends
of fibers)

Superior
labial a.

Mental n.

External
pterygoid
m. (superior
fascicle)

External
pterygoid
m. (inferior
fascicle)

Internal
pterygoid m.

Inferior
alveolar a.

Inferior
alveolar n.

Buccinator
m.

Inferior
alveolar
canal of
mandible

Figure 2-44 Muscles of facial expression have been completely removed from the left half of the face. The lips, mucosa of the oral cavity with its associated glands, and the buccinator muscle have been preserved. The ramus of the mandible, the masseter, and temporal muscles, and the zygomatic arch have been cut away. The contents of the infratemporal and pterygopalatine fossae are visible. The body of the mandible has been partially resected to demonstrate the course of the inferior alveolar vessels and nerve.

See DISSECTIONS, SECTION 2, PP. 13 AND 14

See PRINCIPLES, FIG. 2-56

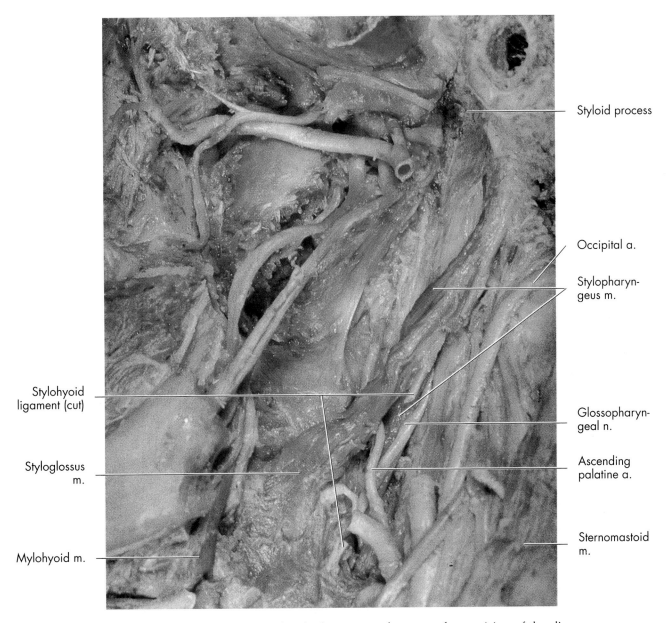

Styloid process

Occipital a.

Stylopharyn-
geus m.

Glossopharyn-
geal n.

Ascending
palatine a.

Sternomastoid
m.

Stylohyoid
ligament (cut)

Styloglossus
m.

Mylohyoid m.

Figure 2-45   Stylopharyngeus and styloglossus muscles seen after excision of the digastric stylohyoid and the middle portion of the stylohyoid ligament.

SEE DISSECTIONS, SECTION 2, P. 16

SEE PRINCIPLES, FIG. 2-80, *B*

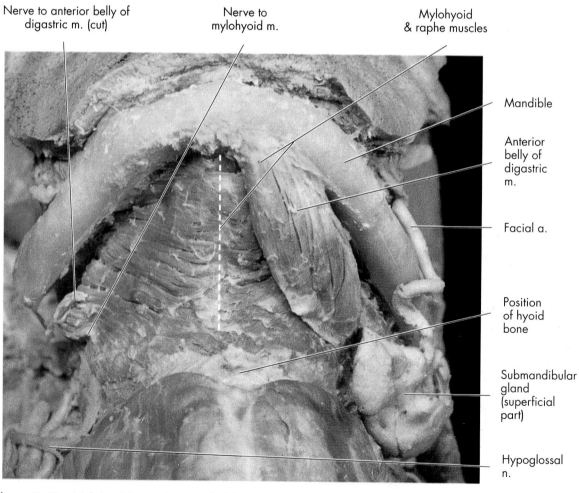

Nerve to anterior belly of
digastric m. (cut)

Nerve to
mylohyoid m.

Mylohyoid
& raphe muscles

Mandible

Anterior
belly of
digastric
m.

Facial a.

Position
of hyoid
bone

Submandibular
gland
(superficial
part)

Hypoglossal
n.

Figure 2-46   Mylohyoid muscle revealed by removal of the right anterior belly of the digastric and the superficial part of the submandibular gland.

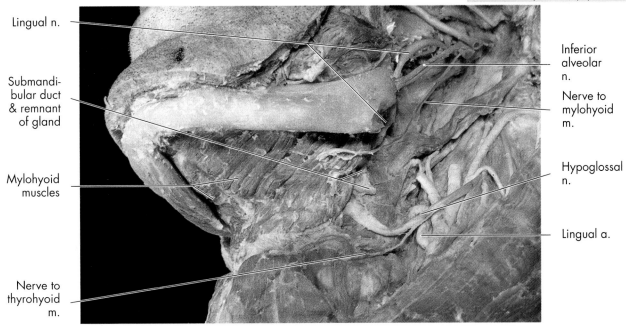

Lingual n.

Submandibular duct & remnant of gland

Mylohyoid muscles

Nerve to thyrohyoid m.

Inferior alveolar n.

Nerve to mylohyoid m.

Hypoglossal n.

Lingual a.

Figure 2-47 Hypoglossal nerve, lingual nerve, and submandibular duct passing above the mylohyoid muscle. *The submandibular (submaxillary) gland is subject to inflammation and swelling when stones form and partially block the submandibular duct. Surgical removal of the gland requires special attention to the mandibular (marginal) branch of the facial nerve, which is subject to injury resulting in facial asymmetry from paralysis of the depressors at the angle of the mouth. The duct runs in close proximity to the hypoglossal nerve, which, if injured, results in paralysis and atrophy of one side of the tongue. If the tongue is protruded, it points toward the side of injury. The lingual nerve is also in close relationship to the duct, and injury to the nerve results in numbness of the tongue subjecting it to unrecognized injury. Taste is lost on the anterior two thirds of the tongue but is compensated for by taste on the contralateral side*

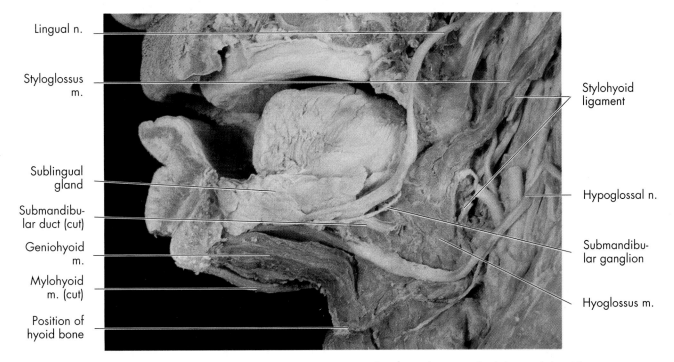

Lingual n.

Styloglossus m.

Sublingual gland

Submandibular duct (cut)

Geniohyoid m.

Mylohyoid m. (cut)

Position of hyoid bone

Stylohyoid ligament

Hypoglossal n.

Submandibular ganglion

Hyoglossus m.

Figure 2-48 Structures deep to mylohyoid seen after partial removal of the mylohyoid and the mandible. The submandibular ganglion is elongated in this specimen.

See DISSECTIONS, Section 2, pp. 18 and 20
See PRINCIPLES, Fig. 2-125

Foramen cecum   Sulcus terminalis

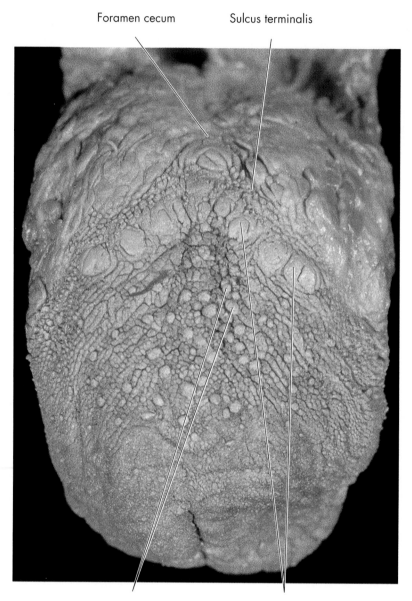

Fungiform papillae   Circumvallate papillae

Figure 2-49   Surface features of the tongue.

See **DISSECTIONS, Section 2, p. 17**

See **PRINCIPLES, Fig. 2-128, _A_**

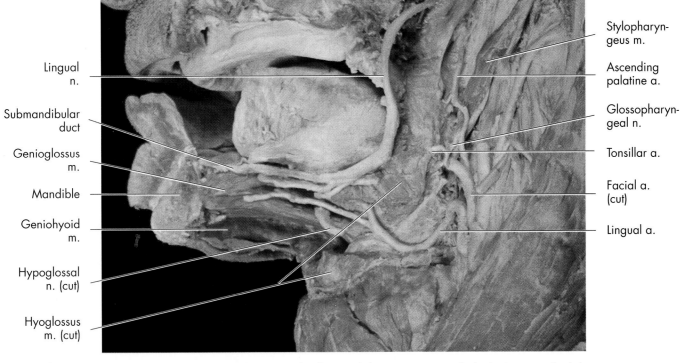

Lingual n.

Submandibular duct

Genioglossus m.

Mandible

Geniohyoid m.

Hypoglossal n. (cut)

Hyoglossus m. (cut)

Stylopharyngeus m.

Ascending palatine a.

Glossopharyngeal n.

Tonsillar a.

Facial a. (cut)

Lingual a.

Figure 2-50   Deeper structures in the base of the tongue revealed after removal of the sublingual gland and part of the hyoglossus muscle.

SEE **DISSECTIONS**, SECTION 2, PP. 17 AND 18

SEE **PRINCIPLES**, FIG. 2-118, *A*

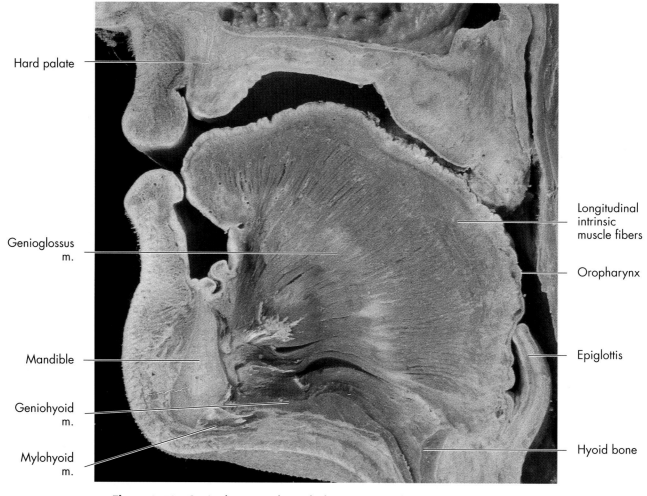

Hard palate

Genioglossus m.

Mandible

Geniohyoid m.

Mylohyoid m.

Longitudinal intrinsic muscle fibers

Oropharynx

Epiglottis

Hyoid bone

Figure 2-51   Sagittal section through the tongue and surrounding structures.

Foramen for zygomatico-
facial n.

Inferior
orbital fissure

Pterygo-
palatine fossa

Zygomatic
arch

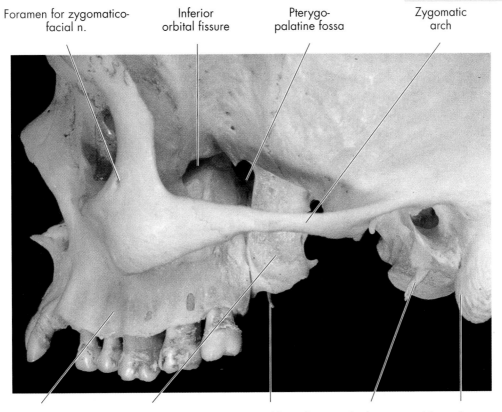

Maxilla   Lateral pterygoid plate   Pterygoid hamulus   Styloid process   Mastoid process

Figure 2-52   Pterygopalatine fossa bounded by the maxilla and lateral pterygoid plate.

Infraorbital n.   Fibers to lacrimal gland   Zygomatic n.   Zygomaticotemporal n.

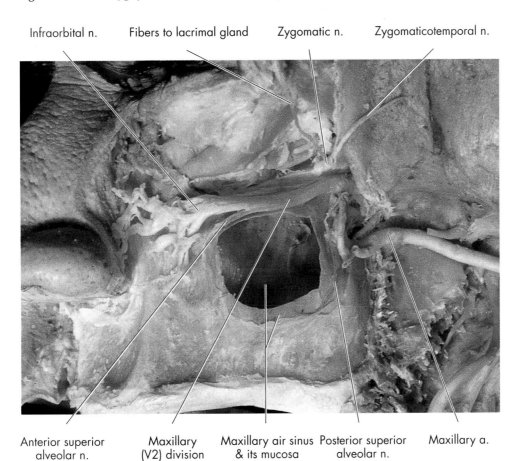

Anterior superior
alveolar n.

Maxillary
(V2) division

Maxillary air sinus
& its mucosa

Posterior superior
alveolar n.

Maxillary a.

Figure 2-53   Maxillary nerve and artery seen after excision of part of the lateral walls of the orbit and maxillary air sinus.

SEE DISSECTIONS, SECTION 2, P. 21

SEE PRINCIPLES, FIGS. 2-106, C; 2-113, A; 2-116

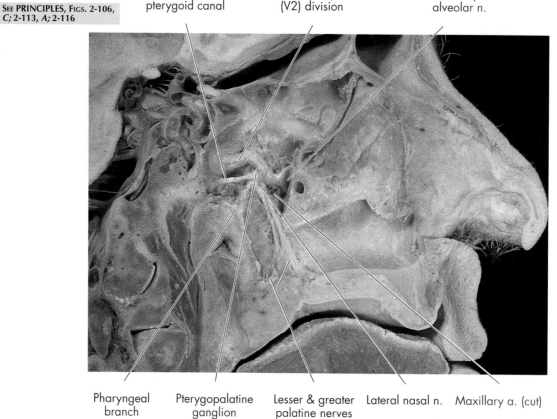

Nerve of pteryoid canal

Maxillary (V2) division

Posterior superior alveolar n.

Pharyngeal branch

Pterygopalatine ganglion

Lesser & greater palatine nerves

Lateral nasal n.

Maxillary a. (cut)

Figure 2-54 Medial view of the contents of the pterygopalatine fossa revealed by removal of bone from the lateral wall of the nose.

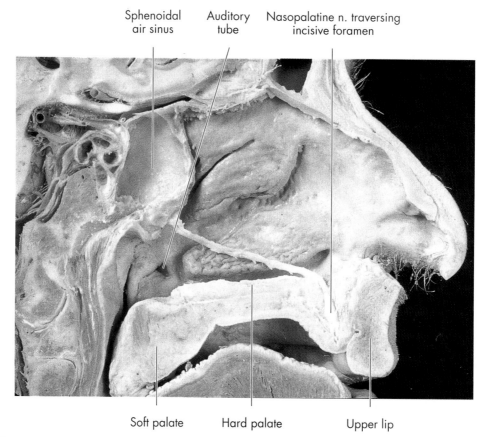

Sphenoidal air sinus

Auditory tube

Nasopalatine n. traversing incisive foramen

Soft palate

Hard palate

Upper lip

Figure 2-55 Sagittal section showing the left nasopalatine nerve in situ after removal of the nasal septum.

See **DISSECTIONS**, Section 2, p. 21

See **PRINCIPLES**, Fig. 2-113, *B*

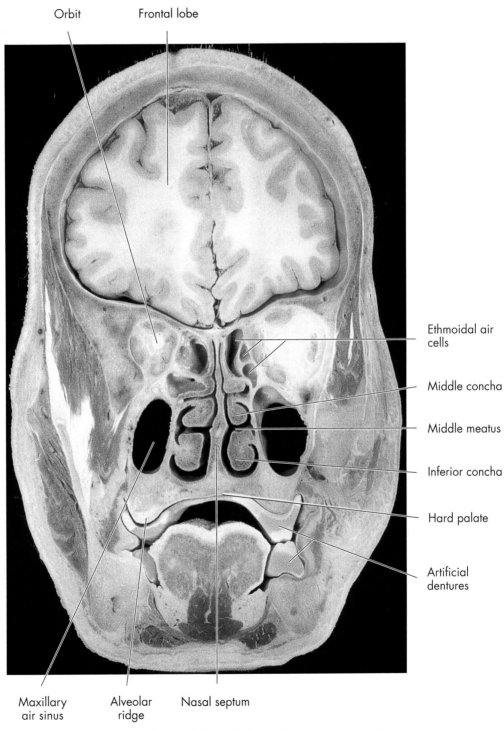

Orbit

Frontal lobe

Ethmoidal air cells

Middle concha

Middle meatus

Inferior concha

Hard palate

Artificial dentures

Maxillary air sinus

Alveolar ridge

Nasal septum

Figure 2-56   Section of the head through the orbits and nasal cavities.

See **PRINCIPLES**, Fig. 2-114, *C*

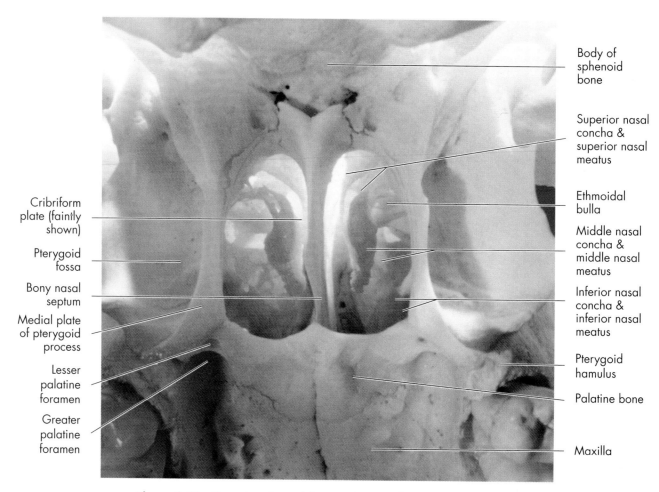

Body of
sphenoid
bone

Superior nasal
concha &
superior nasal
meatus

Ethmoidal
bulla

Middle nasal
concha &
middle nasal
meatus

Inferior nasal
concha &
inferior nasal
meatus

Pterygoid
hamulus

Palatine bone

Maxilla

Cribriform
plate (faintly
shown)

Pterygoid
fossa

Bony nasal
septum

Medial plate
of pterygoid
process

Lesser
palatine
foramen

Greater
palatine
foramen

Figure 2-57   Posterior view of the nasal cavity through the choanae.

See Dissections, Section 2, p. 21

See Principles, Fig. 2-113, *A*

Superior concha   Cribriform plate   Crista galli   Middle concha

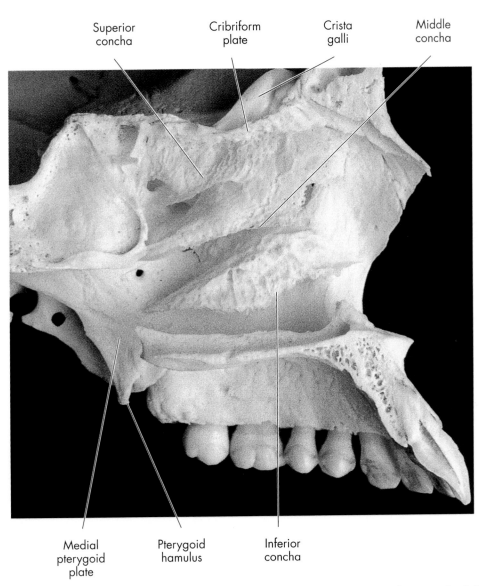

Medial pterygoid plate   Pterygoid hamulus   Inferior concha

Figure 2-58   Bony lateral wall of nasal cavity after sagittal section and removal of the septum.

See **DISSECTIONS**, Section 2, p. 21

See **PRINCIPLES**, Fig. 2-115, *A* and *B*

Posterior border of septum   Sphenoethmoidal recess   Frontal air sinus

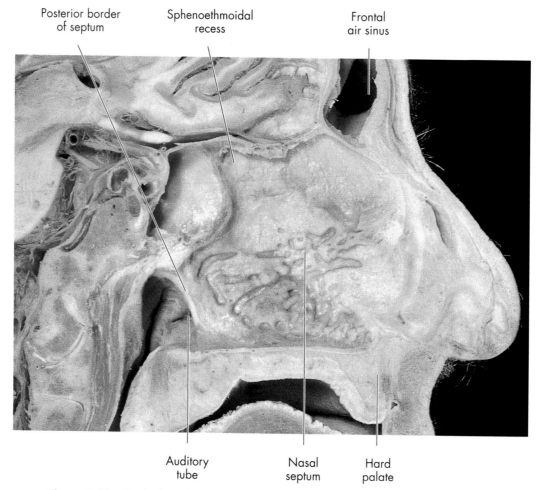

Auditory tube   Nasal septum   Hard palate

Figure 2-59   Sagittal section just to right of midline with an intact nasal septum.

See **Principles**, Fig. 2-14

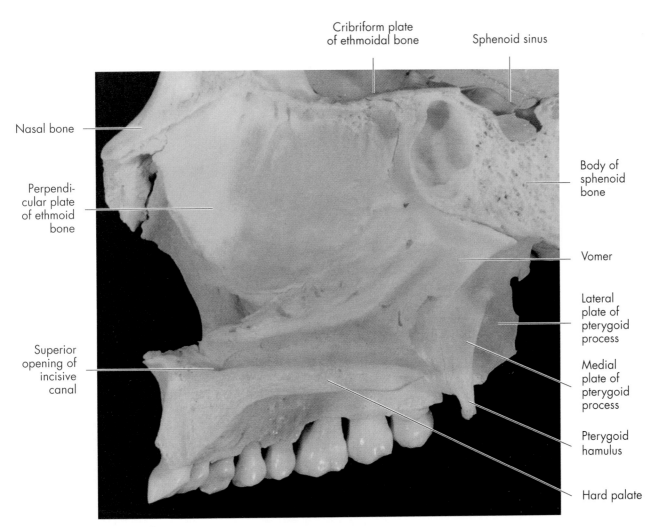

Cribriform plate
of ethmoidal bone

Sphenoid sinus

Nasal bone

Perpendi-
cular plate
of ethmoid
bone

Body of
sphenoid
bone

Vomer

Lateral
plate of
pterygoid
process

Superior
opening of
incisive
canal

Medial
plate of
pterygoid
process

Pterygoid
hamulus

Hard palate

Figure 2-60   Skull cut in a parasagittal plane slightly to the left of the midline to show the bony nasal septum.

SEE DISSECTIONS, SECTION 2, P. 21
SEE PRINCIPLES, FIG. 2-114, C

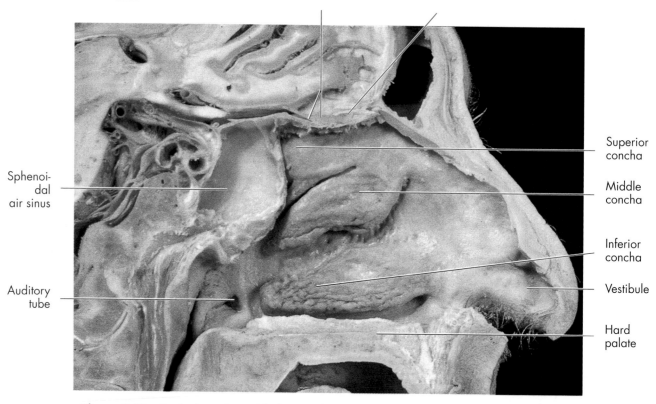

Olfactory bulb & nerve   Cribriform plate

Superior concha

Middle concha

Inferior concha

Vestibule

Hard palate

Sphenoidal air sinus

Auditory tube

Figure 2-61 Sagittal section with the nasal septum removed to show the lateral wall of the nasal cavity.

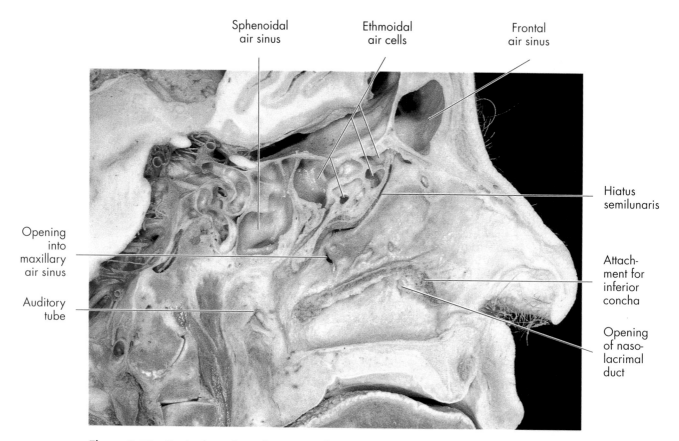

Sphenoidal air sinus   Ethmoidal air cells   Frontal air sinus

Hiatus semilunaris

Attachment for inferior concha

Opening of nasolacrimal duct

Opening into maxillary air sinus

Auditory tube

Figure 2-62 Sagittal section after removal of the conchae, the ethmoid bulla, and the upper part of the lateral nasal wall.

SEE PRINCIPLES, FIG. 2-114, *A* AND *B*

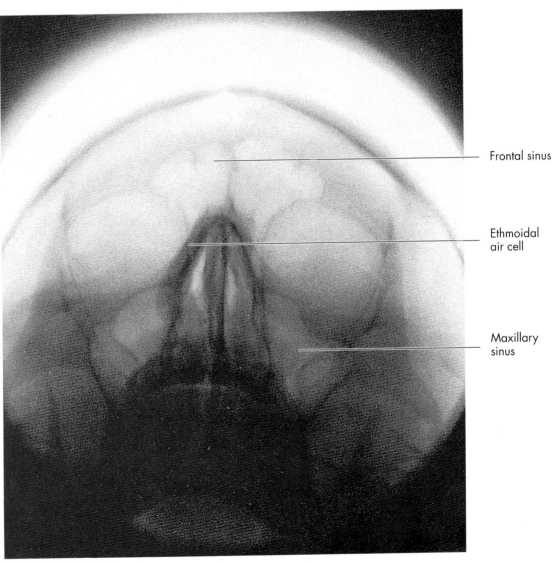

Frontal sinus

Ethmoidal
air cell

Maxillary
sinus

Figure 2-63   Occipitomental radiograph showing paranasal air sinuses.

SEE PRINCIPLES, FIG. 2-114, *A* AND *B*

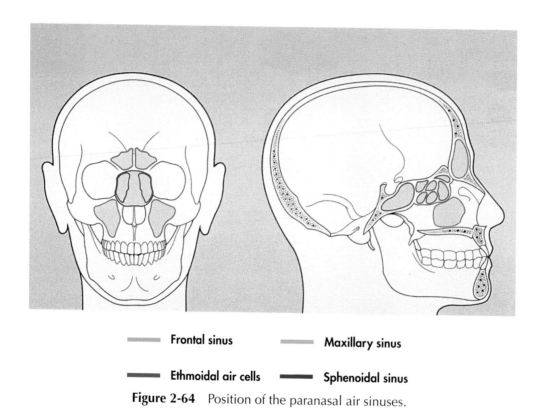

——— Frontal sinus   ——— Maxillary sinus

——— Ethmoidal air cells   ——— Sphenoidal sinus

Figure 2-64   Position of the paranasal air sinuses.

See DISSECTIONS, Section 2, p. 21

See PRINCIPLES, Fig. 2-122

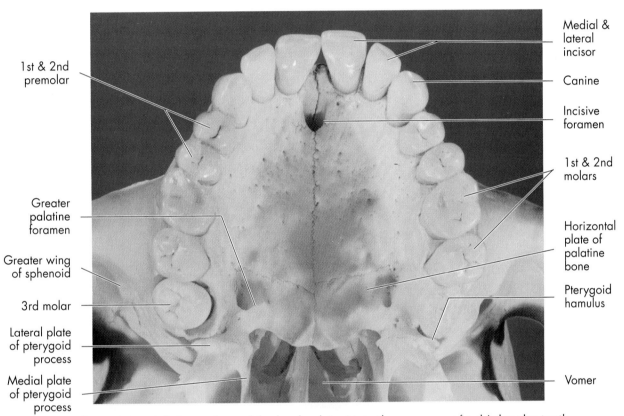

1st & 2nd premolar

Greater palatine foramen

Greater wing of sphenoid

3rd molar

Lateral plate of pterygoid process

Medial plate of pterygoid process

Medial & lateral incisor

Canine

Incisive foramen

1st & 2nd molars

Horizontal plate of palatine bone

Pterygoid hamulus

Vomer

Figure 2-65   Inferior surface of the hard palate. Note the presence of a third molar tooth on the right only. The posterior tips of the conchae are visible through the choanae.

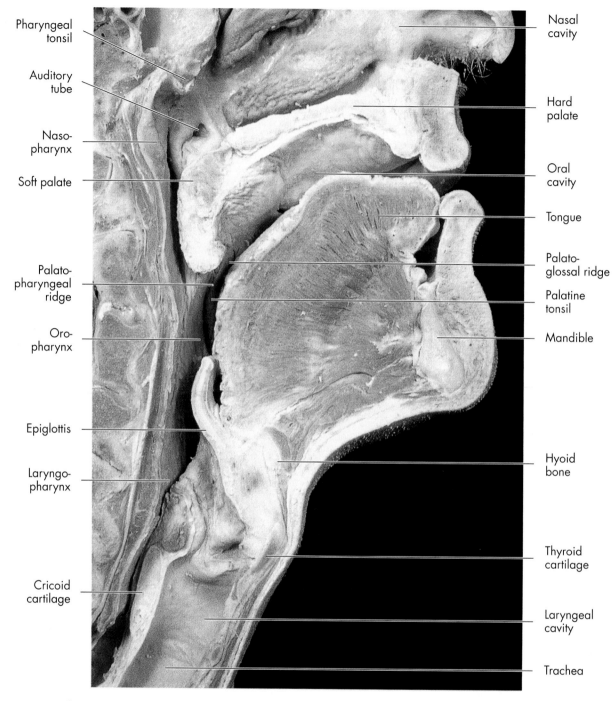

Pharyngeal tonsil

Auditory tube

Naso-pharynx

Soft palate

Palato-pharyngeal ridge

Oro-pharynx

Epiglottis

Laryngo-pharynx

Cricoid cartilage

Nasal cavity

Hard palate

Oral cavity

Tongue

Palato-glossal ridge

Palatine tonsil

Mandible

Hyoid bone

Thyroid cartilage

Laryngeal cavity

Trachea

Figure 2-66 Sagittal section through the palate and pharynx showing communication with the nasal, oral, and laryngeal cavities. *Failure of fusion of the secondary palate during development produces a cleft palate, resulting in an open communication between the oral and nasal cavities. Problems produced by this defect include nasal admission of air with speech, liquid taken orally coming out of the nose, and inefficient sucking or blowing because of an air leak through the nose. Repair of a cleft palate is a common procedure that requires elevation of the mucosa with its fascia and periosteum (mucoperiosteal flap) from the lateral bony palate shelves. The mucoperiosteal flaps thus developed are pulled together in the midline after appropriate relaxing incisions are made. The descending palatine artery and greater palatine nerves are preserved as they emerge from the palatine canal.*

See DISSECTIONS, Section 2, p. 20

See PRINCIPLES, Figs. 2-119, 2-120

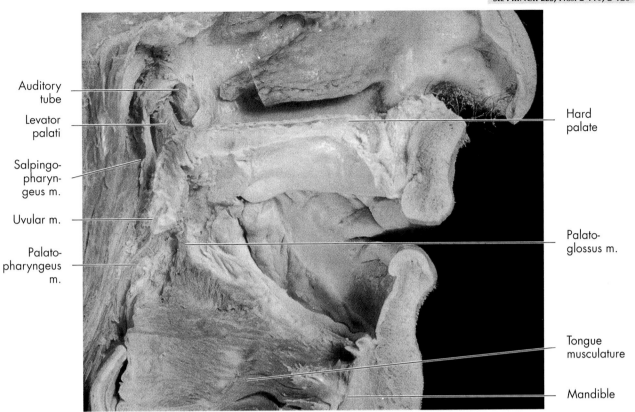

Auditory tube

Levator palati

Salpingo-pharyngeus m.

Uvular m.

Palato-pharyngeus m.

Hard palate

Palato-glossus m.

Tongue musculature

Mandible

Figure 2-67   Further dissection showing some of the muscles of the soft palate.

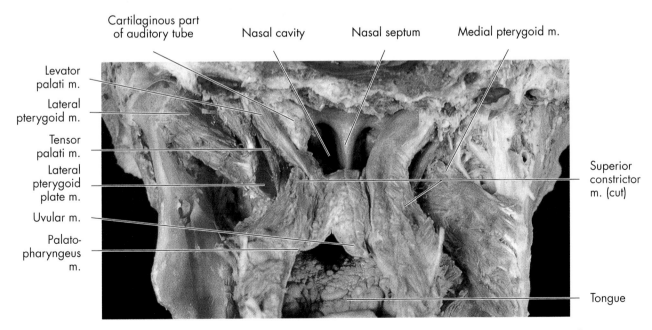

Cartilaginous part of auditory tube

Nasal cavity

Nasal septum

Medial pterygoid m.

Levator palati m.

Lateral pterygoid m.

Tensor palati m.

Lateral pterygoid plate m.

Uvular m.

Palato-pharyngeus m.

Superior constrictor m. (cut)

Tongue

Figure 2-68   Posterior view of soft palate after removal of cervical vertebral column and posterior wall of pharynx. On the left side, the medial pterygoid and the mucosa of the soft palate have been removed to reveal the muscles.

See **DISSECTIONS**, Section 2, pp. 18 and 20

See **PRINCIPLES**, Fig. 2-132, *A*

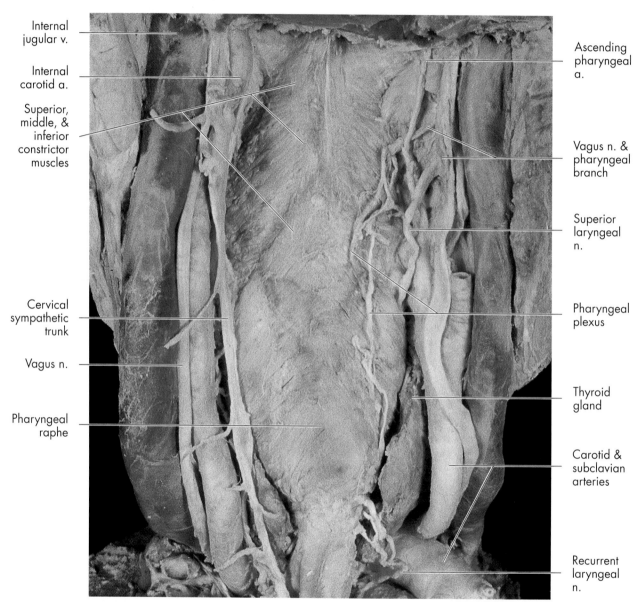

Internal jugular v.

Internal carotid a.

Superior, middle, & inferior constrictor muscles

Cervical sympathetic trunk

Vagus n.

Pharyngeal raphe

Ascending pharyngeal a.

Vagus n. & pharyngeal branch

Superior laryngeal n.

Pharyngeal plexus

Thyroid gland

Carotid & subclavian arteries

Recurrent laryngeal n.

Figure 2-69 Posterior view of pharyngeal musculature after removal of cervical vertebral column, posterior part of the skull, right sympathetic trunk, and part of the right internal carotid artery.

See **DISSECTIONS**, Section 2, pp. 18 and 20

See **PRINCIPLES**, Fig. 2-132, *A*

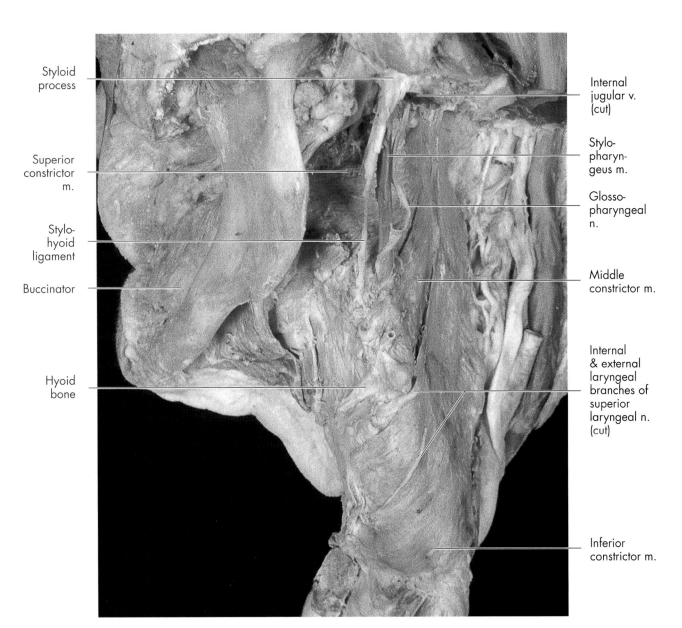

Styloid process

Superior constrictor m.

Stylo-hyoid ligament

Buccinator

Hyoid bone

Internal jugular v. (cut)

Stylo-pharyn-geus m.

Glosso-pharyngeal n.

Middle constrictor m.

Internal & external laryngeal branches of superior laryngeal n. (cut)

Inferior constrictor m.

Figure 2-70   Oblique posterior view of pharyngeal musculature.

See DISSECTIONS, Section 2, p. 18

See PRINCIPLES, Fig. 2-138

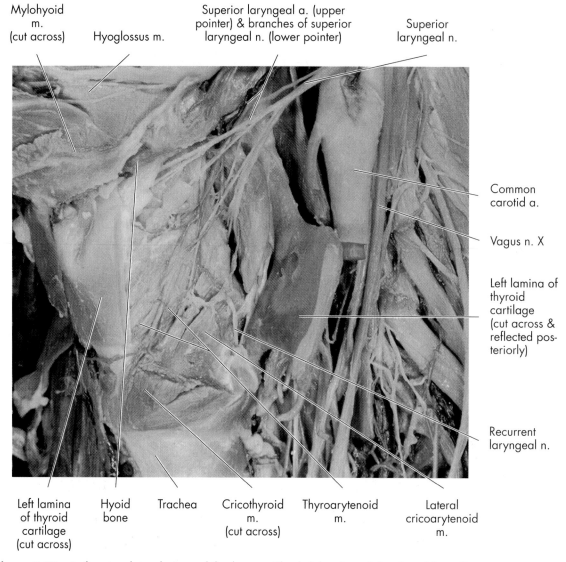

Mylohyoid m. (cut across)

Hyoglossus m.

Superior laryngeal a. (upper pointer) & branches of superior laryngeal n. (lower pointer)

Superior laryngeal n.

Common carotid a.

Vagus n. X

Left lamina of thyroid cartilage (cut across & reflected posteriorly)

Recurrent laryngeal n.

Left lamina of thyroid cartilage (cut across)

Hyoid bone

Trachea

Cricothyroid m. (cut across)

Thyroarytenoid m.

Lateral cricoarytenoid m.

Figure 2-71   Left anterolateral view of the larynx. The left lamina of the thyroid cartilage has been cut and reflected posteriorly, and the left cricothyroid joint has been opened. A thick layer of fibrous tissue has been removed to expose the hyoid bone.

See DISSECTIONS, Section 2, pp. 20 and 22

See PRINCIPLES, Fig. 2-137

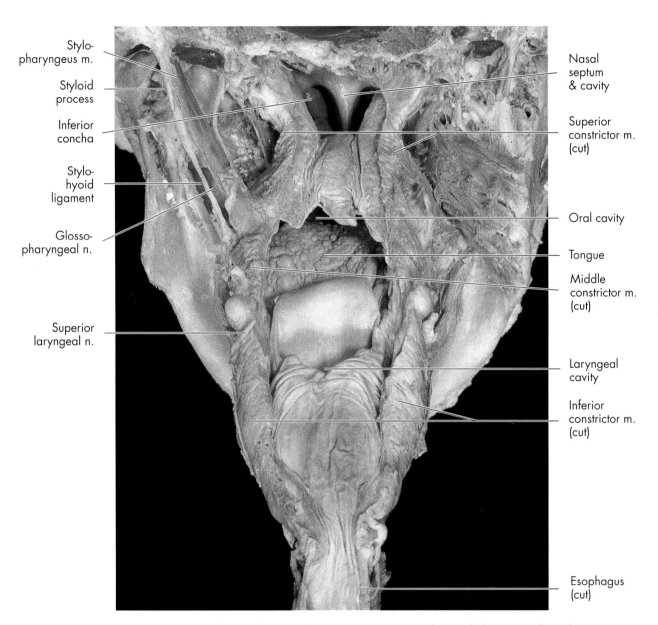

Stylo-
pharyngeus m.

Styloid
process

Inferior
concha

Stylo-
hyoid
ligament

Glosso-
pharyngeal n.

Superior
laryngeal n.

Nasal
septum
& cavity

Superior
constrictor m.
(cut)

Oral cavity

Tongue

Middle
constrictor m.
(cut)

Laryngeal
cavity

Inferior
constrictor m.
(cut)

Esophagus
(cut)

Figure 2-72   Interior of the pharynx. This specimen retains the medial pterygoid on the
right and the styloid apparatus on the left.

See DISSECTIONS, SECTION 2, p. 22

See PRINCIPLES, FIG. 2-137

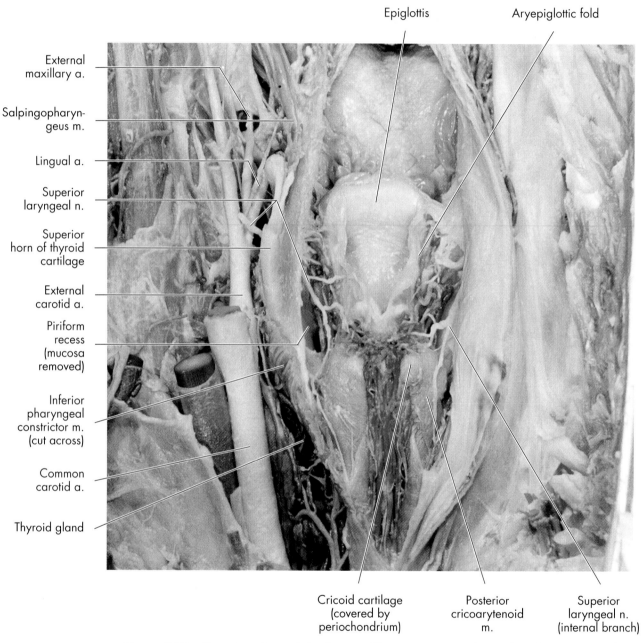

Epiglottis   Aryepiglottic fold

External
maxillary a.

Salpingopharyn-
geus m.

Lingual a.

Superior
laryngeal n.

Superior
horn of thyroid
cartilage

External
carotid a.

Piriform
recess
(mucosa
removed)

Inferior
pharyngeal
constrictor m.
(cut across)

Common
carotid a.

Thyroid gland

Cricoid cartilage   Posterior   Superior
(covered by   cricoarytenoid   laryngeal n.
periochondrium)   m.   (internal branch)

Figure 2-73 Posterior view of the larynx. The mucous membrane has been removed from the piriform recesses and anterior wall of the esophagus. The right superior laryngeal nerve has been retracted to expose branches of the superior laryngeal artery and vein.

See **DISSECTIONS, Section 2, p. 22**

See **PRINCIPLES, Fig. 2-137**

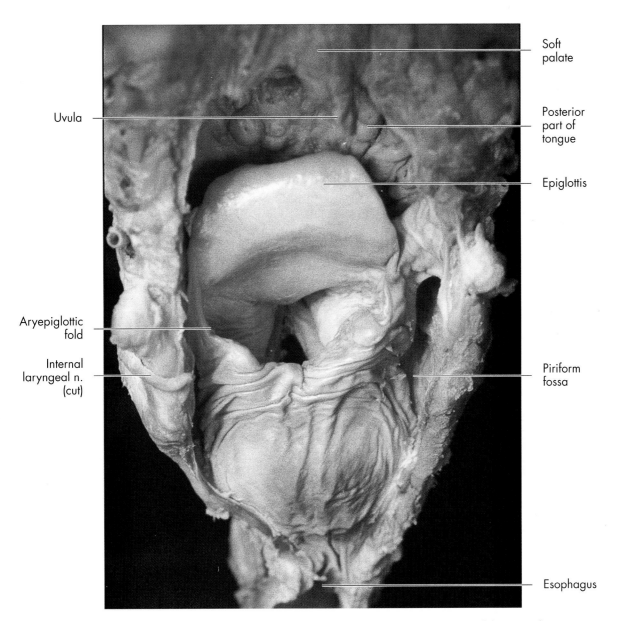

Soft palate

Uvula

Posterior part of tongue

Epiglottis

Aryepiglottic fold

Internal laryngeal n. (cut)

Piriform fossa

Esophagus

Figure 2-74   Posterosuperior view of the larynx seen through the opened laryngopharynx. The lumen of the larynx is visible through the laryngeal inlet.

See DISSECTIONS, Section 2, p. 22

See PRINCIPLES, Fig. 2-136

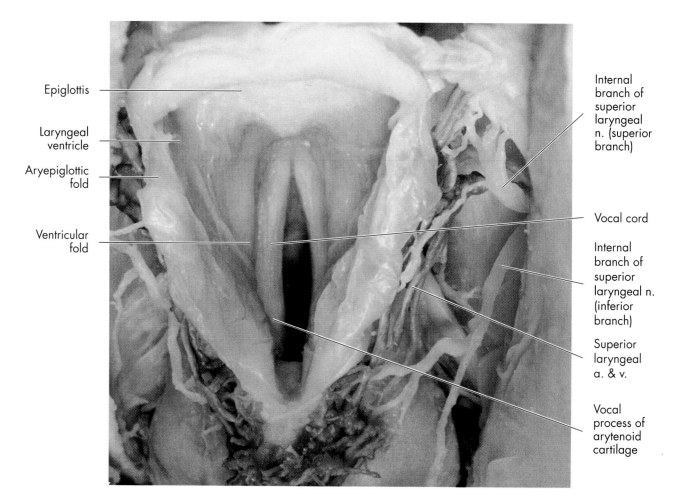

Epiglottis

Laryngeal
ventricle

Aryepiglottic
fold

Ventricular
fold

Internal
branch of
superior
laryngeal
n. (superior
branch)

Vocal cord

Internal
branch of
superior
laryngeal n.
(inferior
branch)

Superior
laryngeal
a. & v.

Vocal
process of
arytenoid
cartilage

Figure 2-75 Superior view of the cavity of the larynx. Superior and inferior sensory branches of the internal branch of the superior laryngeal branch of the vagus nerve are seen. *Anesthesiologists regularly pass a breathing tube through the mouth or nose into the oropharynx behind the epiglottis and through the larynx between the vocal cords into the trachea. One may view the vocal folds and cords through a laryngoscope passed through the mouth, behind the epiglottis.*

SEE DISSECTIONS, SECTION 2, P. 22

SEE PRINCIPLES, FIG. 2-137

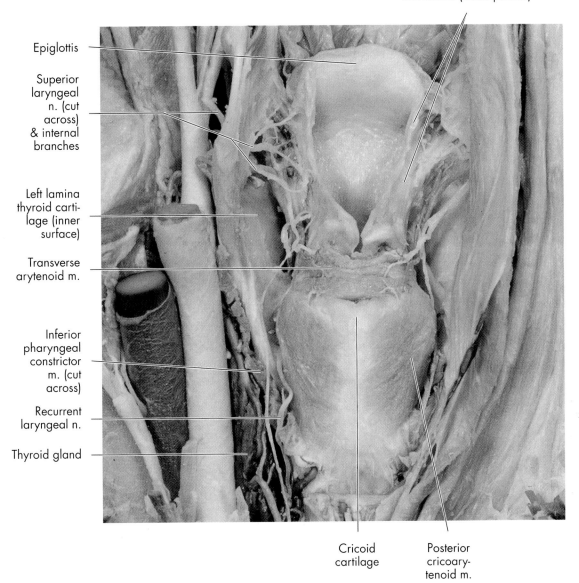

Aryepiglottic fold (upper pointer) & quadrangular membrane (lower pointer)

Epiglottis

Superior laryngeal n. (cut across) & internal branches

Left lamina thyroid cartilage (inner surface)

Transverse arytenoid m.

Inferior pharyngeal constrictor m. (cut across)

Recurrent laryngeal n.

Thyroid gland

Cricoid cartilage

Posterior cricoarytenoid m.

Figure 2-76 Posterior view of the larynx with the mucous membrane removed. The attachment of the cervical part of the esophagus to the cricoid cartilage has been cut and the esophagus sectioned transversely below the inferior margin of the cricoid cartilage. The quadrangular membrane has been exposed by the removal of the aryepiglottic muscle.

See DISSECTIONS, Section 2, p. 22

See PRINCIPLES, Fig. 2-131

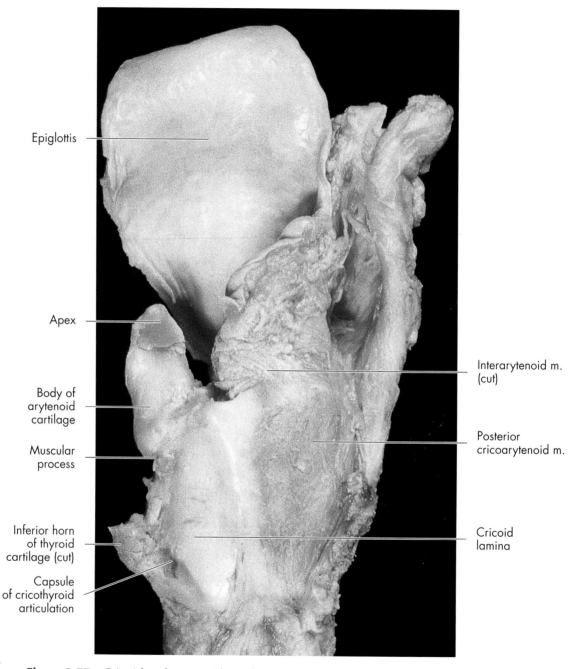

Epiglottis

Apex

Body of
arytenoid
cartilage

Muscular
process

Inferior horn
of thyroid
cartilage (cut)

Capsule
of cricothyroid
articulation

Interarytenoid m.
(cut)

Posterior
cricoarytenoid m.

Cricoid
lamina

Figure 2-77   Cricoid and artyenoid cartilages exposed by removal of most of the soft tissues on the left of the larynx.

Sᴇᴇ DISSECTIONS, Sᴇᴄᴛɪᴏɴ 2, ᴘ. 22

Sᴇᴇ PRINCIPLES, Fɪɢ. 2-133

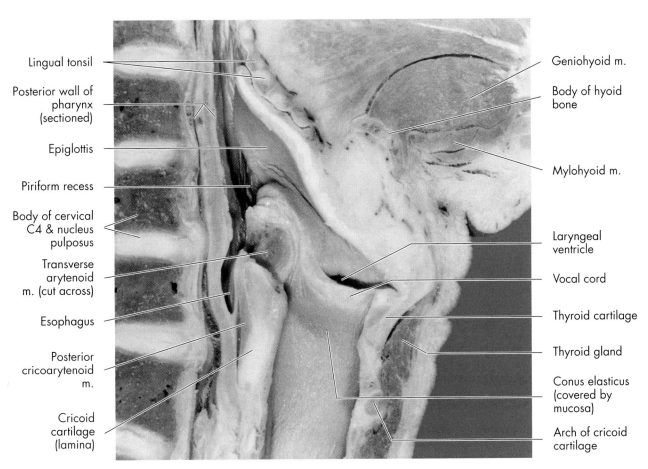

Lingual tonsil

Posterior wall of
pharynx
(sectioned)

Epiglottis

Piriform recess

Body of cervical
C4 & nucleus
pulposus

Transverse
arytenoid
m. (cut across)

Esophagus

Posterior
cricoarytenoid
m.

Cricoid
cartilage
(lamina)

Geniohyoid m.

Body of hyoid
bone

Mylohyoid m.

Laryngeal
ventricle

Vocal cord

Thyroid cartilage

Thyroid gland

Conus elasticus
(covered by
mucosa)

Arch of cricoid
cartilage

Figure 2-78 Sagittal section of the neck shows medial aspect of the larynx as viewed
from the right side.

SEE DISSECTIONS, SECTION 2, P. 22

SEE PRINCIPLES, FIG. 2-133

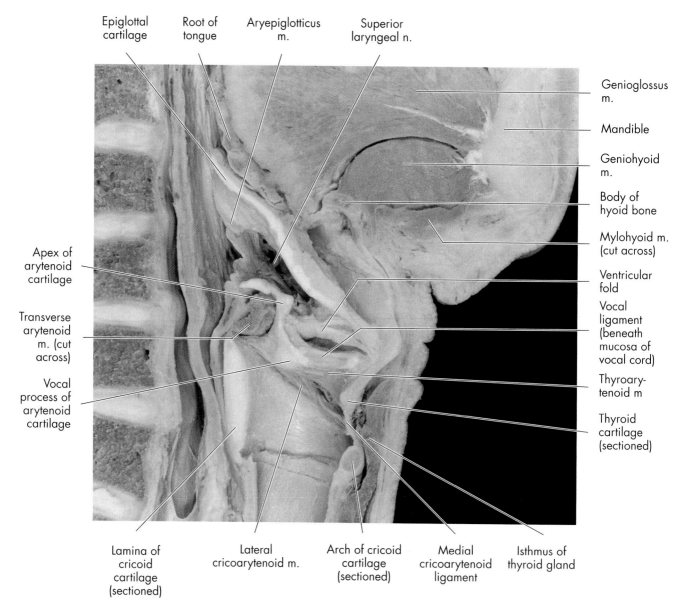

Epiglottal cartilage

Root of tongue

Aryepiglotticus m.

Superior laryngeal n.

Genioglossus m.

Mandible

Geniohyoid m.

Body of hyoid bone

Mylohyoid m. (cut across)

Ventricular fold

Vocal ligament (beneath mucosa of vocal cord)

Thyroary-tenoid m

Thyroid cartilage (sectioned)

Apex of arytenoid cartilage

Transverse arytenoid m. (cut across)

Vocal process of arytenoid cartilage

Lamina of cricoid cartilage (sectioned)

Lateral cricoarytenoid m.

Arch of cricoid cartilage (sectioned)

Medial cricoarytenoid ligament

Isthmus of thyroid gland

Figure 2-79   Medial view of a sagittal section of the neck with dissection of the left half of the larynx. The mucosa of the larynx has been cut away except for that which lines the ventricle and a narrow rim that remains on the vocal and ventricular folds. The elastic cone (conus elasticus) and the quadrangular membrane have been removed. *Cricothyroidotomy and tracheostomy give access from the neck to the trachea for treating laryngopharyngeal obstruction of the airway. Cricothyroidotomy may be achieved using a large bore needle or a knife inserted between the thyroid and cricoid cartilages through the cricothyroid membrane. This allows entry into the larynx below the vocal cords. Tracheostomy requires incision through the neck skin and platysma, then a vertical separation of the strap muscles to expose the upper trachea. Sometimes the thyroid isthmus must be divided. Entry is made at the level of the second or third tracheal ring and a tracheostomy tube is inserted.*

SEE PRINCIPLES, FIG. 2-131

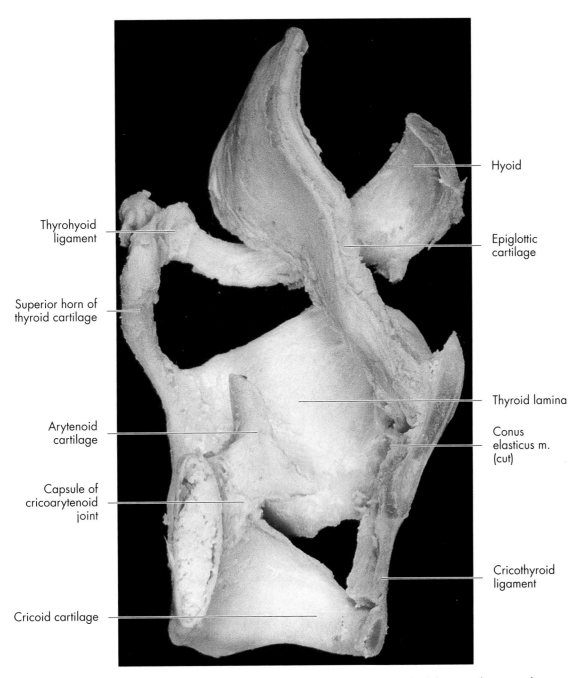

Figure 2-80   Bisected skeleton of the larynx revealed by removal of the membranes. The cricothyroid ligament is the site for emergency cricothyroidotomy for airway obstruction.

See DISSECTIONS, Section 2, p. 22

See PRINCIPLES, Fig. 2-135

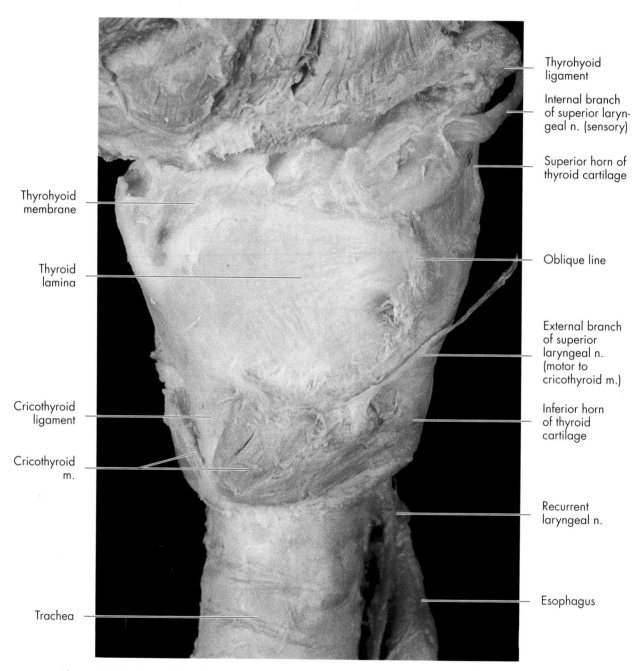

Thyrohyoid ligament

Internal branch of superior laryngeal n. (sensory)

Superior horn of thyroid cartilage

Thyrohyoid membrane

Thyroid lamina

Oblique line

Cricothyroid ligament

External branch of superior laryngeal n. (motor to cricothyroid m.)

Cricothyroid m.

Inferior horn of thyroid cartilage

Recurrent laryngeal n.

Esophagus

Trachea

Figure 2-81   Anterolateral view of the larynx. Note recurrent laryngeal nerve, which is motor to all intrinsic muscles of larynx except the cricothyroid muscle.

See DISSECTIONS, Section 2, p. 22

See PRINCIPLES, Fig. 2-134

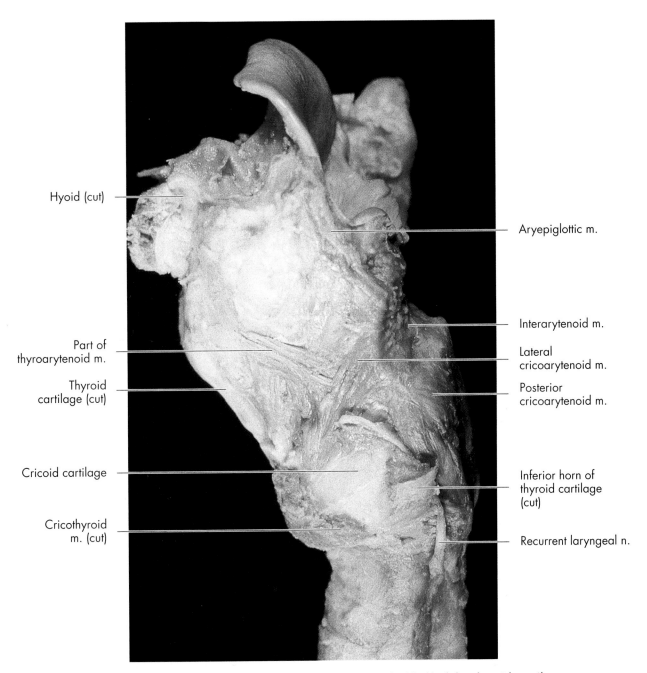

Hyoid (cut)

Aryepiglottic m.

Interarytenoid m.

Part of
thyroarytenoid m.

Lateral
cricoarytenoid m.

Thyroid
cartilage (cut)

Posterior
cricoarytenoid m.

Cricoid cartilage

Inferior horn of
thyroid cartilage
(cut)

Cricothyroid
m. (cut)

Recurrent laryngeal n.

Figure 2-82   Deeper intrinsic muscles seen after removal of half of the thyroid cartilage and the hyoid bone. All are innervated by the recurrent laryngeal nerve except the cricothyroid muscle.

SEE DISSECTIONS, SECTION 2, P. 22

SEE PRINCIPLES, FIG. 2-134

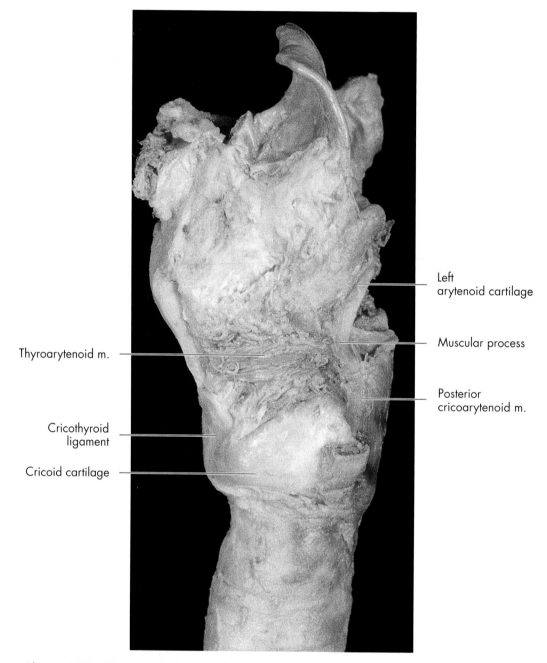

Left
arytenoid cartilage

Muscular process

Posterior
cricoarytenoid m.

Thyroarytenoid m.

Cricothyroid
ligament

Cricoid cartilage

Figure 2-83 Thyroarytenoid and the arytenoid cartilage after excision of the lateral cricoarytenoid, interarytenoid, and aryepiglottic muscles.

SEE **DISSECTIONS**, SECTION 2, P. 22

SEE **PRINCIPLES**, FIG. 2-134

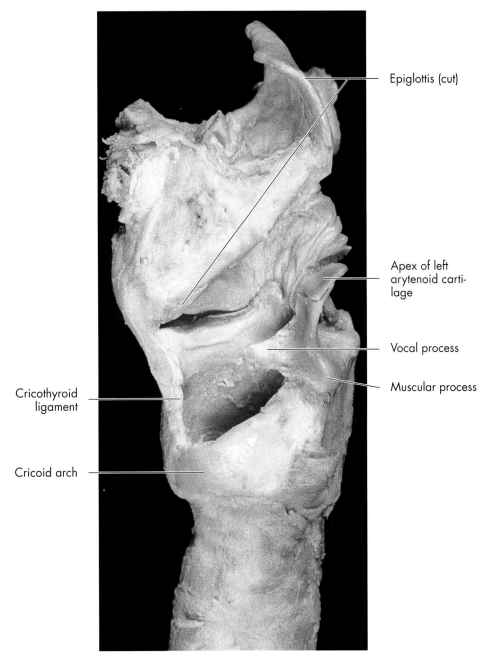

— Epiglottis (cut)

Apex of left
arytenoid carti-
lage

Vocal process

Muscular process

Cricothyroid
ligament

Cricoid arch

Figure 2-84   Cartilages of the larynx revealed by removal of muscles and membranes on the left side.

See DISSECTIONS, Section 2, p. 2

See PRINCIPLES, Fig. 2-1, A

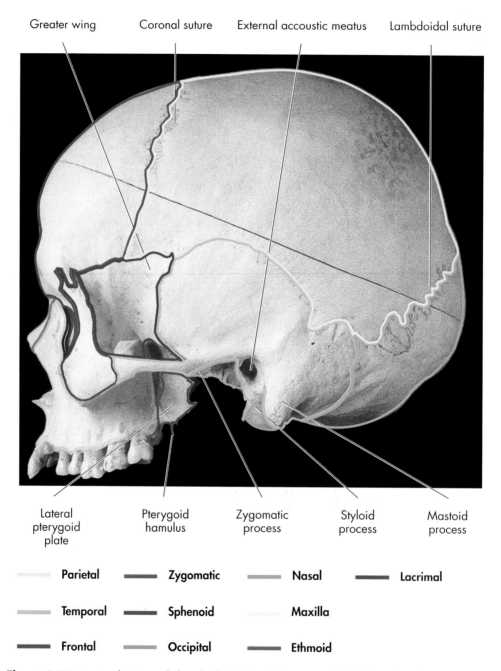

Greater wing   Coronal suture   External accoustic meatus   Lambdoidal suture

Lateral pterygoid plate   Pterygoid hamulus   Zygomatic process   Styloid process   Mastoid process

Parietal   Zygomatic   Nasal   Lacrimal

Temporal   Sphenoid   Maxilla

Frontal   Occipital   Ethmoid

Figure 2-85   Lateral view of the skull (without the mandible) showing the component bones.

Sᴇᴇ **DISSECTIONS, Sᴇᴄᴛɪᴏɴ 2, ᴘ. 5**
Sᴇᴇ **PRINCIPLES, Fɪɢ. 2-15**

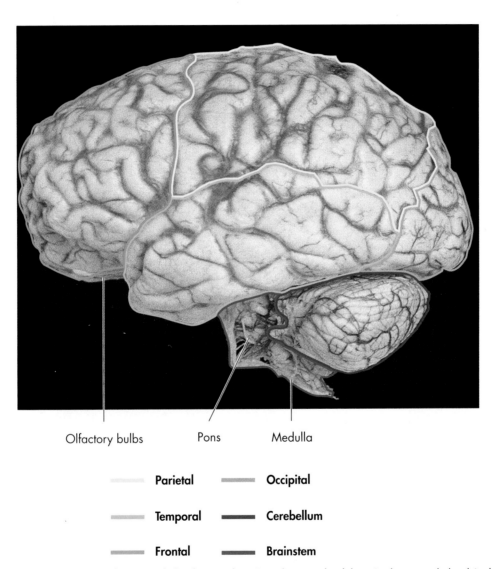

Olfactory bulbs   Pons   Medulla

══ **Parietal**   ══ **Occipital**

══ **Temporal**   ━━ **Cerebellum**

══ **Frontal**   ━━ **Brainstem**

Figure 2-86 Lateral view of the brain showing the cerebral hemisphere and the hindbrain.

See DISSECTIONS, Section 2, p. 5
See PRINCIPLES, Fig. 2-29

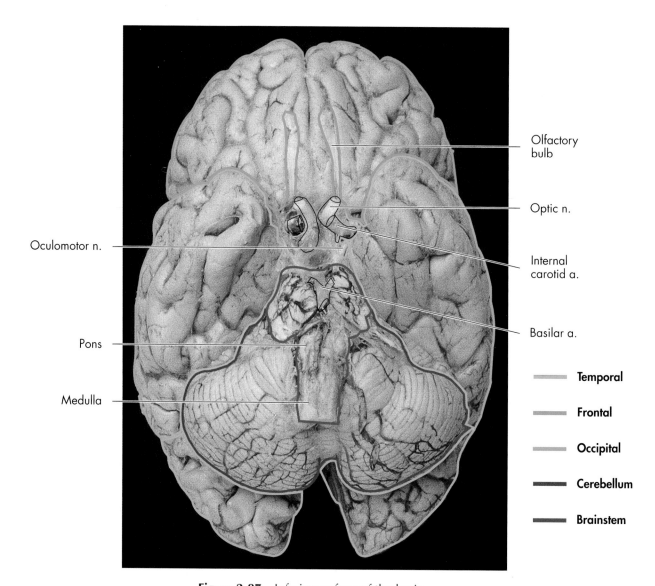

Olfactory bulb

Optic n.

Oculomotor n.

Internal carotid a.

Pons

Basilar a.

Medulla

Temporal

Frontal

Occipital

Cerebellum

Brainstem

Figure 2-87   Inferior surface of the brain.

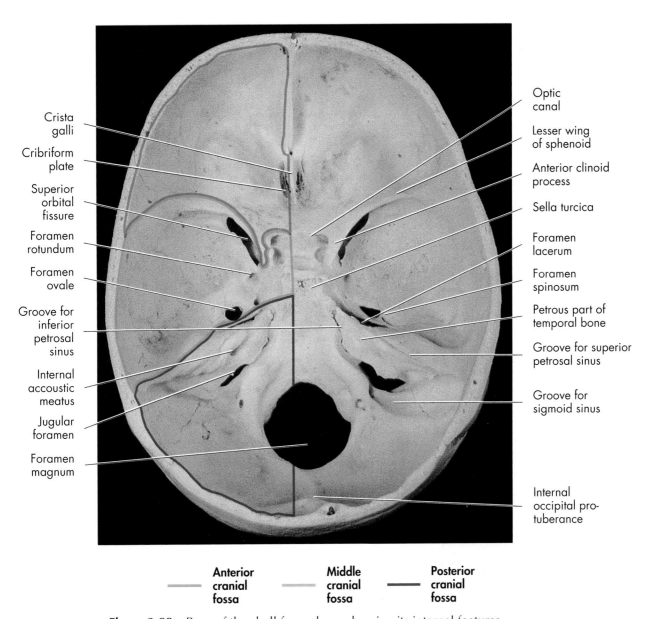

Crista
galli

Cribriform
plate

Superior
orbital
fissure

Foramen
rotundum

Foramen
ovale

Groove for
inferior
petrosal
sinus

Internal
accoustic
meatus

Jugular
foramen

Foramen
magnum

Optic
canal

Lesser wing
of sphenoid

Anterior clinoid
process

Sella turcica

Foramen
lacerum

Foramen
spinosum

Petrous part of
temporal bone

Groove for superior
petrosal sinus

Groove for
sigmoid sinus

Internal
occipital pro-
tuberance

Anterior
cranial
fossa

Middle
cranial
fossa

Posterior
cranial
fossa

Figure 2-88   Base of the skull from above showing its internal features.

See PRINCIPLES, FIG. 2-14, *B*

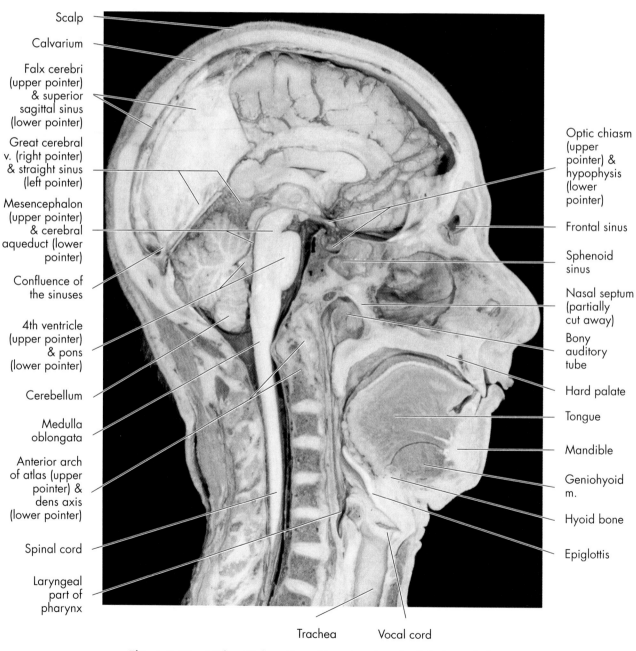

Scalp

Calvarium

Falx cerebri
(upper pointer)
& superior
sagittal sinus
(lower pointer)

Great cerebral
v. (right pointer)
& straight sinus
(left pointer)

Mesencephalon
(upper pointer)
& cerebral
aqueduct (lower
pointer)

Confluence of
the sinuses

4th ventricle
(upper pointer)
& pons
(lower pointer)

Cerebellum

Medulla
oblongata

Anterior arch
of atlas (upper
pointer) &
dens axis
(lower pointer)

Spinal cord

Laryngeal
part of
pharynx

Optic chiasm
(upper
pointer) &
hypophysis
(lower
pointer)

Frontal sinus

Sphenoid
sinus

Nasal septum
(partially
cut away)

Bony
auditory
tube

Hard palate

Tongue

Mandible

Geniohyoid
m.

Hyoid bone

Epiglottis

Trachea   Vocal cord

Figure 2-89   Midsagittal section of head and neck, right lateral view.

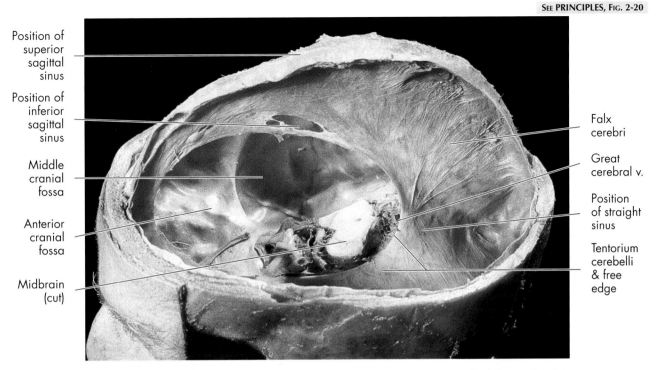

Position of superior sagittal sinus

Position of inferior sagittal sinus

Middle cranial fossa

Anterior cranial fossa

Midbrain (cut)

Falx cerebri

Great cerebral v.

Position of straight sinus

Tentorium cerebelli & free edge

Figure 2-90 Falx cerebri and tentorium cerebelli revealed by removal of the vault of the cranium, associated dura, and the cerebral hemisphere.

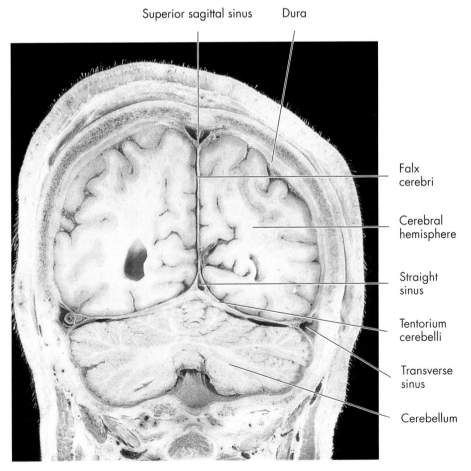

Superior sagittal sinus   Dura

Falx cerebri

Cerebral hemisphere

Straight sinus

Tentorium cerebelli

Transverse sinus

Cerebellum

Figure 2-91 Coronal section through the posterior cranial fossa, showing the dura and its folds and venous sinuses.

SEE PRINCIPLES, FIG. 2-6

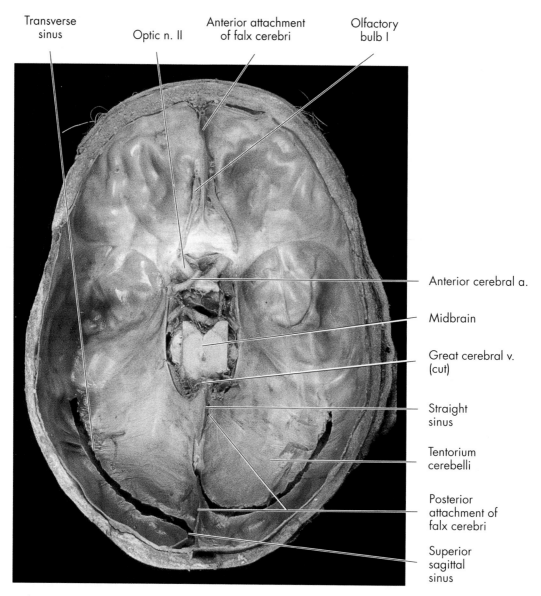

Transverse sinus

Optic n. II

Anterior attachment of falx cerebri

Olfactory bulb I

Anterior cerebral a.

Midbrain

Great cerebral v. (cut)

Straight sinus

Tentorium cerebelli

Posterior attachment of falx cerebri

Superior sagittal sinus

Figure 2-92 Superior view of the tentorium cerebelli after removal of the falx cerebri and cerebral hemispheres. The venous sinuses have been opened. The straight sinus turns to the right and the superior sagittal sinus to the left in this specimen.

See DISSECTIONS, Section 2, p. 6

See PRINCIPLES, Figs. 2-6, 2-23

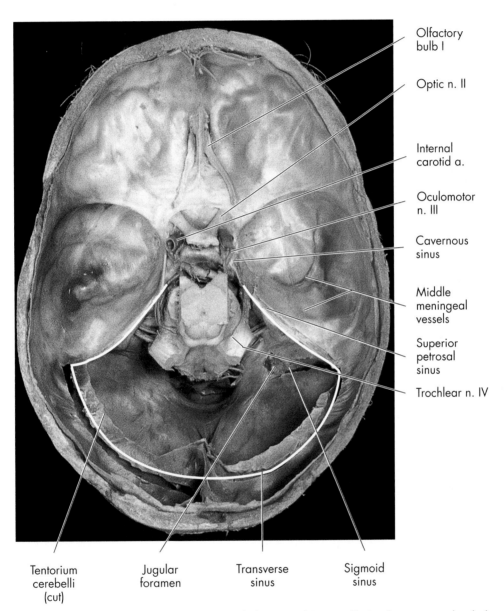

Olfactory bulb I

Optic n. II

Internal carotid a.

Oculomotor n. III

Cavernous sinus

Middle meningeal vessels

Superior petrosal sinus

Trochlear n. IV

Tentorium cerebelli (cut)

Jugular foramen

Transverse sinus

Sigmoid sinus

Figure 2-93 Interior of posterior cranial fossa (*white outline*) after removal of the tentorium cerebelli and cerebellum. The venous sinuses have been further opened.

See DISSECTIONS, Section 2, p. 6
See PRINCIPLES, Fig. 2-27

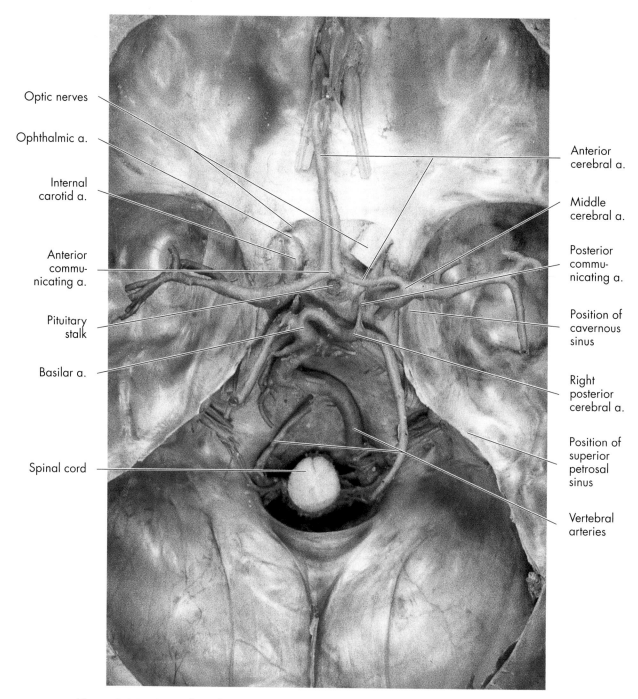

Optic nerves

Ophthalmic a.

Internal
carotid a.

Anterior
commu-
nicating a.

Pituitary
stalk

Basilar a.

Spinal cord

Anterior
cerebral a.

Middle
cerebral a.

Posterior
commu-
nicating a.

Position of
cavernous
sinus

Right
posterior
cerebral a.

Position of
superior
petrosal
sinus

Vertebral
arteries

Figure 2-94 Arterial circle, exposed by complete removal of the brain. The basilar and vertebral arteries are asymmetric in this specimen.

See DISSECTIONS, SECTION 2, P. 7
See PRINCIPLES, FIG. 2-22

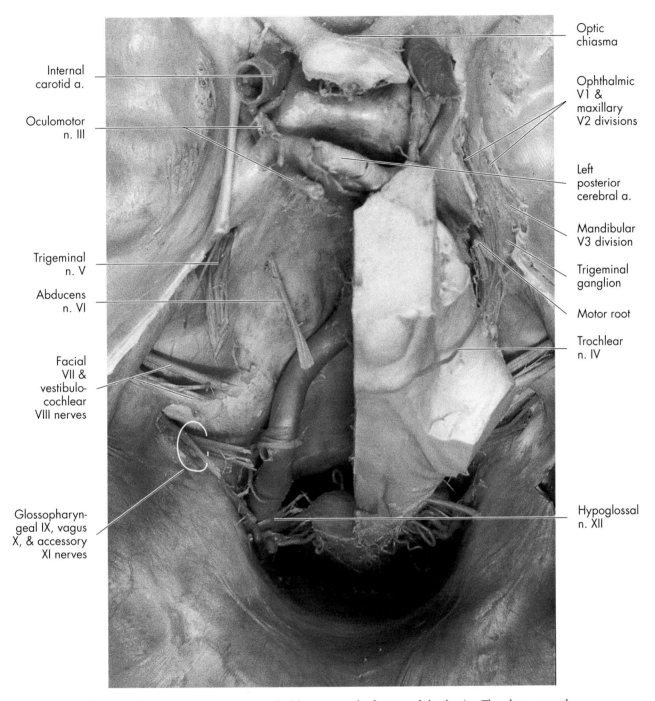

Figure 2-95 Cranial nerves revealed by removal of most of the brain. The dura over the right trigeminal ganglion has been excised.

See PRINCIPLES, FIG. 2-9

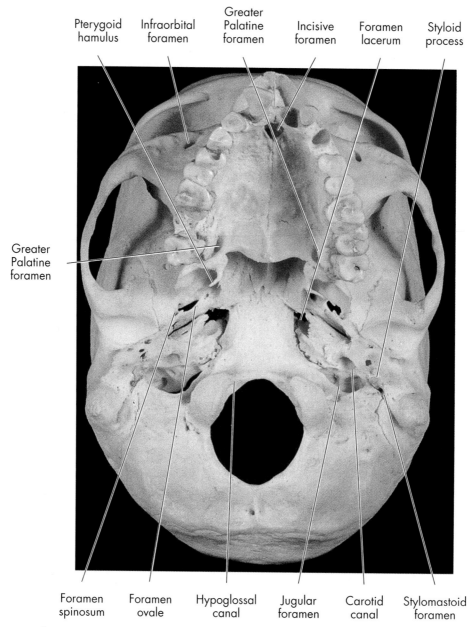

Pterygoid hamulus

Infraorbital foramen

Greater Palatine foramen

Incisive foramen

Foramen lacerum

Styloid process

Greater Palatine foramen

Foramen spinosum

Foramen ovale

Hypoglossal canal

Jugular foramen

Carotid canal

Stylomastoid foramen

Figure 2-96   Inferior view of the base of the skull showing the principal foramina.

SEE **PRINCIPLES, FIG. 2-2**

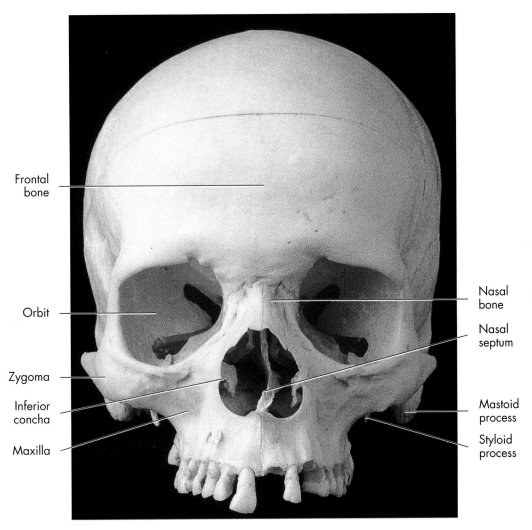

Frontal
bone

Orbit

Zygoma

Inferior
concha

Maxilla

Nasal
bone

Nasal
septum

Mastoid
process

Styloid
process

Figure 2-97   Anterior view of the skull without the mandible.

SEE **PRINCIPLES**, FIG. 2-114, *C*

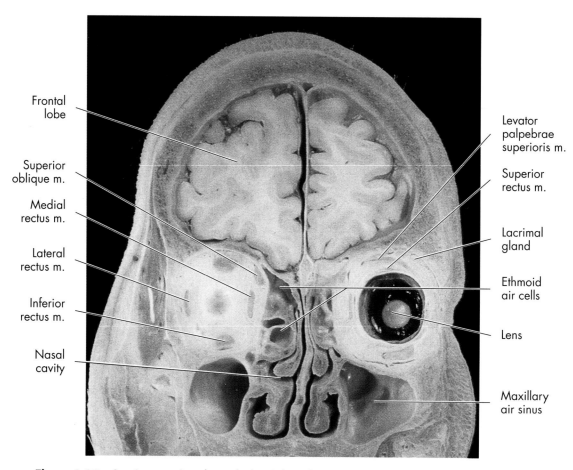

Frontal lobe

Superior oblique m.

Medial rectus m.

Lateral rectus m.

Inferior rectus m.

Nasal cavity

Levator palpebrae superioris m.

Superior rectus m.

Lacrimal gland

Ethmoid air cells

Lens

Maxillary air sinus

Figure 2-98   Section passing through the right orbit, more anteriorly than the left, showing the extraocular muscles and relations of the orbits. Note the nasal conchae.

See **DISSECTIONS**, Section 2, p. 8
See **PRINCIPLES**, Figs. 2-93, *A;* 2-96

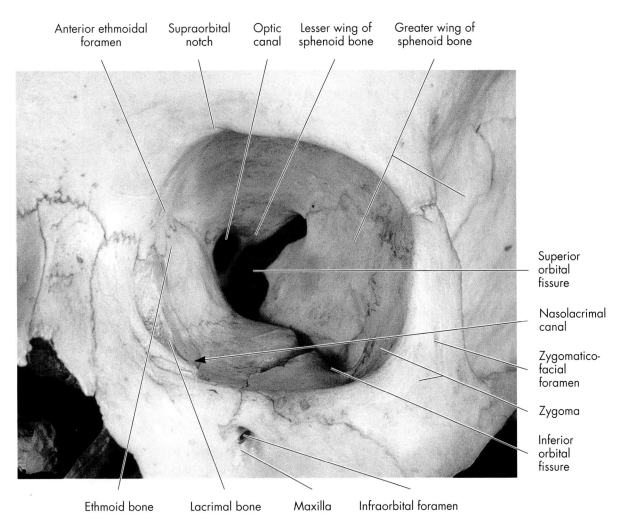

Anterior ethmoidal foramen

Supraorbital notch

Optic canal

Lesser wing of sphenoid bone

Greater wing of sphenoid bone

Superior orbital fissure

Nasolacrimal canal

Zygomatico-facial foramen

Zygoma

Inferior orbital fissure

Ethmoid bone   Lacrimal bone   Maxilla   Infraorbital foramen

Figure 2-99   Bony walls, fissures, and foramina of the left orbit.

See PRINCIPLES, Fig. 2-108

Lacrimal
caruncle

Superior
lacrimal
duct
(opened)

Lacrimal sac

Lacrimal
puncta

External nasal
branches of
anterior
ethmoidal n.

Inferior
lacrimal duct
(opened)

Edge of
maxilla (cut)

Periosteal
lining of
nasolacrimal
canal

Inferior
oblique m.

Septal
cartilage

Infraorbital
a. & n.

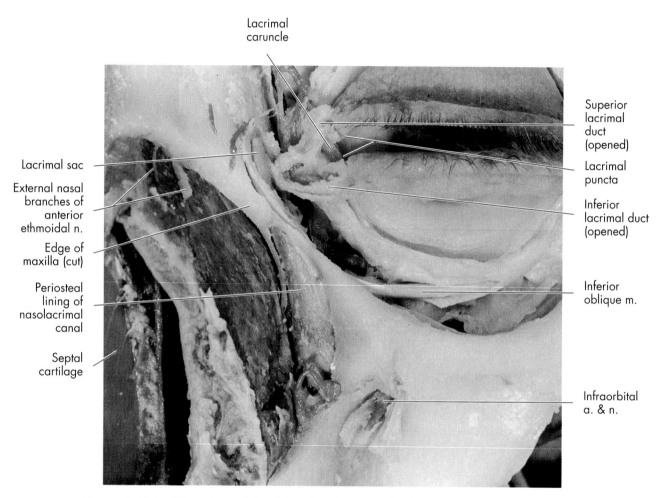

Figure 2-100   Dissection of the left orbit showing the lacrimal sac and bony naso-lacrimal canal, which has been opened. The lacrimal sac has been uncovered by removal of the medial palpebral ligament and reflection of the lacrimal fascia. The lacrimal canaliculi converge toward a common opening through the lateral wall of the sac. The periosteal lining of the nasolacrimal canal is undisturbed.

See PRINCIPLES, Fig. 2-108

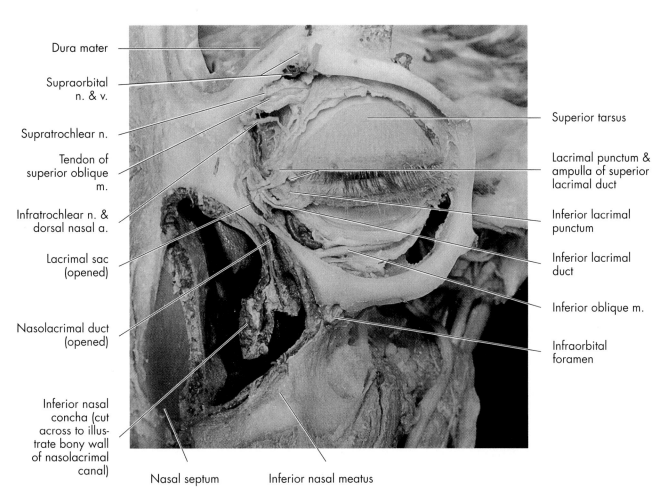

Dura mater

Supraorbital n. & v.

Supratrochlear n.

Tendon of superior oblique m.

Infratrochlear n. & dorsal nasal a.

Lacrimal sac (opened)

Nasolacrimal duct (opened)

Inferior nasal concha (cut across to illustrate bony wall of nasolacrimal canal)

Superior tarsus

Lacrimal punctum & ampulla of superior lacrimal duct

Inferior lacrimal punctum

Inferior lacrimal duct

Inferior oblique m.

Infraorbital foramen

Nasal septum   Inferior nasal meatus

Figure 2-101   Dissection of the left orbit from an anterior approach to expose the lacrimal sac and nasolacrimal duct. The tendon of the superior oblique muscle has been exposed within the trochlea, and its relation to the insertion of the levator palpebrae superioris muscle is displayed.

162   Clinical Anatomy Atlas

See DISSECTIONS, Section 2, p. 10
See PRINCIPLES, Fig. 2-103

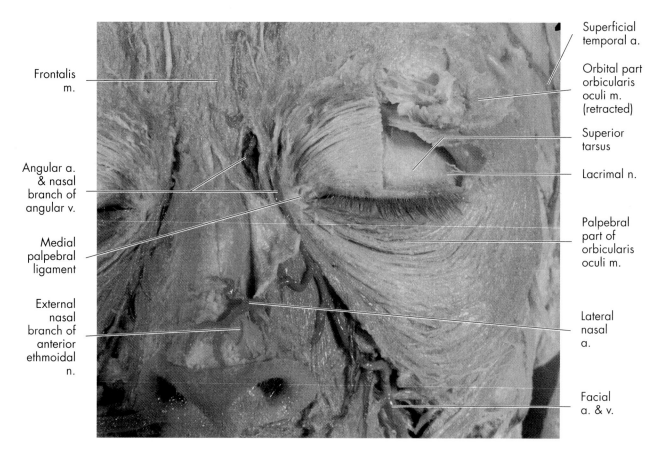

Frontalis m.

Angular a. & nasal branch of angular v.

Medial palpebral ligament

External nasal branch of anterior ethmoidal n.

Superficial temporal a.

Orbital part orbicularis oculi m. (retracted)

Superior tarsus

Lacrimal n.

Palpebral part of orbicularis oculi m.

Lateral nasal a.

Facial a. & v.

Figure 2-102   Orbicularis oculi muscle incised vertically and retracted to expose deeper structures in the upper eyelid.

See DISSECTIONS, Section 2, p. 10
See PRINCIPLES, Fig. 2-103

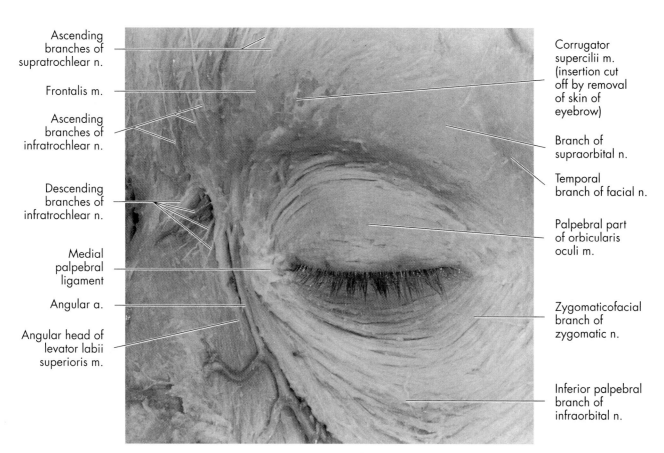

Ascending branches of supratrochlear n.

Frontalis m.

Ascending branches of infratrochlear n.

Descending branches of infratrochlear n.

Medial palpebral ligament

Angular a.

Angular head of levator labii superioris m.

Corrugator supercilii m. (insertion cut off by removal of skin of eyebrow)

Branch of supraorbital n.

Temporal branch of facial n.

Palpebral part of orbicularis oculi m.

Zygomaticofacial branch of zygomatic n.

Inferior palpebral branch of infraorbital n.

Figure 2-103 Dissection of the left orbit from an anterior approach showing the orbicularis oculi muscle and superficial nerves and blood vessels. The skin and subcutaneous tissue have been removed except for a narrow margin retained at the edges of the eyelids.

See PRINCIPLES, FIG. 2-103

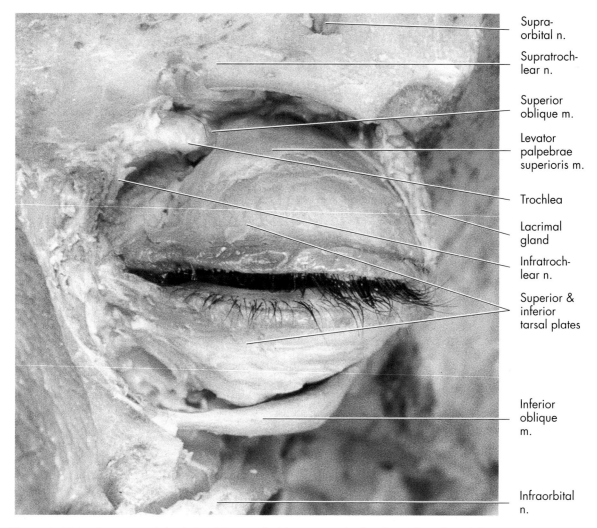

Figure 2-104 Contents of the left orbit revealed by removal of its lateral wall and floor and parts of the eyelids. The supraorbital nerve lies in a canal in the frontal bone.

See **DISSECTIONS**, Section 2, p. 8
See **PRINCIPLES**, Figs. 2-106, 2-109

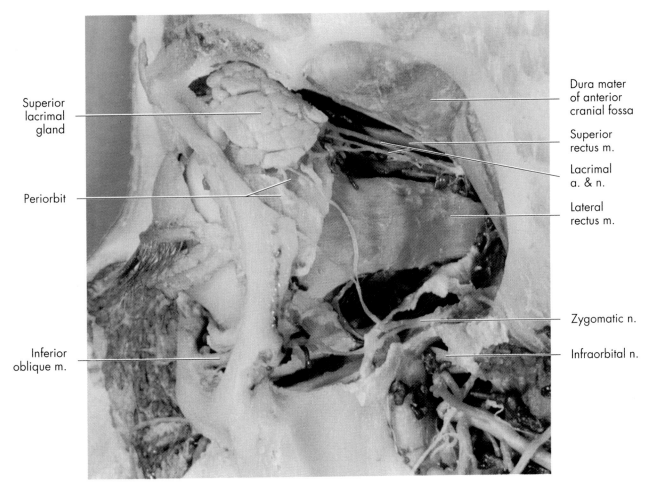

Superior lacrimal gland

Periorbit

Inferior oblique m.

Dura mater of anterior cranial fossa

Superior rectus m.

Lacrimal a. & n.

Lateral rectus m.

Zygomatic n.

Infraorbital n.

Figure 2-105   Dissection of the left orbit from a lateral approach. The fascia of the lateral rectus muscle is intact but is thin through most of its extent. Anteriorly the fascia thickens rapidly and has a broad attachment to the orbital tubercle of the zygomatic bone to form the lateral check ligament. The periorbit is split into two layers to enclose the lacrimal gland.

See DISSECTIONS, Section 2, p. 8

See PRINCIPLES, Fig. 2-106

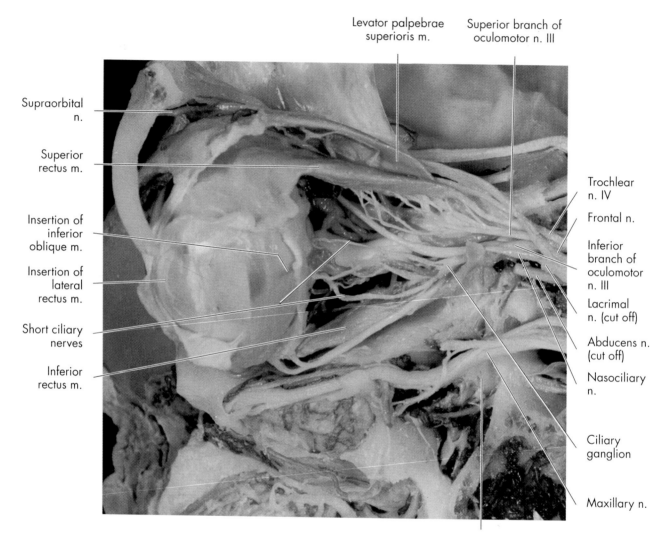

Figure 2-106   Dissection of the left orbit from a lateral approach showing the nerve supply to the superior rectus and levator palpebrae superioris muscles. The muscles have been elevated and branches of the superior division of the oculomotor nerve enter the superior rectus muscle. Branches of the nerve also pass through the muscle and along its medial border to reach the inferior surface of the levator palpebrae superioris muscle.

See DISSECTIONS, Section 2, p. 8
See PRINCIPLES, Figs. 2-105, 2-106, *A*

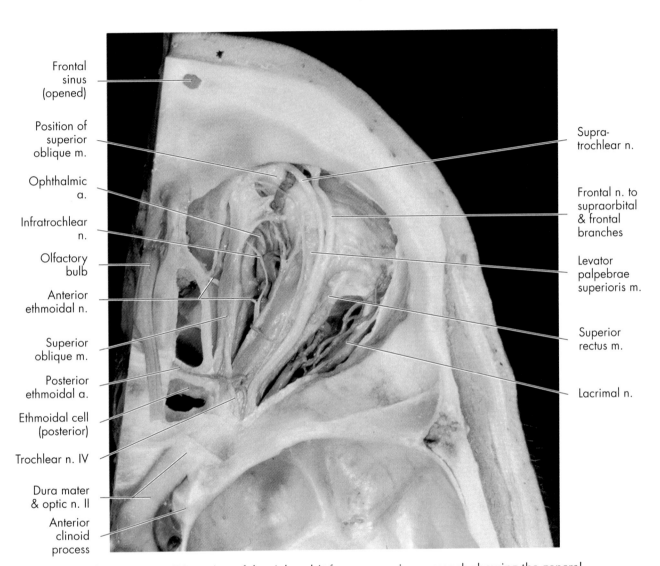

Frontal sinus (opened)

Position of superior oblique m.

Ophthalmic a.

Infratrochlear n.

Olfactory bulb

Anterior ethmoidal n.

Superior oblique m.

Posterior ethmoidal a.

Ethmoidal cell (posterior)

Trochlear n. IV

Dura mater & optic n. II

Anterior clinoid process

Supra-trochlear n.

Frontal n. to supraorbital & frontal branches

Levator palpebrae superioris m.

Superior rectus m.

Lacrimal n.

Figure 2-107   Dissection of the right orbit from a superior approach showing the general relation of structures within orbit. Bone has been cut away from the roof of the orbit, and the ethmoidal sinuses have been opened. Supraorbital and frontal branches of frontal nerve are not separated.

See DISSECTIONS, Section 2, p. 8

See PRINCIPLES, Figs. 2-105, 2-106, A

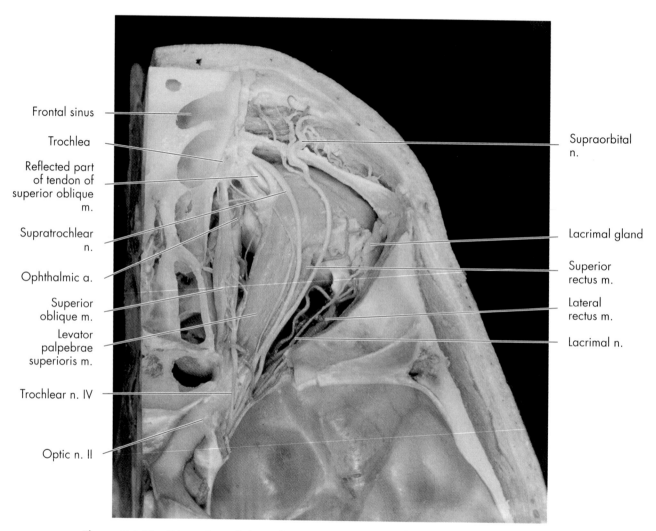

Frontal sinus

Trochlea

Reflected part of tendon of superior oblique m.

Supratrochlear n.

Ophthalmic a.

Superior oblique m.

Levator palpebrae superioris m.

Trochlear n. IV

Optic n. II

Supraorbital n.

Lacrimal gland

Superior rectus m.

Lateral rectus m.

Lacrimal n.

Figure 2-108 Dissection of the right orbit from a superior approach showing the relation of the aponeurosis of the levator palpebrae superioris muscle to the tendon of the superior oblique muscle and lacrimal gland. The thick fascia that surrounds the tendon of the superior oblique muscle blends with fascia of the levator and superior rectus muscles as well as with the fascia bulb.

SEE DISSECTIONS, SECTION 2, P. 8
SEE PRINCIPLES, FIGS. 2-104, 2-105

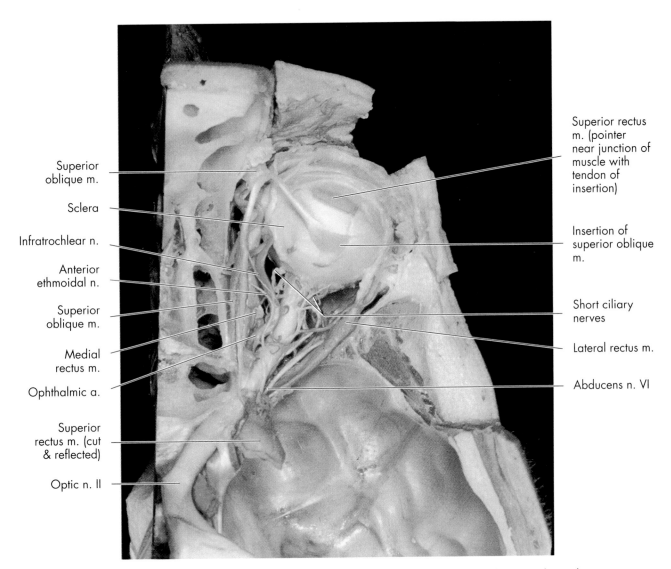

Superior oblique m.

Sclera

Infratrochlear n.

Anterior ethmoidal n.

Superior oblique m.

Medial rectus m.

Ophthalmic a.

Superior rectus m. (cut & reflected)

Optic n. II

Superior rectus m. (pointer near junction of muscle with tendon of insertion)

Insertion of superior oblique m.

Short ciliary nerves

Lateral rectus m.

Abducens n. VI

Figure 2-109 Dissection of the right orbit from a superior approach showing the ophthalmic artery, ciliary nerves and arteries, sheath of optic nerve, and insertion of the superior oblique muscle. The superior rectus muscle has been cut and reflected to expose underlying structures. The fascia of the bulb (Tenon's capsule) has been partially cut away. In this specimen, the ophthalmic artery passes beneath the optic nerve rather than above it; this is a rather common variation.

SEE DISSECTIONS, SECTION 2, P. 8

SEE PRINCIPLES, FIG. 2-109

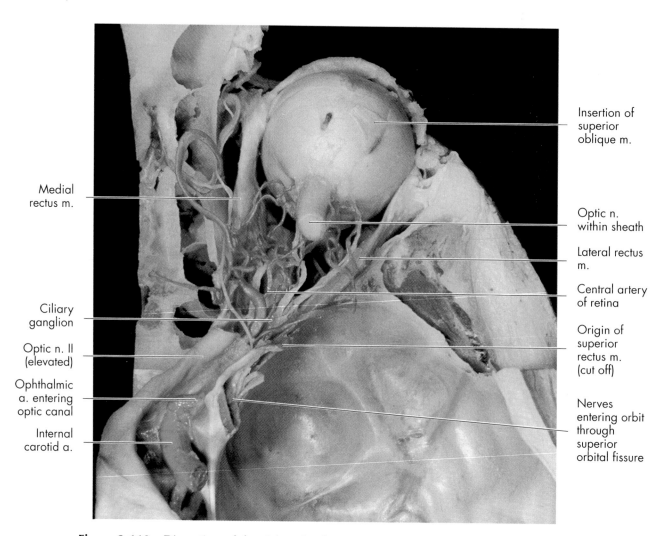

Medial
rectus m.

Ciliary
ganglion

Optic n. II
(elevated)

Ophthalmic
a. entering
optic canal

Internal
carotid a.

Insertion of
superior
oblique m.

Optic n.
within sheath

Lateral rectus
m.

Central artery
of retina

Origin of
superior
rectus m.
(cut off)

Nerves
entering orbit
through
superior
orbital fissure

Figure 2-110   Dissection of the right orbit from a superior approach showing branches of the ophthalmic artery. The optic nerve has been cut and the eye turned anteriorly. The central end of the optic nerve has been displaced from the optic canal to illustrate the course of the ophthalmic artery in a separate dural investment inferior to the nerve.

See **DISSECTIONS**, **SECTION 2**, P. 8

See **PRINCIPLES**, FIG. 2-106, *B*

Ophthalmic a.

Anterior
ethmoidal a.

Short ciliary
nerves

Medial
rectus m.

Branches of
oculomotor n.
III to medial
rectus m.

Superior
oblique m.
(cut off)

Ciliary
ganglion

Nasociliary
n. (cut off)

Ophthalmic a.

Trochlear n.
IV (cut off)

Ophthalmic
n. (cut off)

Branch of
oculomotor
n. III to
inferior
oblique m.

Inferior rectus
m.

Lateral rectus
m.

Branch of
oculomotor
n. III to
inferior rectus
m.

Abducens
VI n.

Branch of
oculomotor
n. III to
superior rectus
m. (cut off)

Middle
cranial
fossa

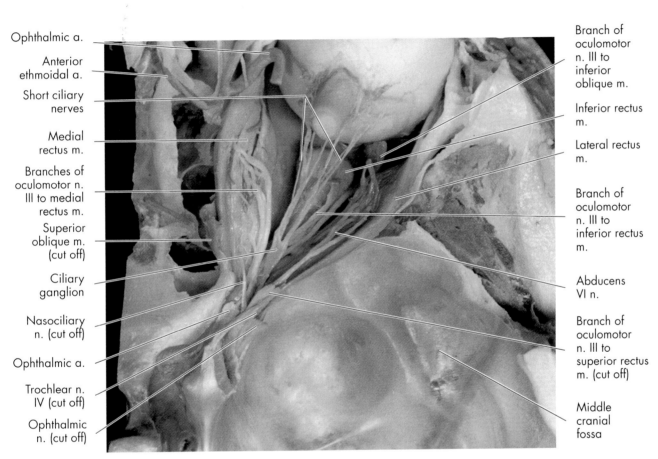

Figure 2-111   Dissection of the right orbit from a superior approach showing the ciliary ganglion and its connections as well as the nerve supply to medial, inferior, and lateral rectus muscles. The ophthalmic artery and its branches have been cut away to reveal the ciliary nerves and ganglion as well as the nerves that enter the rectus muscles. A filament from the ophthalmic sympathetic plexus joins the ciliary ganglion.

SEE PRINCIPLES, FIG. 2-97

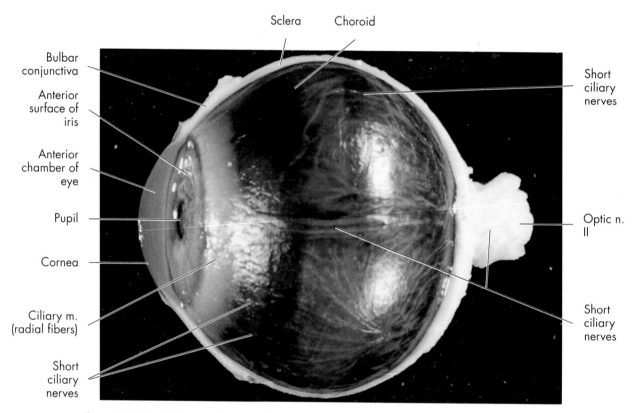

Sclera

Choroid

Bulbar
conjunctiva

Anterior
surface of
iris

Anterior
chamber of
eye

Pupil

Cornea

Ciliary m.
(radial fibers)

Short
ciliary
nerves

Short
ciliary
nerves

Optic n.
II

Short
ciliary
nerves

Figure 2-112   Sclera and cornea have been cut away on the medial side of the right eye
to show the anterior chamber, iris, ciliary body, and outer surface of the choroid.

SEE PRINCIPLES, FIG. 2-102

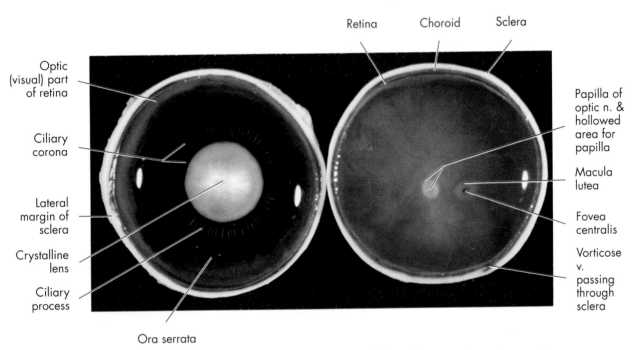

Retina   Choroid   Sclera

Optic (visual) part of retina

Ciliary corona

Lateral margin of sclera

Crystalline lens

Ciliary process

Ora serrata

Papilla of optic n. & hollowed area for papilla

Macula lutea

Fovea centralis

Vorticose v. passing through sclera

Figure 2-113   Interior of the left eye cut in a frontal plane just anterior to its equator.

See PRINCIPLES, Fig. 2-97

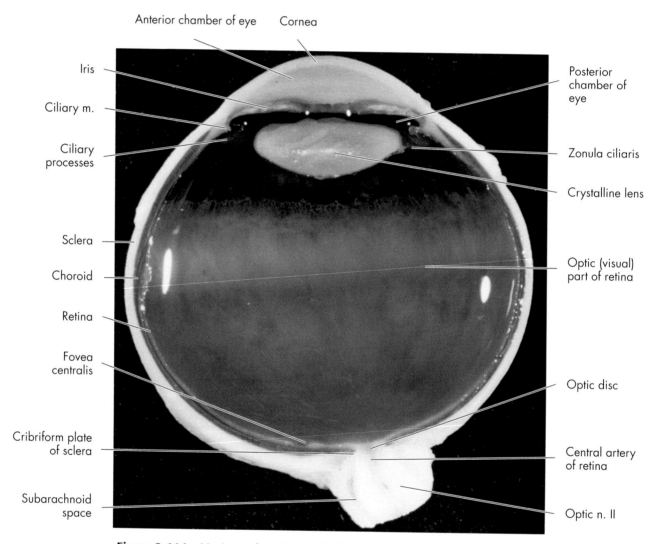

Anterior chamber of eye   Cornea

Iris

Ciliary m.

Ciliary processes

Sclera

Choroid

Retina

Fovea centralis

Cribriform plate of sclera

Subarachnoid space

Posterior chamber of eye

Zonula ciliaris

Crystalline lens

Optic (visual) part of retina

Optic disc

Central artery of retina

Optic n. II

Figure 2-114   Horizontal section of the left eye through the fovea centralis.

Sᴇᴇ PRINCIPLES, Fɪɢs. 2-98, 2-101

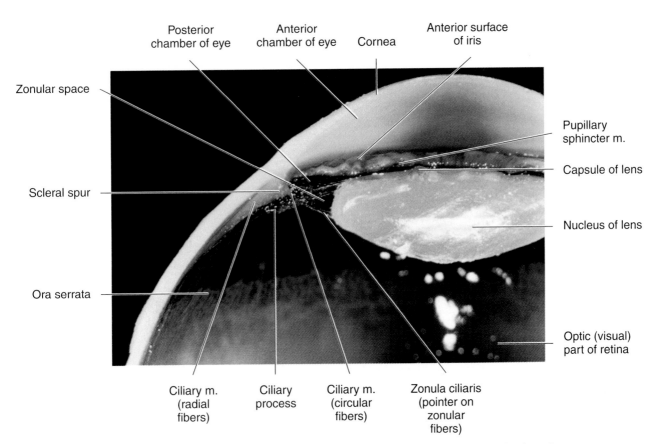

Posterior
chamber of eye

Anterior
chamber of eye

Cornea

Anterior surface
of iris

Zonular space

Pupillary
sphincter m.

Capsule of lens

Scleral spur

Nucleus of lens

Ora serrata

Optic (visual)
part of retina

Ciliary m.
(radial
fibers)

Ciliary
process

Ciliary m.
(circular
fibers)

Zonula ciliaris
(pointer on
zonular
fibers)

Figure 2-115   Horizontal section through the left eye showing the ciliary body, ciliary zonule, and lens.

SEE PRINCIPLES, FIG. 2-102

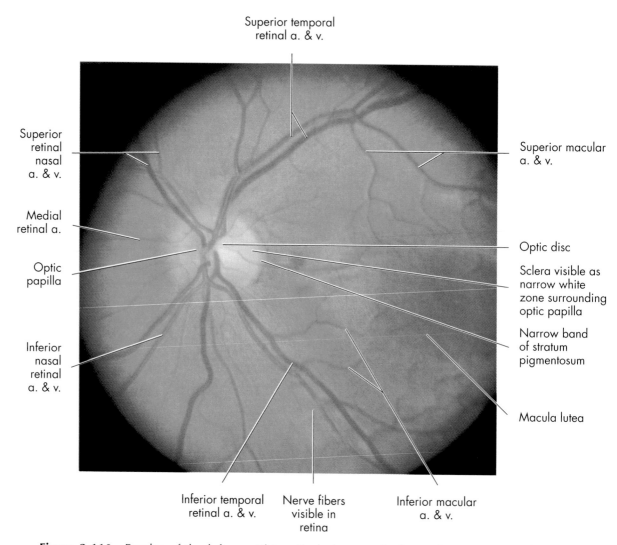

Superior temporal
retinal a. & v.

Superior
retinal
nasal
a. & v.

Superior macular
a. & v.

Medial
retinal a.

Optic disc

Optic
papilla

Sclera visible as
narrow white
zone surrounding
optic papilla

Narrow band
of stratum
pigmentosum

Inferior
nasal
retinal
a. & v.

Macula lutea

Inferior temporal
retinal a. & v.

Nerve fibers
visible in
retina

Inferior macular
a. & v.

Figure 2-116   Fundus of the left eye. This retinal photograph shows the narrower and paler retinal arteries when compared to their corresponding veins.

See DISSECTIONS, Section 2, p. 9
See PRINCIPLES, Fig. 2-85

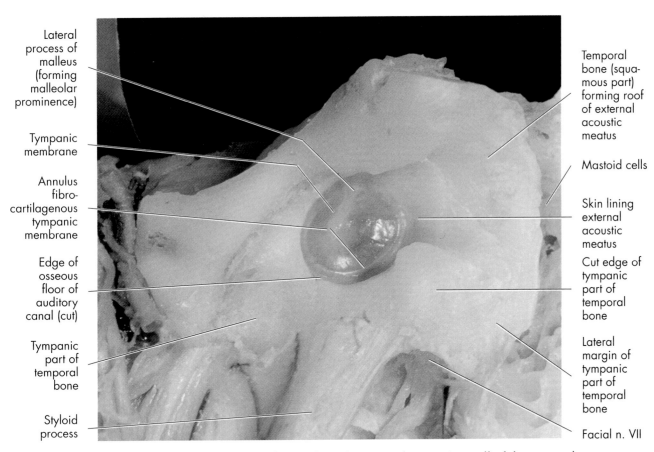

Lateral process of malleus (forming malleolar prominence)

Tympanic membrane

Annulus fibro-cartilagenous tympanic membrane

Edge of osseous floor of auditory canal (cut)

Tympanic part of temporal bone

Styloid process

Temporal bone (squa-mous part) forming roof of external acoustic meatus

Mastoid cells

Skin lining external acoustic meatus

Cut edge of tympanic part of temporal bone

Lateral margin of tympanic part of temporal bone

Facial n. VII

Figure 2-117   Left tympanic membrane, lateral aspect. The anterior wall of the external auditory canal has been removed. The manubrium of the malleus is visible through the drum.

See DISSECTIONS, Section 2, p. 9

See PRINCIPLES, Fig. 2-87

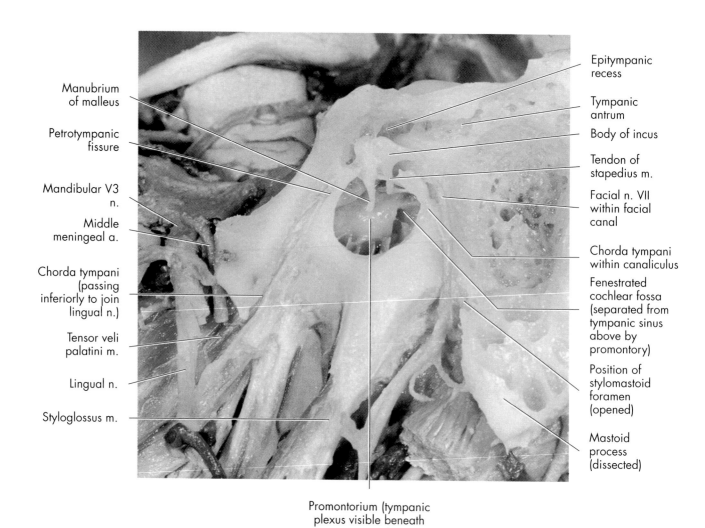

Manubrium of malleus

Petrotympanic fissure

Mandibular V3 n.

Middle meningeal a.

Chorda tympani (passing inferiorly to join lingual n.)

Tensor veli palatini m.

Lingual n.

Styloglossus m.

Epitympanic recess

Tympanic antrum

Body of incus

Tendon of stapedius m.

Facial n. VII within facial canal

Chorda tympani within canaliculus

Fenestrated cochlear fossa (separated from tympanic sinus above by promontory)

Position of stylomastoid foramen (opened)

Mastoid process (dissected)

Promontorium (tympanic plexus visible beneath mucosa)

Figure 2-118 Middle ear cavity, lateral view. The tympanic membrane (eardrum) has been removed, and the facial nerve and its chorda tympani branch are visible.

See **DISSECTIONS, Section 2, p. 9**
See **PRINCIPLES, Figs. 2-88, 2-89**

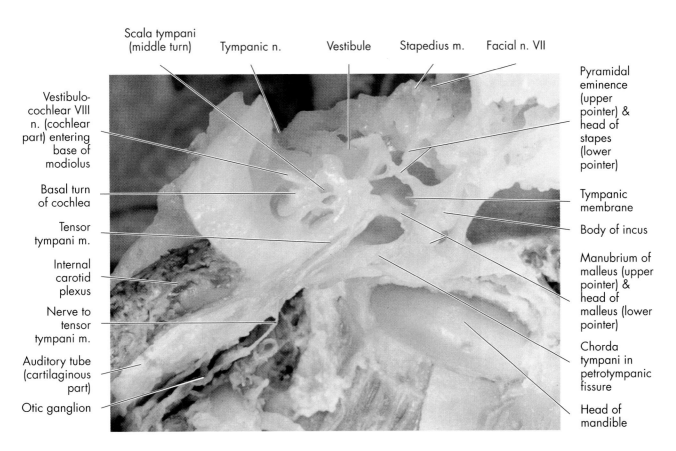

Scala tympani (middle turn)   Tympanic n.   Vestibule   Stapedius m.   Facial n. VII

Pyramidal eminence (upper pointer) & head of stapes (lower pointer)

Vestibulo-cochlear VIII n. (cochlear part) entering base of modiolus

Basal turn of cochlea

Tensor tympani m.

Internal carotid plexus

Nerve to tensor tympani m.

Auditory tube (cartilaginous part)

Otic ganglion

Tympanic membrane

Body of incus

Manubrium of malleus (upper pointer) & head of malleus (lower pointer)

Chorda tympani in petrotympanic fissure

Head of mandible

Figure 2-119   Dissection of the left temporal bone from the superior aspect to show the cochlea and ear ossicles in situ. The upper margin of the vestibular window has been removed so that the entire stapes is visible.

See DISSECTIONS, Section 2, p. 9
See PRINCIPLES, Fig. 2-89

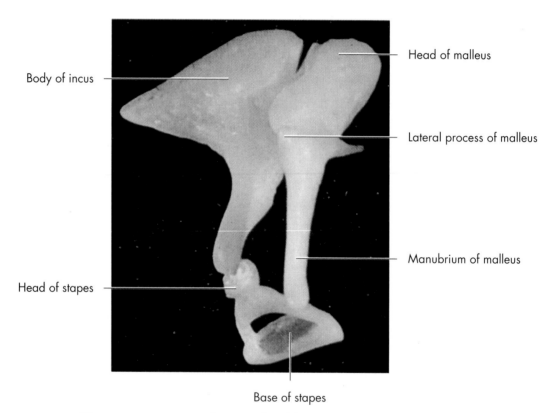

Body of incus

Head of malleus

Lateral process of malleus

Manubrium of malleus

Head of stapes

Base of stapes

Figure 2-120   Ear ossicles articulated from the lateral aspect.

SECTION THREE

Upper Limb

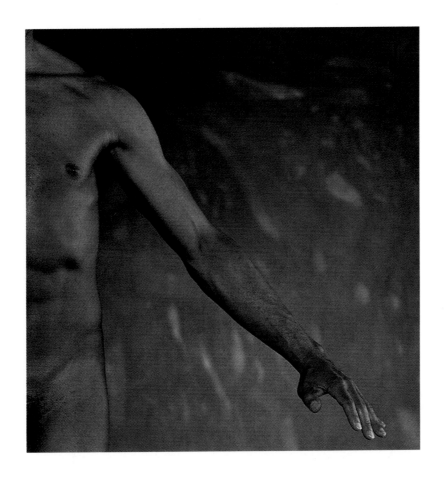

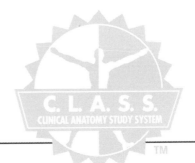

See **PRINCIPLES**, **FIG. 3-1**

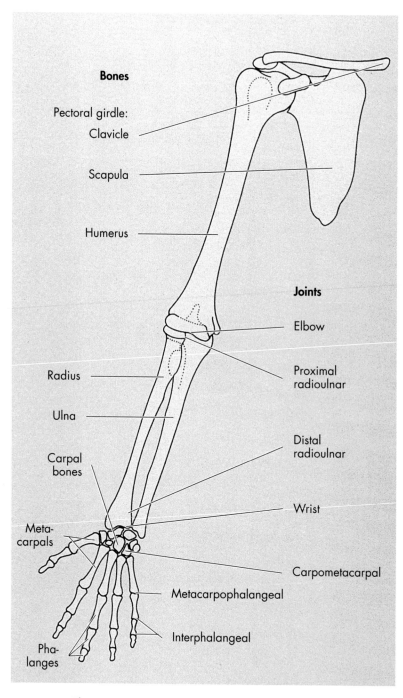

Bones

Pectoral girdle:

Clavicle

Scapula

Humerus

Radius

Ulna

Carpal
bones

Meta-
carpals

Pha-
langes

Joints

Elbow

Proximal
radioulnar

Distal
radioulnar

Wrist

Carpometacarpal

Metacarpophalangeal

Interphalangeal

Figure 3-1   Bones and joints of the upper limb.

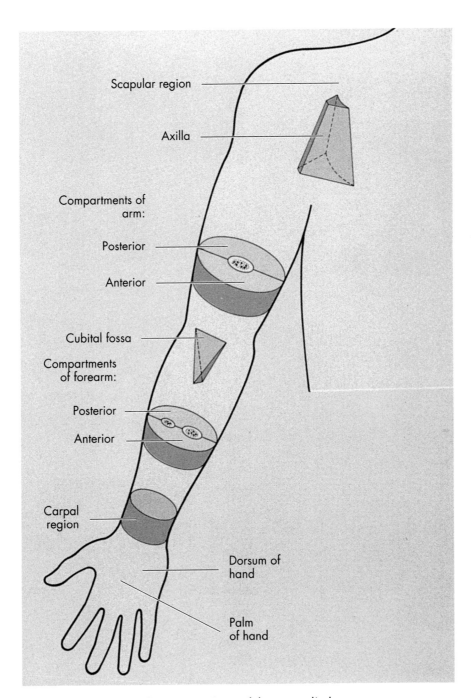

Scapular region

Axilla

Compartments of arm:

Posterior

Anterior

Cubital fossa

Compartments of forearm:

Posterior

Anterior

Carpal region

Dorsum of hand

Palm of hand

Figure 3-2   Parts of the upper limb.

SEE **PRINCIPLES**, FIG. 3-29

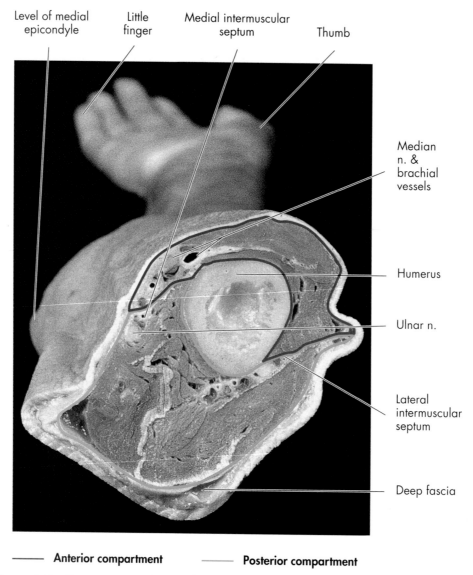

Level of medial epicondyle

Little finger

Medial intermuscular septum

Thumb

Median n. & brachial vessels

Humerus

Ulnar n.

Lateral intermuscular septum

Deep fascia

——— **Anterior compartment** ——— **Posterior compartment**

Figure 3-3 Transverse section midway between shoulder and elbow joints showing compartments of the arm.

SEE PRINCIPLES, FIG. 3-37

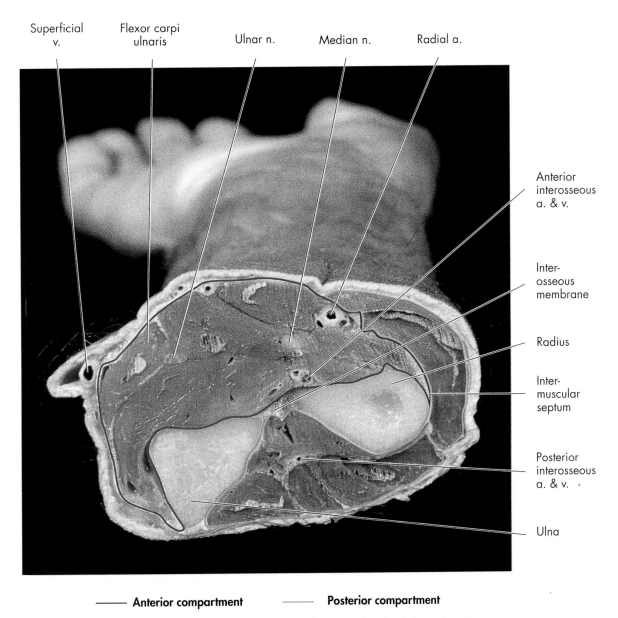

Superficial v.

Flexor carpi ulnaris

Ulnar n.

Median n.

Radial a.

Anterior interosseous a. & v.

Inter-osseous membrane

Radius

Inter-muscular septum

Posterior interosseous a. & v.

Ulna

—— **Anterior compartment**   —— **Posterior compartment**

Figure 3-4   Transverse section midway between elbow and wrist joints showing compartments of the forearm.

SEE **PRINCIPLES,** FIG. 3-48

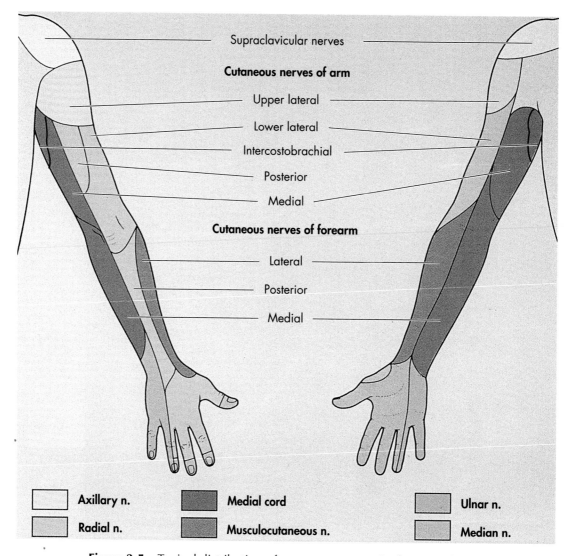

Supraclavicular nerves

Cutaneous nerves of arm

Upper lateral

Lower lateral

Intercostobrachial

Posterior

Medial

Cutaneous nerves of forearm

Lateral

Posterior

Medial

Axillary n.	Medial cord	Ulnar n.
Radial n.	Musculocutaneous n.	Median n.

Figure 3-5   Typical distribution of cutaneous nerves in the upper limb.

See PRINCIPLES, FIG. 3-48

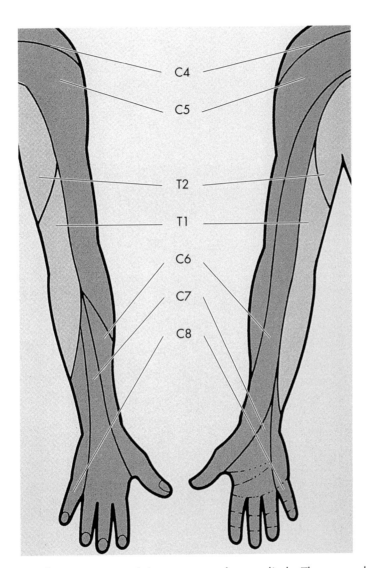

Figure 3-6   Typical arrangement of dermatomes of upper limb. There may be considerable overlap of areas supplied.

See PRINCIPLES, FIG. 3-23

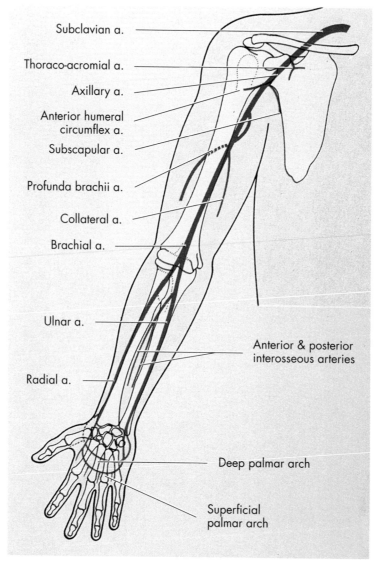

Subclavian a.

Thoraco-acromial a.

Axillary a.

Anterior humeral
circumflex a.

Subscapular a.

Profunda brachii a.

Collateral a.

Brachial a.

Ulnar a.

Radial a.

Anterior & posterior
interosseous arteries

Deep palmar arch

Superficial
palmar arch

Figure 3-7 Principal arteries of the upper limb. No muscular branches are shown. Posterior humeral circumflex artery is hidden behind the axillary artery.

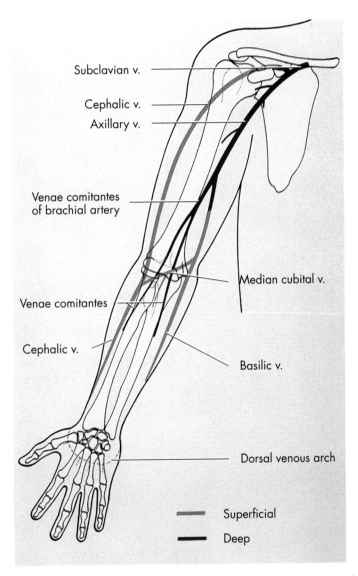

Figure 3-8 Typical arrangement of the principal veins of the upper limb. For clarity, venae comitantes are illustrated as single channels.

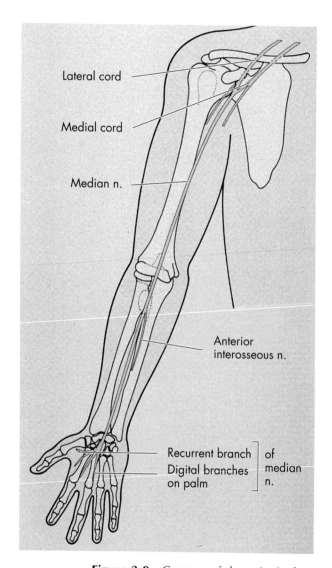

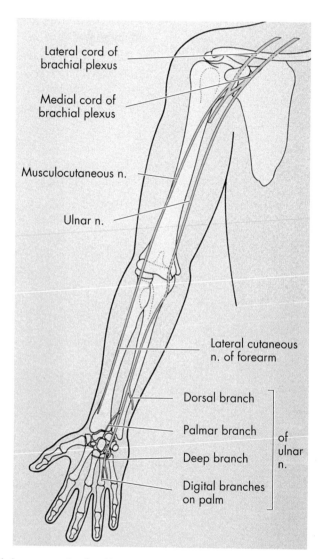

Figure 3-9   Courses of the principal nerves of the upper limb. Illustrations from left to right: median nerve, musculocutaneous and ulnar nerves, radial and axillary nerves (*opposite page*).

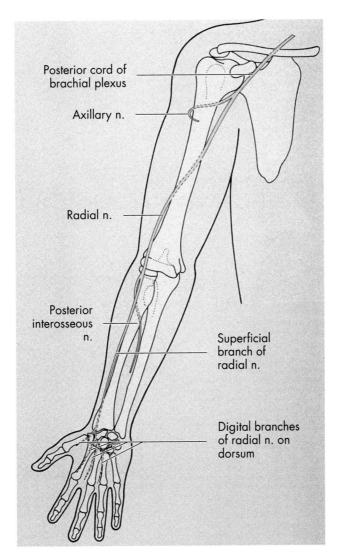

Posterior cord of
brachial plexus

Axillary n.

Radial n.

Posterior
interosseous
n.

Superficial
branch of
radial n.

Digital branches
of radial n. on
dorsum

Figure 3-9—cont'd   For legend, see opposite page.

See DISSECTIONS, Section 3, p. 3
See PRINCIPLES, Fig. 3-18

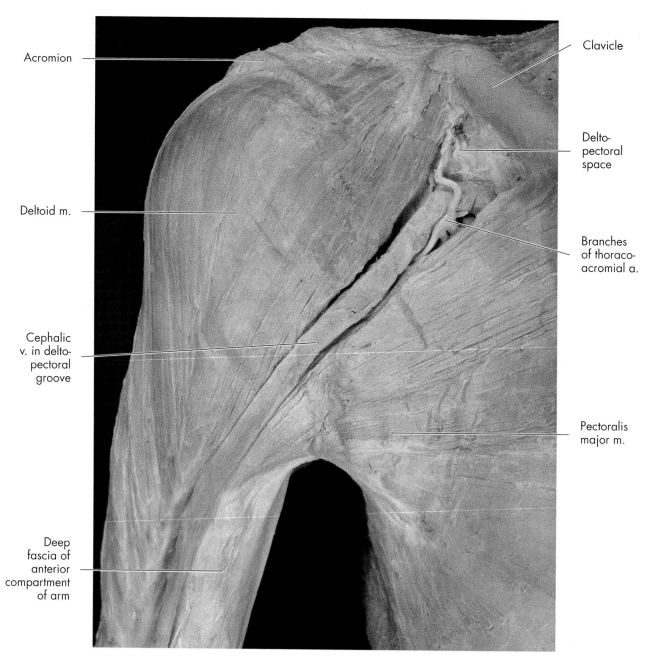

Acromion

Deltoid m.

Cephalic
v. in delto-
pectoral
groove

Deep
fascia of
anterior
compartment
of arm

Clavicle

Delto-
pectoral
space

Branches
of thoraco-
acromial a.

Pectoralis
major m.

Figure 3-10   Anterior view of the deltoid. The cephalic vein lies in the deltopectoral groove. Deformity of the clavicle is due to a healed fracture.

See **DISSECTIONS**, Section 3, p. 3
See **PRINCIPLES**, Fig. 3-18

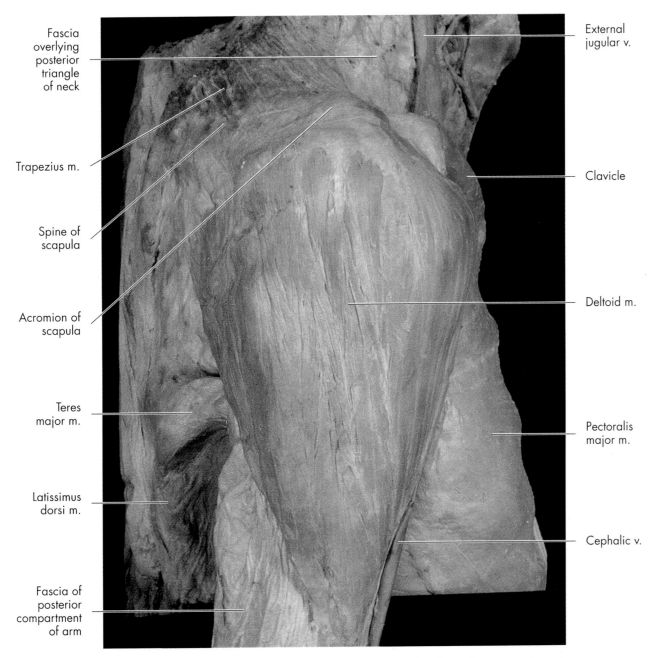

Fascia overlying posterior triangle of neck

Trapezius m.

Spine of scapula

Acromion of scapula

Teres major m.

Latissimus dorsi m.

Fascia of posterior compartment of arm

External jugular v.

Clavicle

Deltoid m.

Pectoralis major m.

Cephalic v.

Figure 3-11 Lateral view. The deltoid has continuous proximal attachments to the spine, to the acromion of the scapula, and to the lateral part of the clavicle.

See **PRINCIPLES, Fig. 3-20**

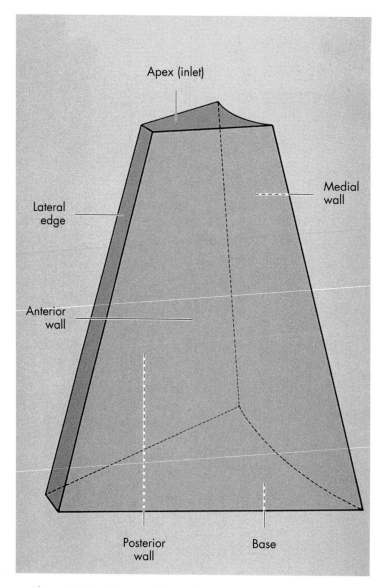

Figure 3-12   Shape of the axilla in the anatomic position.

See **PRINCIPLES, Fig. 3-20**

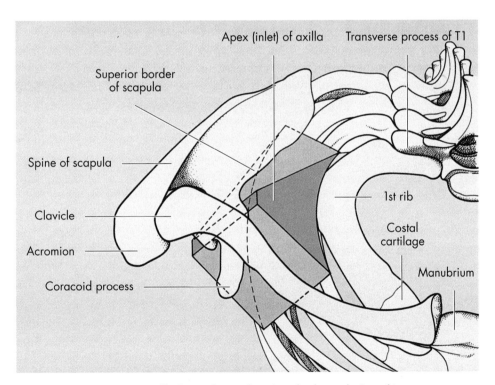

Figure 3-13   Axilla from above showing the boundaries of its apex.

See DISSECTIONS, Section 3, p. 3
See PRINCIPLES, Fig. 3-18

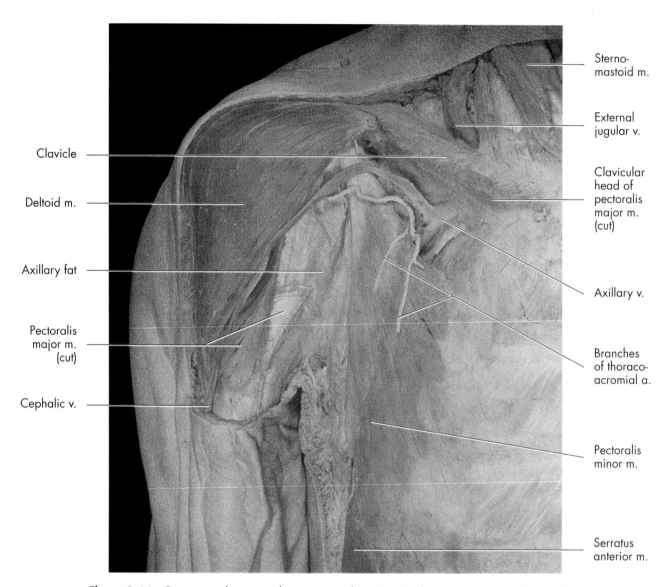

Clavicle

Deltoid m.

Axillary fat

Pectoralis
major m.
(cut)

Cephalic v.

Sterno-
mastoid m.

External
jugular v.

Clavicular
head of
pectoralis
major m.
(cut)

Axillary v.

Branches
of thoraco-
acromial a.

Pectoralis
minor m.

Serratus
anterior m.

Figure 3-14   Structures that pass above pectoralis minor in the anterior wall of the axilla.
Pectoralis major and fascia around pectoralis minor have been removed.

SEE **PRINCIPLES**, FIG. 3-20

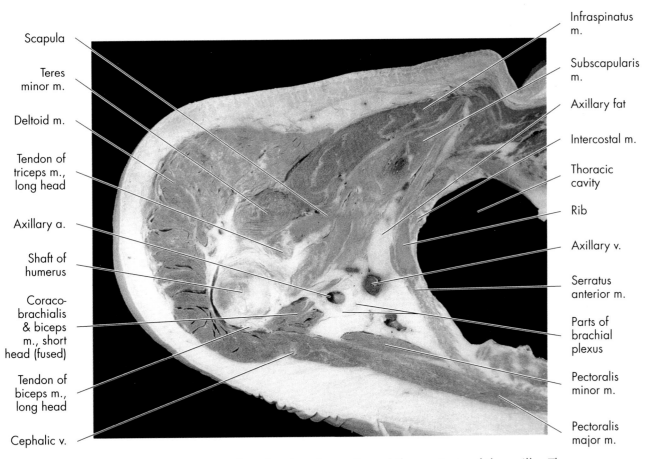

Scapula

Teres
minor m.

Deltoid m.

Tendon of
triceps m.,
long head

Axillary a.

Shaft of
humerus

Coraco-
brachialis
& biceps
m., short
head (fused)

Tendon of
biceps m.,
long head

Cephalic v.

Infraspinatus
m.

Subscapularis
m.

Axillary fat

Intercostal m.

Thoracic
cavity

Rib

Axillary v.

Serratus
anterior m.

Parts of
brachial
plexus

Pectoralis
minor m.

Pectoralis
major m.

Figure 3-15   Transverse section showing the walls and the contents of the axilla. The lung has been removed.

SEE DISSECTIONS, SECTION 3, P. 4

SEE PRINCIPLES, FIG. 3-19

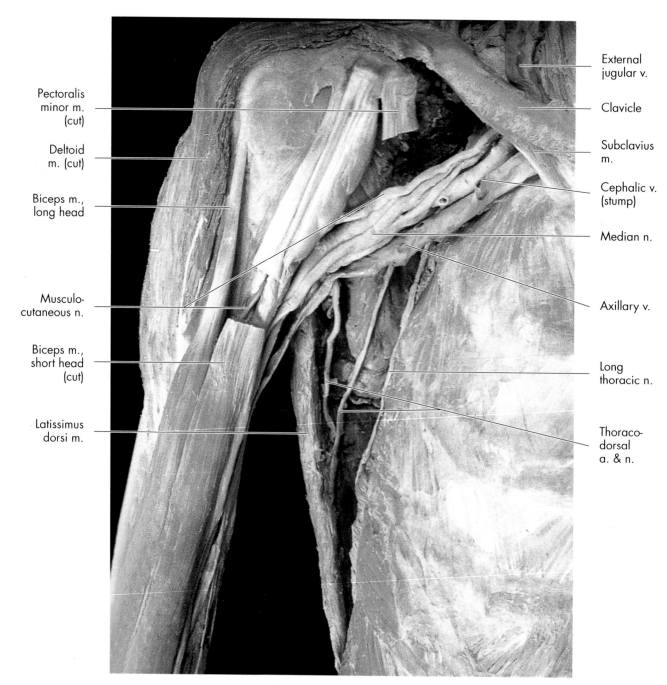

Pectoralis minor m. (cut)

Deltoid m. (cut)

Biceps m., long head

Musculo-cutaneous n.

Biceps m., short head (cut)

Latissimus dorsi m.

External jugular v.

Clavicle

Subclavius m.

Cephalic v. (stump)

Median n.

Axillary v.

Long thoracic n.

Thoraco-dorsal a. & n.

Figure 3-16 Axillary neurovascular bundle, exposed by removal of the pectoral muscles and axillary fat. *The brachial plexus can be effectively anesthetized by injection of a local anesthetic agent into the axillary sheath. With the shoulder abducted, a needle, passed through the axillary skin toward the palpable pulsations of the axillary artery, will penetrate the axillary sheath surrounding the brachial plexus elements, axillary artery, and the vein. The anesthetic agent will spread upward within the axillary sheath to bathe the brachial plexus cords, rendering them anesthetized. The intercostobrachial nerve lies outside the axillary sheath and must be blocked separately if anesthesia of the posterior aspect of the arm just distal to the axilla is required.*

See DISSECTIONS, SECTION 3, P. 4
See PRINCIPLES, FIG. 3-19

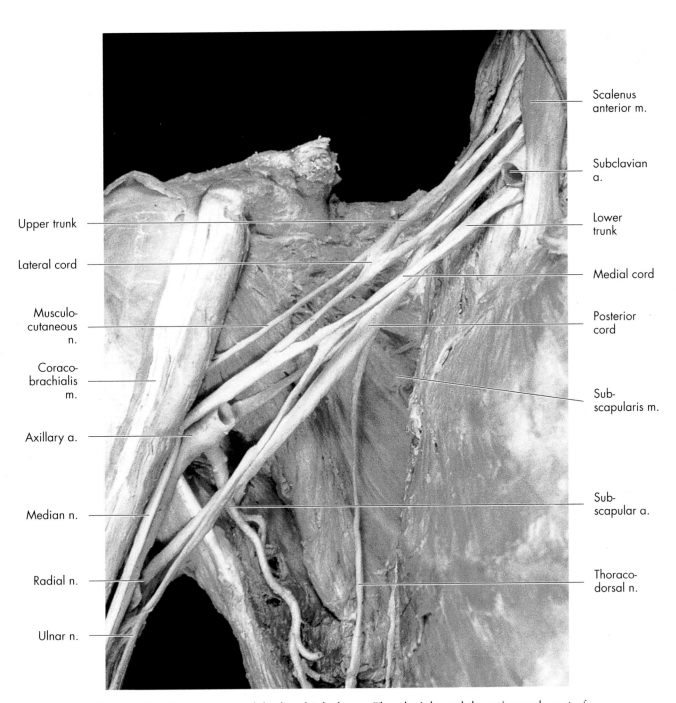

Figure 3-17 Components of the brachial plexus. The clavicle and the veins and most of the axillary artery have been removed.

See DISSECTIONS, SECTION 3, P. 4
See PRINCIPLES, FIG. 3-26

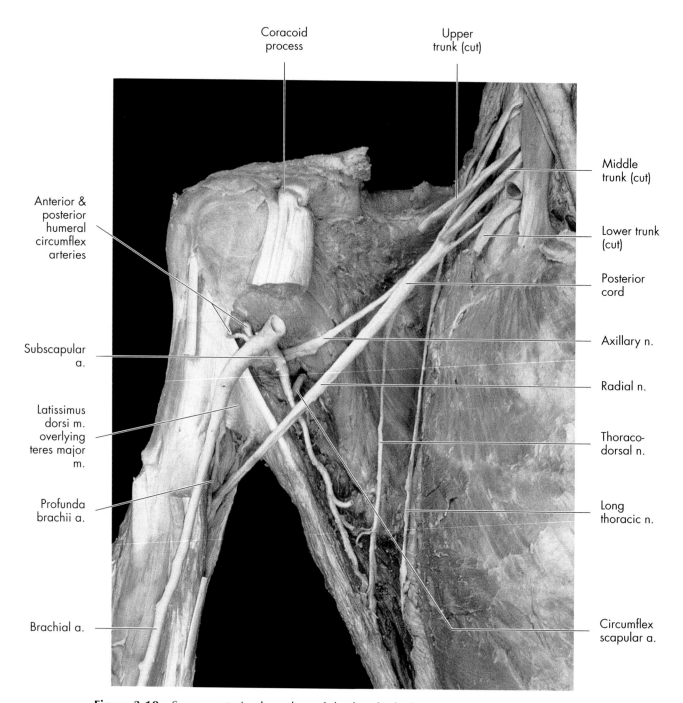

Figure 3-18 Some posterior branches of the brachial plexus seen after removal of the more anterior parts of the plexus. Biceps and coracobrachialis have been excised.

SEE PRINCIPLES, FIG. 3-25

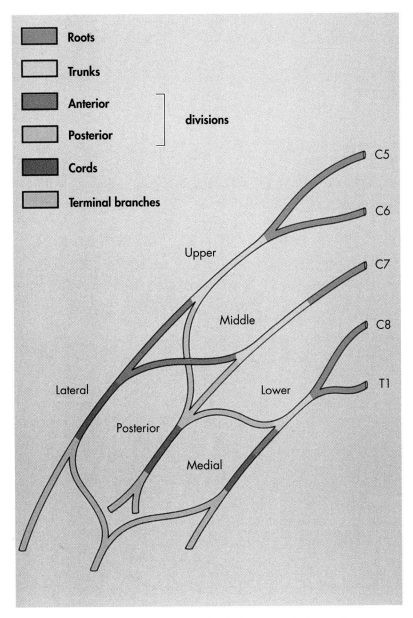

Figure 3-19 Main components of the brachial plexus in their usual arrangement. Note that the medial and lateral cords are derived from anterior divisions, while the posterior cord is made up of all posterior divisions. It is logical to consider the terms *anterolateral* and *anteromedial* to the traditional terms *lateral* and *medial* cords. Terminal motor and sensory distribution from the cords follows the anterior and posterior pattern throughout the limb.

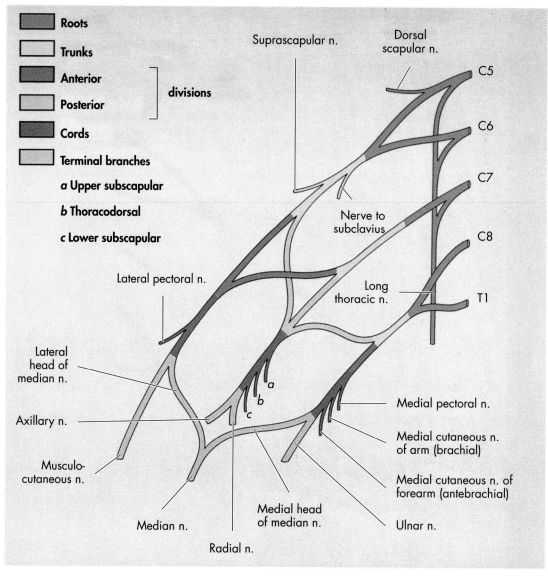

Figure 3-20   Branches of the brachial plexus. The arrangement of these nerves may vary considerably.

See DISSECTIONS, Section 3, pp. 3 and 7

See PRINCIPLES, Fig. 3-29

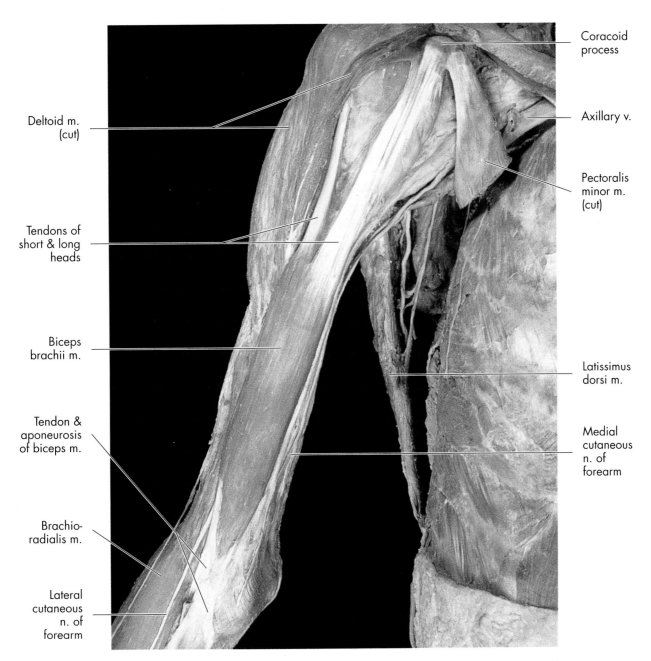

Coracoid process

Axillary v.

Pectoralis minor m. (cut)

Deltoid m. (cut)

Tendons of short & long heads

Biceps brachii m.

Latissimus dorsi m.

Tendon & aponeurosis of biceps m.

Medial cutaneous n. of forearm

Brachio-radialis m.

Lateral cutaneous n. of forearm

Figure 3-21   Anterior view of the biceps after removal of deep fascia and anterior fibers of the deltoid.

See DISSECTIONS, Section 3, p. 3
See PRINCIPLES, Fig. 3-29

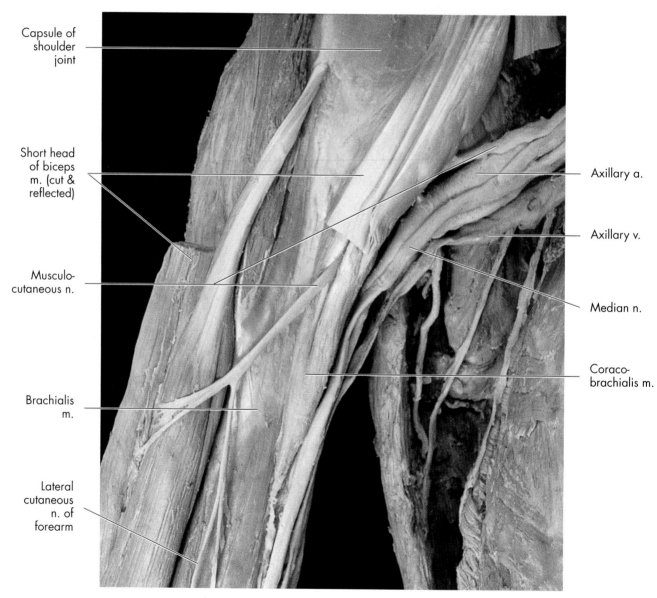

Capsule of shoulder joint

Short head of biceps m. (cut & reflected)

Musculo- cutaneous n.

Brachialis m.

Lateral cutaneous n. of forearm

Axillary a.

Axillary v.

Median n.

Coraco- brachialis m.

Figure 3-22   Musculocutaneous nerve piercing coracobrachialis. The short head of the biceps has been divided and the muscle reflected laterally.

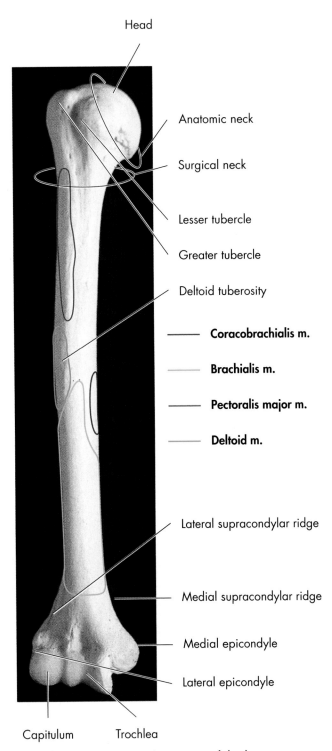

Head

Anatomic neck

Surgical neck

Lesser tubercle

Greater tubercle

Deltoid tuberosity

——— **Coracobrachialis m.**

——— **Brachialis m.**

——— **Pectoralis major m.**

——— **Deltoid m.**

Lateral supracondylar ridge

Medial supracondylar ridge

Medial epicondyle

Lateral epicondyle

Capitulum   Trochlea

Figure 3-23 Anterior aspect of the humerus.

SEE DISSECTIONS, SECTION 3, P. 7
SEE PRINCIPLES, FIG. 3-23

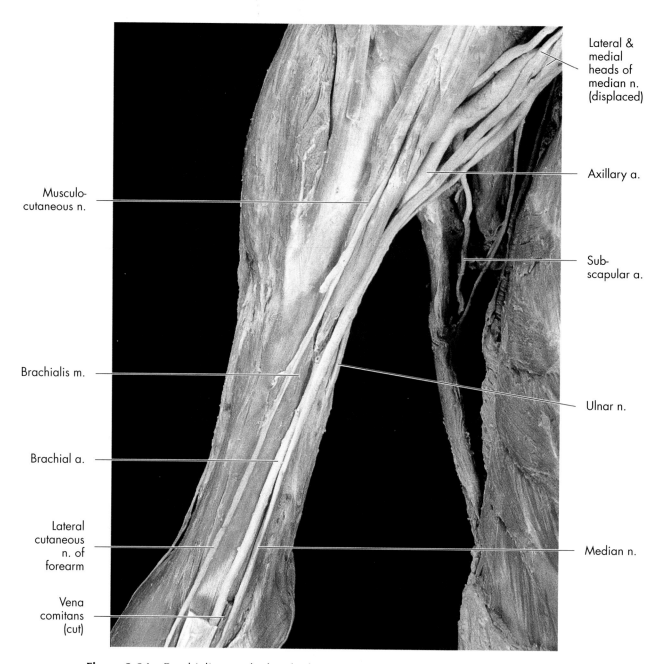

Figure 3-24   Brachialis muscle, brachial artery, and nerves of the anterior compartment. Biceps muscle and most veins have been excised.

See DISSECTIONS, Section 3, p. 7
See PRINCIPLES, Fig. 3-45

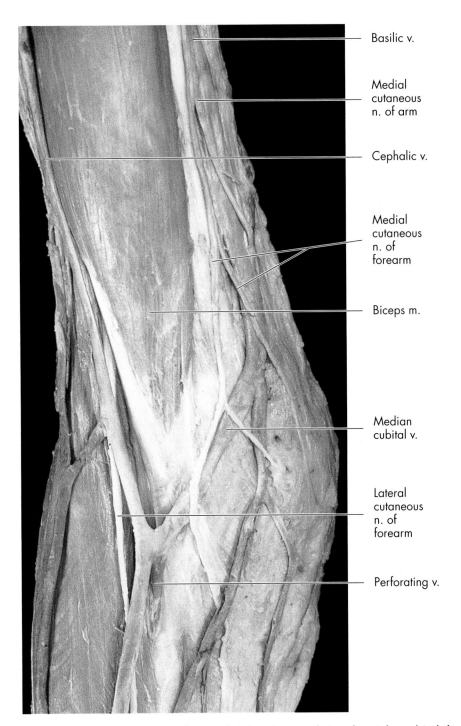

Basilic v.

Medial cutaneous n. of arm

Cephalic v.

Medial cutaneous n. of forearm

Biceps m.

Median cubital v.

Lateral cutaneous n. of forearm

Perforating v.

Figure 3-25 Cutaneous nerves and superficial veins overlying the right cubital fossa. Superficial fascia has been retained medial to the basilic vein.

See DISSECTIONS, Section 3, p. 7

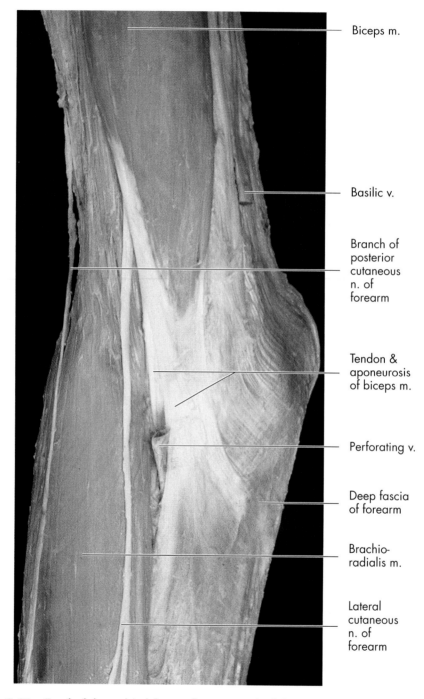

Biceps m.

Basilic v.

Branch of
posterior
cutaneous
n. of
forearm

Tendon &
aponeurosis
of biceps m.

Perforating v.

Deep fascia
of forearm

Brachio-
radialis m.

Lateral
cutaneous
n. of
forearm

Figure 3-26   Roof of the cubital fossa after removal of the superficial fascia, veins, and nerves. A perforation vein communicates with deep veins by passing through the deep fascia.

See **DISSECTIONS, Section** 3, p. 7
See **PRINCIPLES,** Fig. 3-29

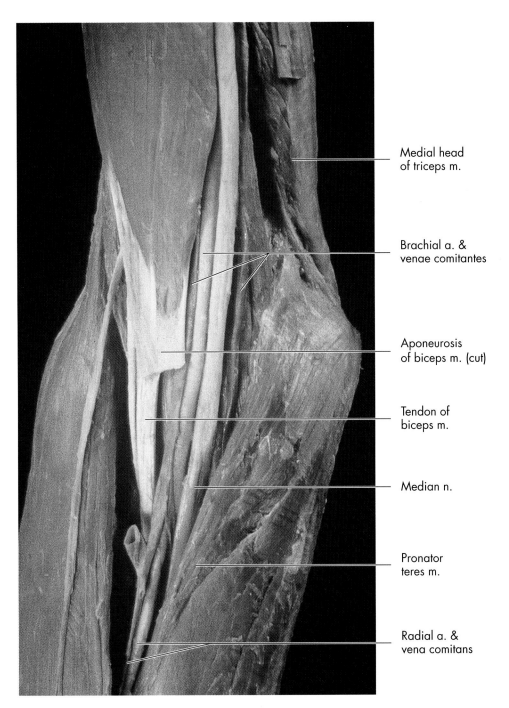

Medial head
of triceps m.

Brachial a. &
venae comitantes

Aponeurosis
of biceps m. (cut)

Tendon of
biceps m.

Median n.

Pronator
teres m.

Radial a. &
vena comitans

Figure 3-27   Contents of the cubital fossa. Aponeurosis of the biceps and the deep fascia
have been removed.

SEE PRINCIPLES, FIG. 3-29

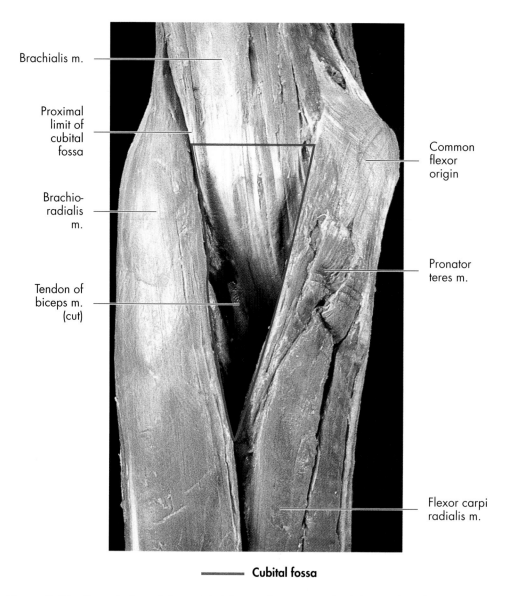

Brachialis m.

Proximal limit of cubital fossa

Brachio-radialis m.

Tendon of biceps m. (cut)

Common flexor origin

Pronator teres m.

Flexor carpi radialis m.

—— Cubital fossa

Figure 3-28   Boundaries of the cubital fossa after removal of the roof and contents are the pronator teres muscle, the brachioradialis muscle, and a line between the medial and lateral epicondyles.

SEE DISSECTIONS, SECTION 3, P. 7
SEE PRINCIPLES, FIG. 3-29

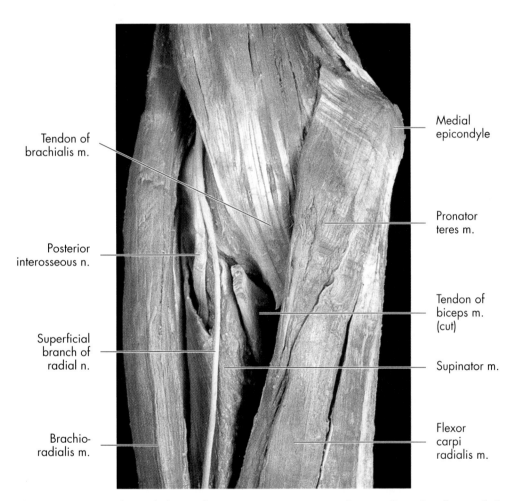

Tendon of
brachialis m.

Posterior
interosseous n.

Superficial
branch of
radial n.

Brachio-
radialis m.

Medial
epicondyle

Pronator
teres m.

Tendon of
biceps m.
(cut)

Supinator m.

Flexor
carpi
radialis m.

Figure 3-29   Brachioradialis and pronator teres retracted, revealing the floor of the cubital fossa and exposing the radial nerve and its posterior interosseous branch passing between the deep and superficial heads of the supinator muscle. *The nerve is sometimes compressed by entrapment at this supinator fibrous arcade.*

See DISSECTIONS, Section 3, p. 10
See PRINCIPLES, Fig. 3-39

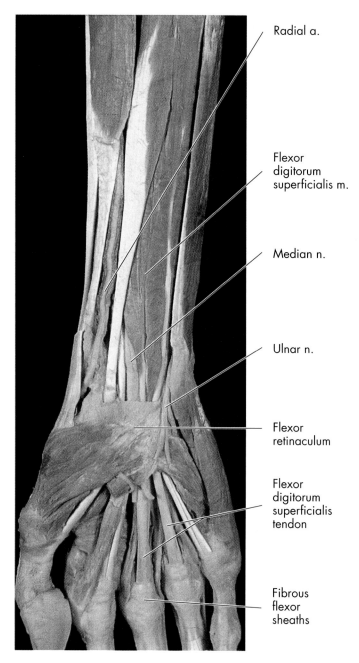

Radial a.

Flexor
digitorum
superficialis m.

Median n.

Ulnar n.

Flexor
retinaculum

Flexor
digitorum
superficialis
tendon

Fibrous
flexor
sheaths

Figure 3-30   Flexor retinaculum revealed by removal of superficial and most of the deep fascia. The retinaculum is partly obscured by some of the intrinsic muscles of the thumb and little finger.

See DISSECTIONS, Section 3, p. 10
See PRINCIPLES, Fig. 3-39

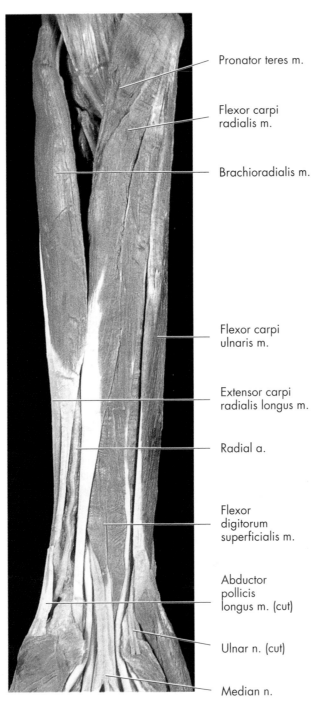

Pronator teres m.

Flexor carpi
radialis m.

Brachioradialis m.

Flexor carpi
ulnaris m.

Extensor carpi
radialis longus m.

Radial a.

Flexor
digitorum
superficialis m.

Abductor
pollicis
longus m. (cut)

Ulnar n. (cut)

Median n.

Figure 3-31   Flexor carpi radialis and flexor carpi ulnaris seen after removal of deep fascia and the flexor retinaculum. This specimen lacks a palmaris longus. The palmaris longus may be absent in 10% to 15% of people.

See **DISSECTIONS**, Section 3, p. 10

See **PRINCIPLES**, Fig. 3-40

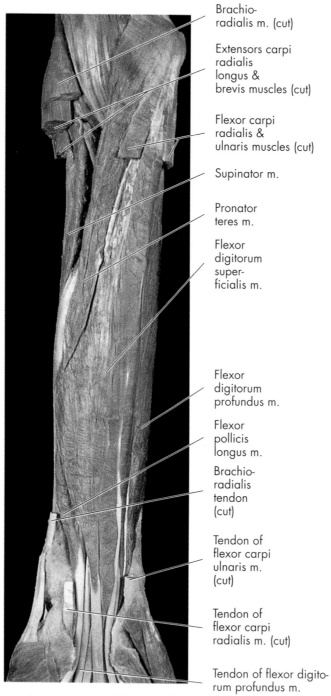

Brachio-
radialis m. (cut)

Extensors carpi
radialis
longus &
brevis muscles (cut)

Flexor carpi
radialis &
ulnaris muscles (cut)

Supinator m.

Pronator
teres m.

Flexor
digitorum
super-
ficialis m.

Flexor
digitorum
profundus m.

Flexor
pollicis
longus m.

Brachio-
radialis
tendon
(cut)

Tendon of
flexor carpi
ulnaris m.
(cut)

Tendon of
flexor carpi
radialis m. (cut)

Tendon of flexor digito-
rum profundus m.

Figure 3-32   Flexor digitorum superficialis and pronator teres revealed by division of the flexor carpi ulnaris and radialis and the brachioradialis. The vessels and nerves in the forearm have been removed.

See **DISSECTIONS,** Section 3, p. 10

See **PRINCIPLES,** Fig. 3-35

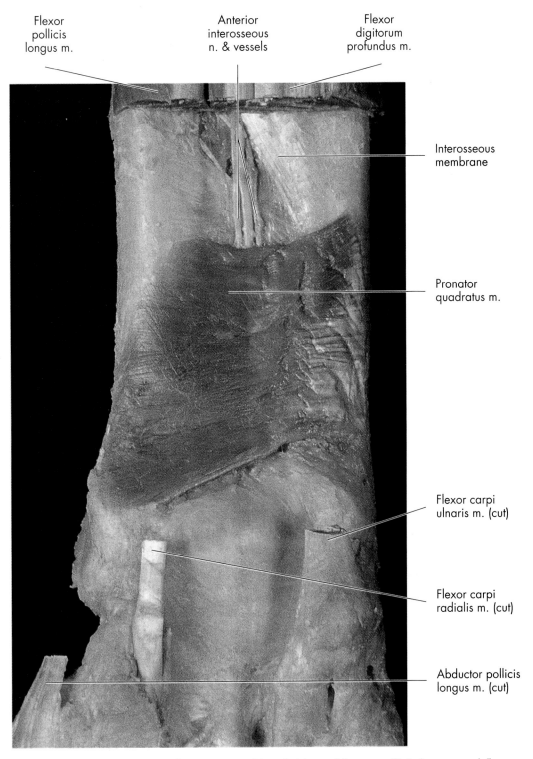

Flexor
pollicis
longus m.

Anterior
interosseous
n. & vessels

Flexor
digitorum
profundus m.

Interosseous
membrane

Pronator
quadratus m.

Flexor carpi
ulnaris m. (cut)

Flexor carpi
radialis m. (cut)

Abductor pollicis
longus m. (cut)

Figure 3-33   Pronator quadratus exposed by division of flexor pollicis longus and flexor digitorum profundus and removal of all superficialis and profundus flexors.

SEE PRINCIPLES, FIG. 3-38

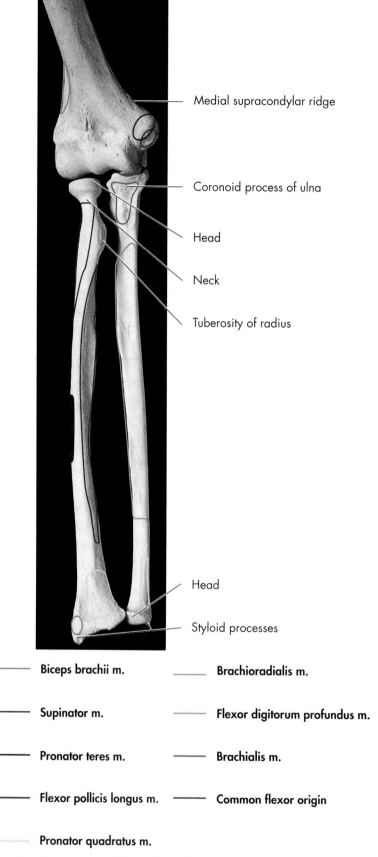

Medial supracondylar ridge

Coronoid process of ulna

Head

Neck

Tuberosity of radius

Head

Styloid processes

—— Biceps brachii m.   —— Brachioradialis m.

—— Supinator m.   —— Flexor digitorum profundus m.

—— Pronator teres m.   —— Brachialis m.

—— Flexor pollicis longus m.   —— Common flexor origin

—— Pronator quadratus m.

Figure 3-34 Anterior aspects of the radius, ulna, and the distal end of the humerus. The bones have been separated slightly.

See DISSECTIONS, Section 3, p. 10

See PRINCIPLES, Fig. 3-40

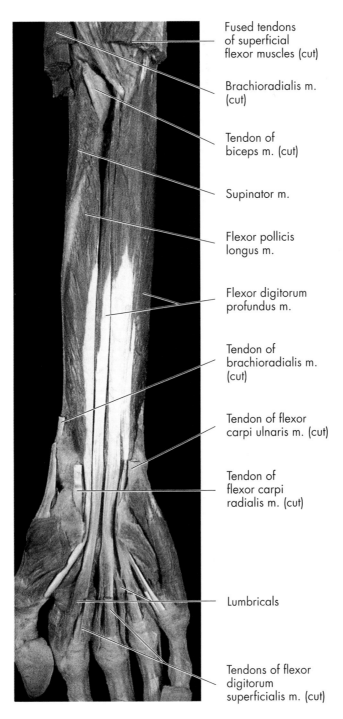

Fused tendons
of superficial
flexor muscles (cut)

Brachioradialis m.
(cut)

Tendon of
biceps m. (cut)

Supinator m.

Flexor pollicis
longus m.

Flexor digitorum
profundus m.

Tendon of
brachioradialis m.
(cut)

Tendon of flexor
carpi ulnaris m. (cut)

Tendon of
flexor carpi
radialis m. (cut)

Lumbricals

Tendons of flexor
digitorum
superficialis m. (cut)

Figure 3-35   Flexor digitorum profundus and flexor pollicis longus exposed by removal of the superficial flexors. As evident in this specimen, the index component of the flexor digitorum profundus is often separate from the rest of the profundus muscles.

SEE DISSECTIONS, SECTION 3, P. 10
SEE PRINCIPLES, FIGS. 3-30, 3-43

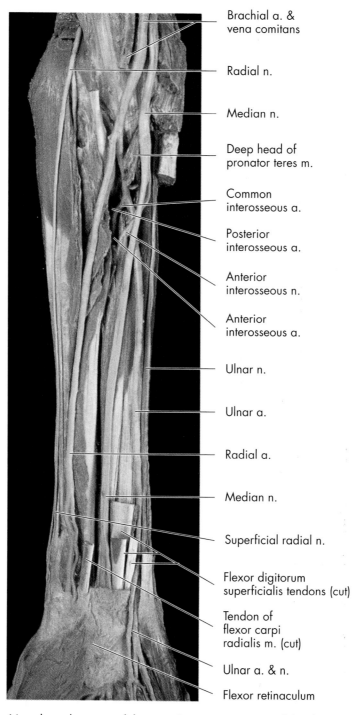

Brachial a. &
vena comitans

Radial n.

Median n.

Deep head of
pronator teres m.

Common
interosseous a.

Posterior
interosseous a.

Anterior
interosseous n.

Anterior
interosseous a.

Ulnar n.

Ulnar a.

Radial a.

Median n.

Superficial radial n.

Flexor digitorum
superficialis tendons (cut)

Tendon of
flexor carpi
radialis m. (cut)

Ulnar a. & n.

Flexor retinaculum

Figure 3-36   Vessels and nerves of the anterior compartment of the forearm. The superficial flexor muscles and the brachioradialis have been divided and most of the venae comitantes have been removed.

See **PRINCIPLES**, Figs. 3-50, 3-57

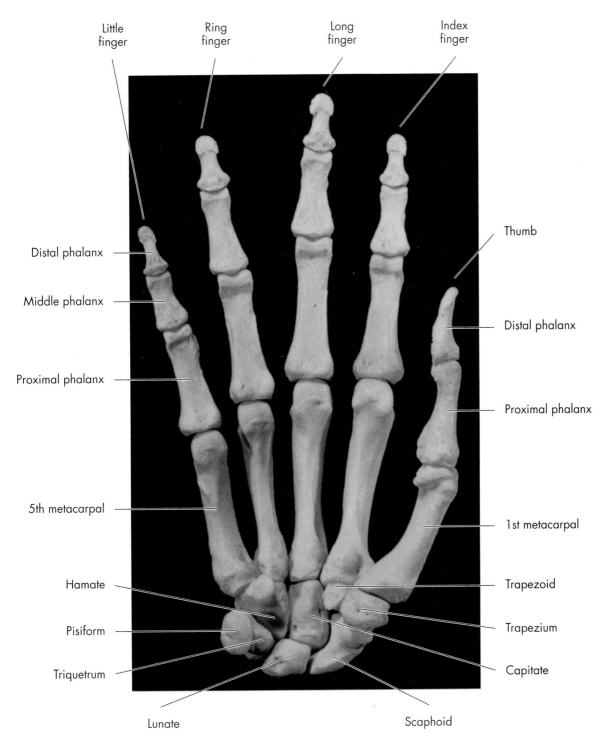

Little finger

Ring finger

Long finger

Index finger

Thumb

Distal phalanx

Middle phalanx

Proximal phalanx

Distal phalanx

Proximal phalanx

5th metacarpal

1st metacarpal

Hamate

Trapezoid

Pisiform

Trapezium

Triquetrum

Capitate

Lunate

Scaphoid

Figure 3-37 Anterior view of articulated bones of the right hand.

See PRINCIPLES, Figs. 3-50, 3-57

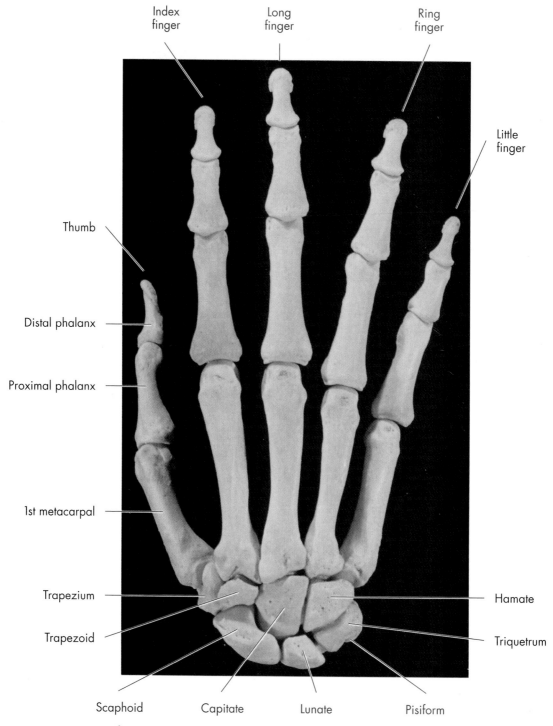

Figure 3-38   Posterior view of articulated bones of the right hand.

See **PRINCIPLES**, Fig. 3-49

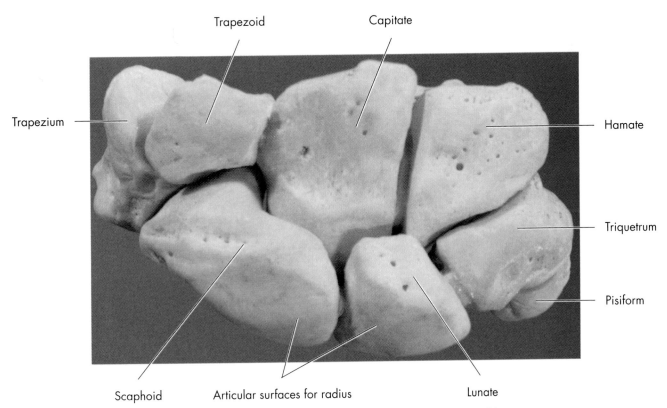

Capitate

Trapezoid

Articular surface for
1st metacarpal

Groove
for tendon
of flexor
carpi
radialis m.

Trapezium

Hamate

Triquetrum

Pisiform

Lunate

Scaphoid

Figure 3-39   Anterior view of articulated right carpal bones. Nutrient foramina are visible on several of the rough nonarticular surfaces of the bones.

Trapezoid

Capitate

Trapezium

Hamate

Triquetrum

Pisiform

Scaphoid

Articular surfaces for radius

Lunate

Figure 3-40   Posterior or dorsal view of articulated right carpal bones.

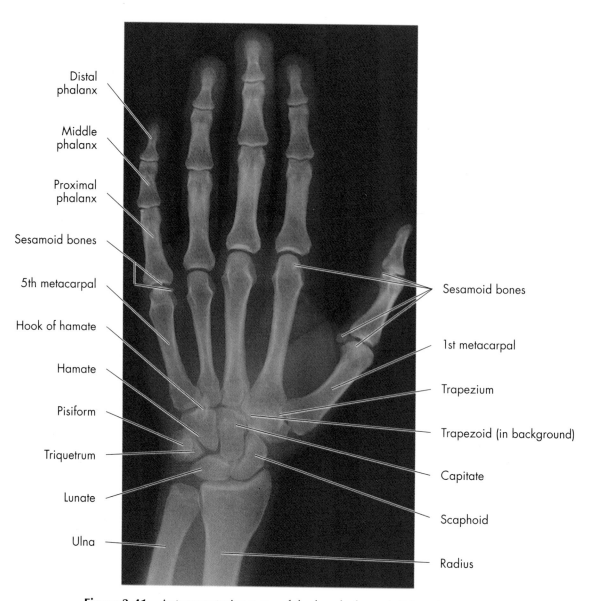

Distal
phalanx

Middle
phalanx

Proximal
phalanx

Sesamoid bones

5th metacarpal

Hook of hamate

Hamate

Pisiform

Triquetrum

Lunate

Ulna

Sesamoid bones

1st metacarpal

Trapezium

Trapezoid (in background)

Capitate

Scaphoid

Radius

Figure 3-41   Anteroposterior x-ray of the hand of an adult female.

See DISSECTIONS, Section 3, p. 11
See PRINCIPLES, P. 382

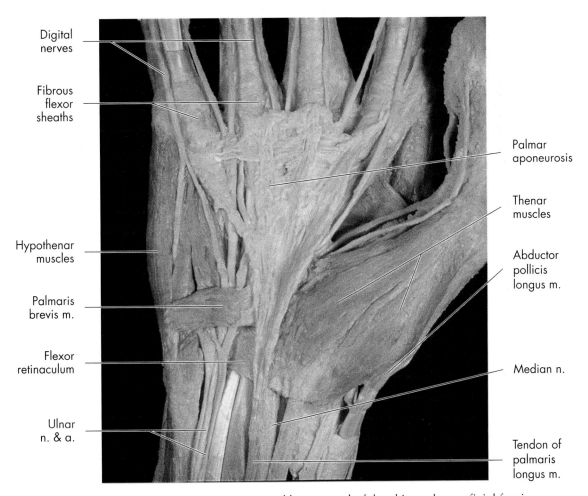

Digital nerves

Fibrous flexor sheaths

Hypothenar muscles

Palmaris brevis m.

Flexor retinaculum

Ulnar n. & a.

Palmar aponeurosis

Thenar muscles

Abductor pollicis longus m.

Median n.

Tendon of palmaris longus m.

Figure 3-42   Palmar aponeurosis exposed by removal of the skin and superficial fascia.

SEE DISSECTIONS, SECTION 3, P. 11

SEE PRINCIPLES, FIG. 3-54

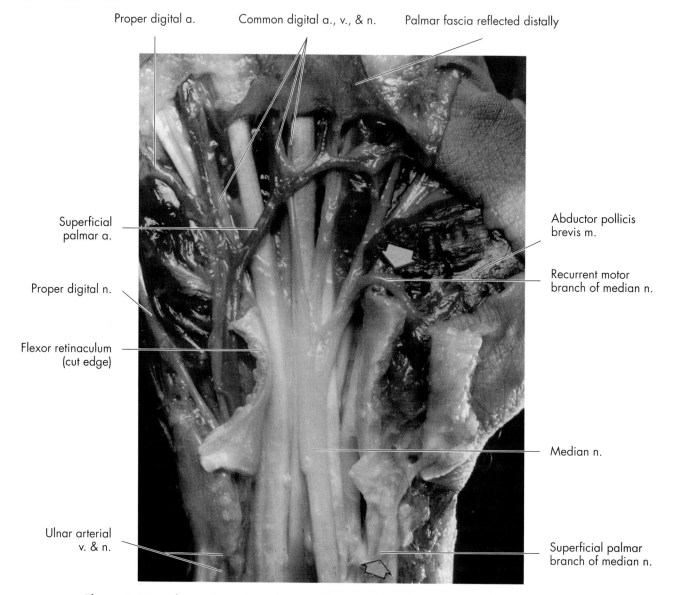

Proper digital a.   Common digital a., v., & n.   Palmar fascia reflected distally

Superficial palmar a.

Proper digital n.

Flexor retinaculum (cut edge)

Ulnar arterial v. & n.

Abductor pollicis brevis m.

Recurrent motor branch of median n.

Median n.

Superficial palmar branch of median n.

Figure 3-43   Palmar view of the hand with the palmar fascia removed and the flexor retinaculum cut and reflected at the wrist (volar carpal ligament) to show the carpal tunnel. *The carpal tunnel at the wrist has a bony floor of carpal bones and a roof formed by the flexor retinaculum (volar carpal ligament). Structures passing from forearm to hand, such as the flexor digitorum superficialis and profundus to all fingers, the flexor pollicis longus to the thumb, and the median nerve pass through this unyielding space. Swelling within the tunnel, such as occurs with inflammation of the synovium around the tendons, may compress the median nerve. The median nerve is the most superficial structure in the tunnel, and, when compressed, it creates tingling and numbness in the palmar aspect of the thumb, index, long, and radial half of the ring fingers. If compression of the nerve is unrelieved, paralysis and atrophy of the muscles innervated by the nerve (abductor pollicis brevis, opponens pollicis, flexor pollicis brevis, and the first and second lumbricals) may occur. Surgical release of the flexor retinaculum is undertaken to remove compression on the median nerve. The large arrows point to the superficial palmar and the recurrent motor branches of the median nerve. These branches are vulnerable to injury in carpal tunnel surgery.*

See DISSECTIONS, Section 3, p. 11
See PRINCIPLES, Fig. 3-66

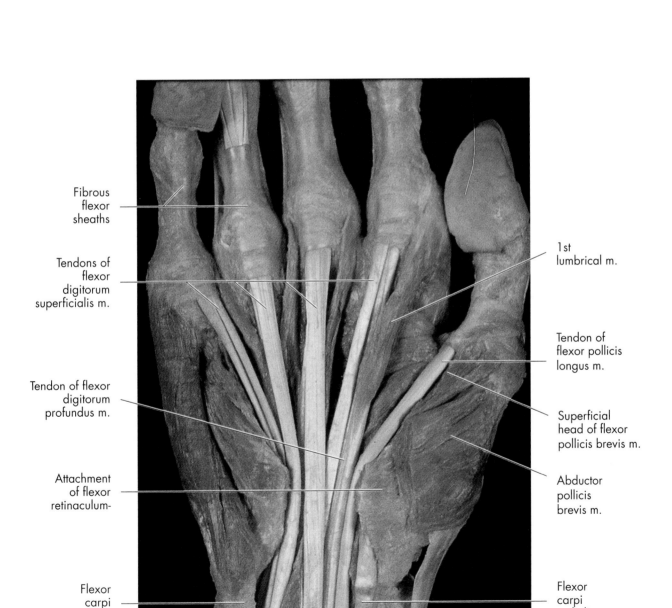

Fibrous
flexor
sheaths

Tendons of
flexor
digitorum
superficialis m.

Tendon of flexor
digitorum
profundus m.

Attachment
of flexor
retinaculum

Flexor
carpi
ulnaris m.

1st
lumbrical m.

Tendon of
flexor pollicis
longus m.

Superficial
head of flexor
pollicis brevis m.

Abductor
pollicis
brevis m.

Flexor
carpi
radialis m.

Figure 3-44   Tendons of flexor digitorum superficialis in the palm. The palmar aponeurosis, flexor retinaculum, and palmar vessels and nerves have been removed.

SEE PRINCIPLES, FIG. 3-65

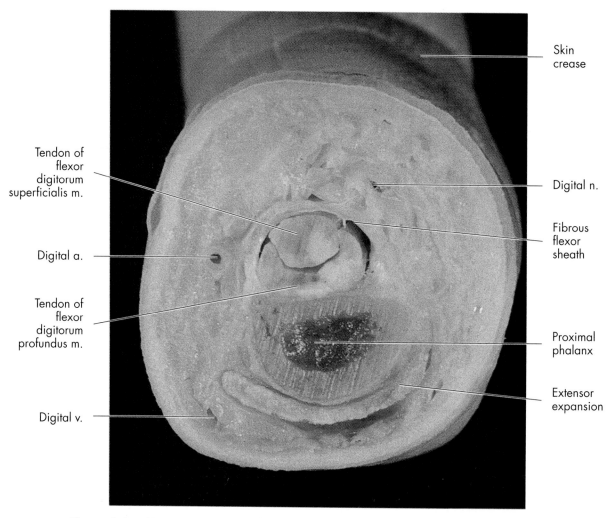

Skin
crease

Tendon of
flexor
digitorum
superficialis m.

Digital n.

Fibrous
flexor
sheath

Digital a.

Tendon of
flexor
digitorum
profundus m.

Proximal
phalanx

Extensor
expansion

Digital v.

Figure 3-45   Transverse section through the index finger at the level of the proximal phalanx.

See **DISSECTIONS**, Section 3, p. 11

See **PRINCIPLES**, Fig. 3-66

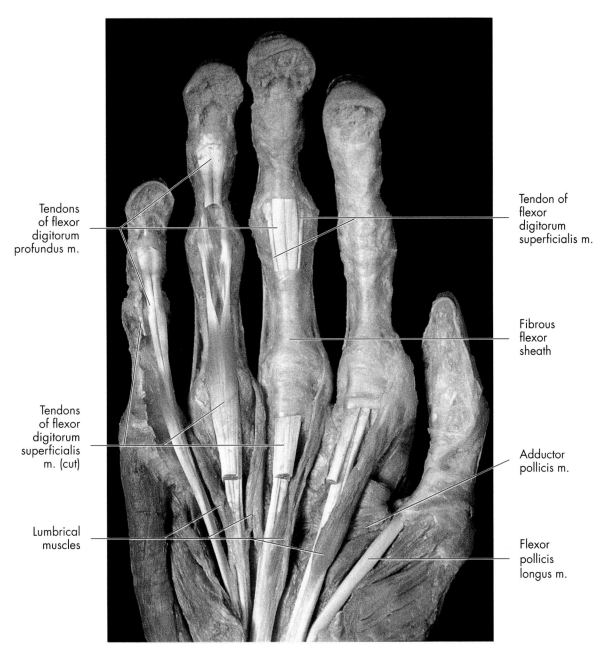

Tendons
of flexor
digitorum
profundus m.

Tendon of
flexor
digitorum
superficialis m.

Fibrous
flexor
sheath

Tendons
of flexor
digitorum
superficialis
m. (cut)

Lumbrical
muscles

Adductor
pollicis m.

Flexor
pollicis
longus m.

Figure 3-46   Digital fibrous flexor sheaths. The partially cut-away synovial sheath and one pulley of the middle finger exposes the tendons of the flexor digitorum superficialis and profundus, whose phalangeal attachments are revealed on the ring and little fingers.

Sᴇᴇ **DISSECTIONS**, Sᴇᴄᴛɪᴏɴ 3, ᴘ. 11

Sᴇᴇ **PRINCIPLES**, Fɪɢ. 3-63

Flexor digitorum
superficialis tendon

Vincula longa

Flexor digitorum
profundus tendon

Insertion of flexor
digitorum superficialis
tendon on middle phalanx

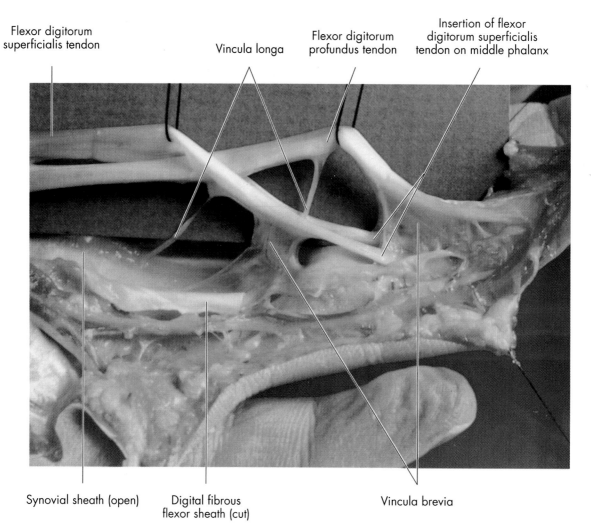

Synovial sheath (open)

Digital fibrous
flexor sheath (cut)

Vincula brevia

Figure 3-47   Flexor digitorum superficialis and profundus tendons elevated from the digital flexor sheath to show their sites of attachment and the vincula.

See **DISSECTIONS**, Section 3, p. 11
See **PRINCIPLES**, Fig. 3-62

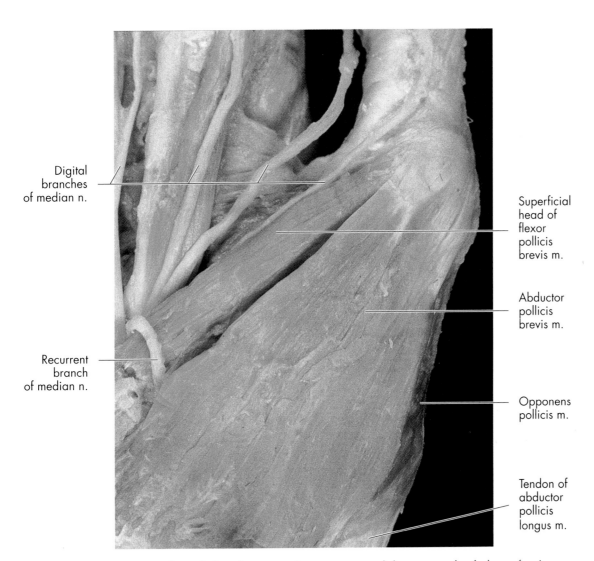

Digital branches of median n.

Recurrent branch of median n.

Superficial head of flexor pollicis brevis m.

Abductor pollicis brevis m.

Opponens pollicis m.

Tendon of abductor pollicis longus m.

Figure 3-48 Muscles of the thenar eminence exposed by removal of deep fascia. Abductor pollicis brevis is superficial to the flexor pollicis brevis and opponens pollicis.

See DISSECTIONS, Section 3, p. 11

See PRINCIPLES, Fig. 3-61

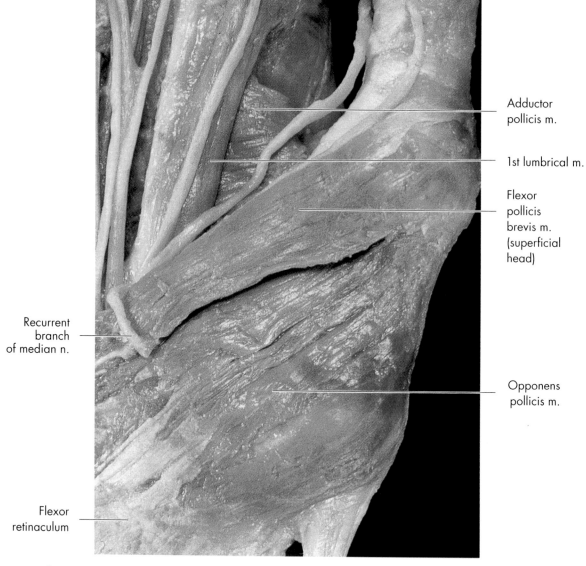

Adductor
pollicis m.

1st lumbrical m.

Flexor
pollicis
brevis m.
(superficial
head)

Recurrent
branch
of median n.

Opponens
pollicis m.

Flexor
retinaculum

Figure 3-49   Opponens pollicis and flexor pollicis brevis exposed by removal of the abductor pollicis brevis.

See DISSECTIONS, Section 3, p. 11
See PRINCIPLES, Fig. 3-61

Digital
branches
of ulnar n.

Abductor
digiti
minimi m.

Opponens
digiti
minimi m.

Flexor
retinaculum

Flexor
digiti
minimi m.

Superficial branch
of ulnar n.

Deep
branch
of ulnar n.

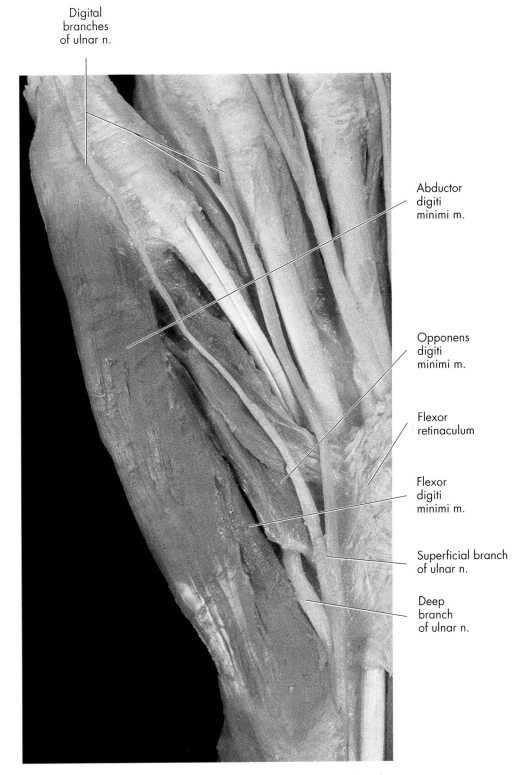

Figure 3-50 Hypothenar muscles exposed by removal of the deep fascia.

See DISSECTIONS, Section 3, p. 11

See PRINCIPLES, Fig. 3-62

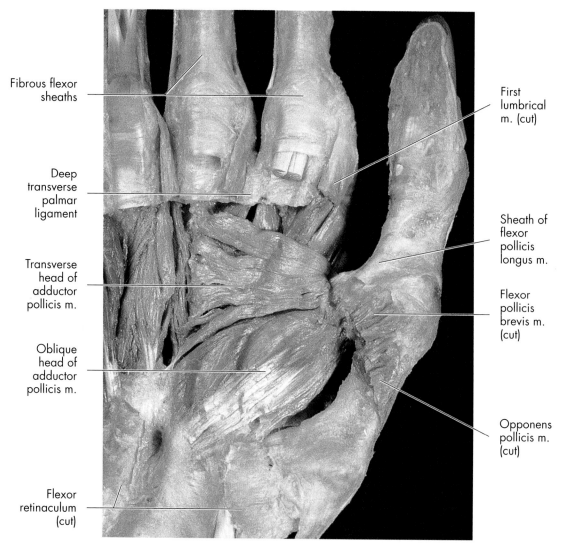

Fibrous flexor sheaths

Deep transverse palmar ligament

Transverse head of adductor pollicis m.

Oblique head of adductor pollicis m.

Flexor retinaculum (cut)

First lumbrical m. (cut)

Sheath of flexor pollicis longus m.

Flexor pollicis brevis m. (cut)

Opponens pollicis m. (cut)

Figure 3-51 Adductor pollicis. The muscles of the thenar eminence, long flexor tendons, and the palmar and digital vessels and nerves have been removed.

See **DISSECTIONS**, Section 3, p. 11
See **PRINCIPLES**, Fig. 3-64

Dorsal
interossei muscles

2nd
lumbrical
m. (cut)

Deep transverse
palmar ligament

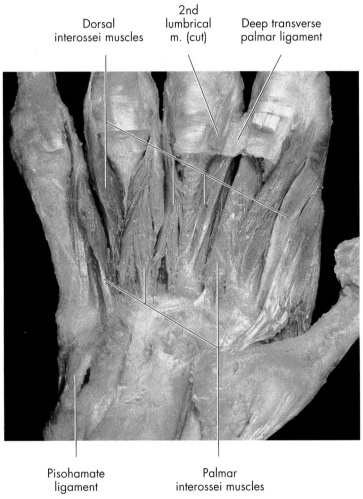

Pisohamate
ligament

Palmar
interossei muscles

Figure 3-52 Palmar and dorsal interossei exposed by removal of the long flexor tendons and the adductor pollicis. The dorsal interossei have much more bulk than the palmar interossei. Note that they pass dorsal to the deep transverse palmar ligament while the lumbricals pass palmar to it.

SEE DISSECTIONS, SECTION 3, P. 11

SEE PRINCIPLES, FIG. 3-64

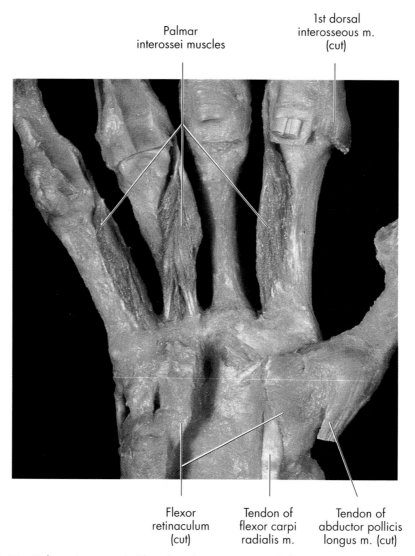

Palmar interossei muscles

1st dorsal interosseous m. (cut)

Flexor retinaculum (cut)

Tendon of flexor carpi radialis m.

Tendon of abductor pollicis longus m. (cut)

Figure 3-53 Palmar interossei. The dorsal interossei and deep transverse palmar ligaments have been excised.

See **DISSECTIONS, Section 3, p. 11**
See **PRINCIPLES, Fig. 3-64**

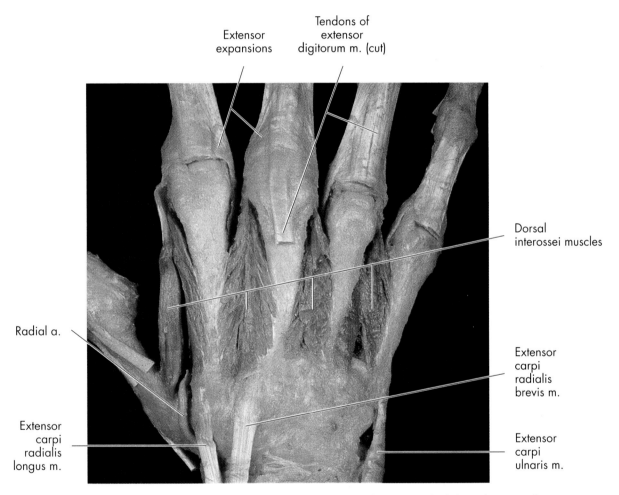

Extensor
expansions

Tendons of
extensor
digitorum m. (cut)

Dorsal
interossei muscles

Extensor
carpi
radialis
brevis m.

Radial a.

Extensor
carpi
radialis
longus m.

Extensor
carpi
ulnaris m.

Figure 3-54   Dorsal view of the dorsal interossei exposed by removal of deep fascia and tendons of the extensor digitorum.

See DISSECTIONS, Section 3, p. 11

See PRINCIPLES, Fig. 3-66

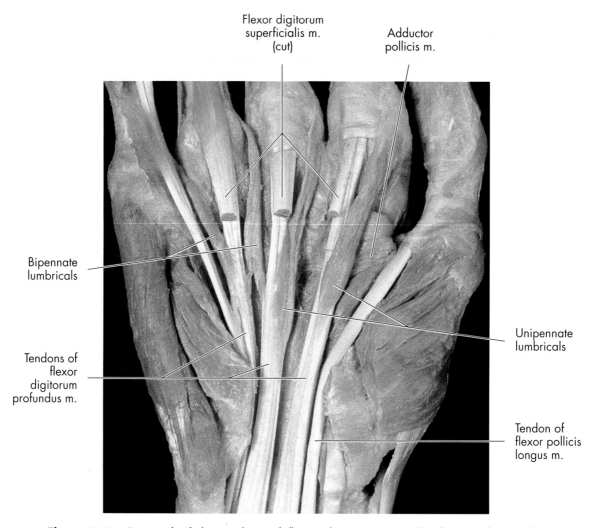

Flexor digitorum
superficialis m.
(cut)

Adductor
pollicis m.

Bipennate
lumbricals

Tendons of
flexor
digitorum
profundus m.

Unipennate
lumbricals

Tendon of
flexor pollicis
longus m.

Figure 3-55   Removal of the tendons of flexor digitorum superficialis reveals attachments of the lumbrical muscles to the tendons of the flexor digitorum profundus.

SEE DISSECTIONS, SECTION 3, P. 9
SEE PRINCIPLES, FIG. 3-63

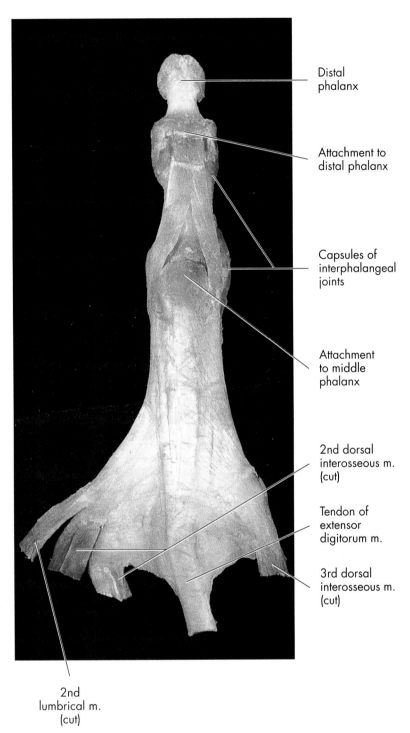

Distal
phalanx

Attachment to
distal phalanx

Capsules of
interphalangeal
joints

Attachment
to middle
phalanx

2nd dorsal
interosseous m.
(cut)

Tendon of
extensor
digitorum m.

3rd dorsal
interosseous m.
(cut)

2nd
lumbrical m.
(cut)

Figure 3-56 Dorsal view of the digital expansion of the middle finger. The extension has been flattened proximally to show the attachments of lumbrical and interosseous muscles.

See DISSECTIONS, Section 3, p. 11

See PRINCIPLES, Fig. 3-44

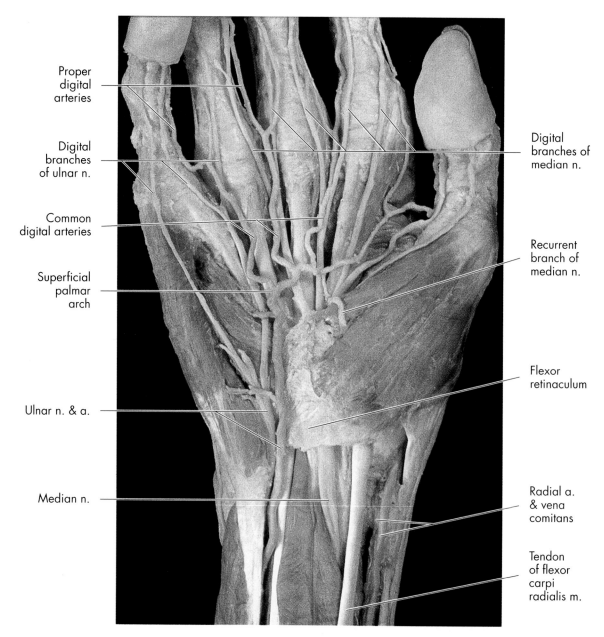

Proper digital arteries

Digital branches of ulnar n.

Common digital arteries

Superficial palmar arch

Ulnar n. & a.

Median n.

Digital branches of median n.

Recurrent branch of median n.

Flexor retinaculum

Radial a. & vena comitans

Tendon of flexor carpi radialis m.

Figure 3-57 Superficial vessels and nerves of the palm. Skin, superficial fascia, and the palmar aponeurosis have been removed.

SEE PRINCIPLES, FIG. 3-44

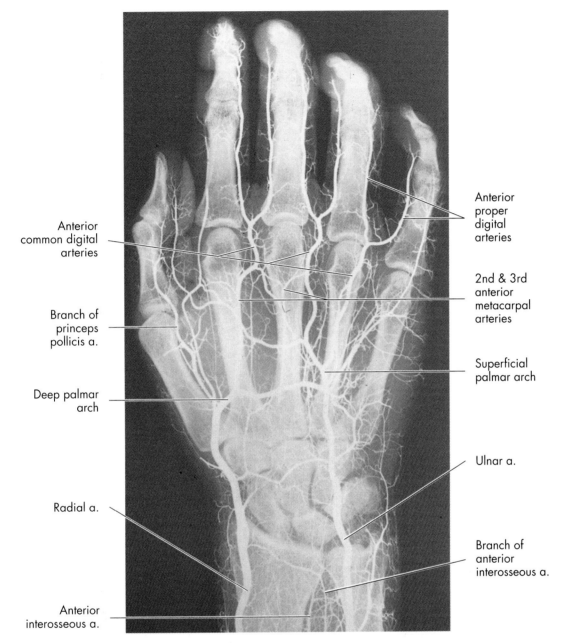

Anterior common digital arteries

Branch of princeps pollicis a.

Deep palmar arch

Radial a.

Anterior interosseous a.

Anterior proper digital arteries

2nd & 3rd anterior metacarpal arteries

Superficial palmar arch

Ulnar a.

Branch of anterior interosseous a.

Figure 3-58   Anteroposterior angiogram of the left hand of an adult male. A frequent variation from the commonly described arrangement of the vessels is present. The superficial palmar branch of the radial artery does not enter into the formation of the superficial palmar arch. *In the hand, the radial and ulnar arteries normally anastomose with one another through a deep palmar arch (primarily radial) and a superficial palmar arch (primarily ulnar). If the ulnar artery is blocked, the radial artery readily provides adequate collateral blood supply so that the whole hand remains viable. The same outcome normally occurs if the radial artery is blocked. This collateral supply is only effective if the arches are intact and competent. One may test that competency by asking the patient to empty the hand of blood by making a tight fist. Before the patient opens the hand, the examiner compresses both the radial and ulnar arteries at the wrist. When the hand is opened, it will be blanched white. By releasing only the ulnar artery one can see the extent to which the flush of color returns to the thumb and index finger. The vascular arch system is competent if all of the fingers and hand have prompt return of color. The test may be repeated releasing only the radial artery (Allen's test).*

See DISSECTIONS, Section 3, p. 11
See PRINCIPLES, Fig. 3-44

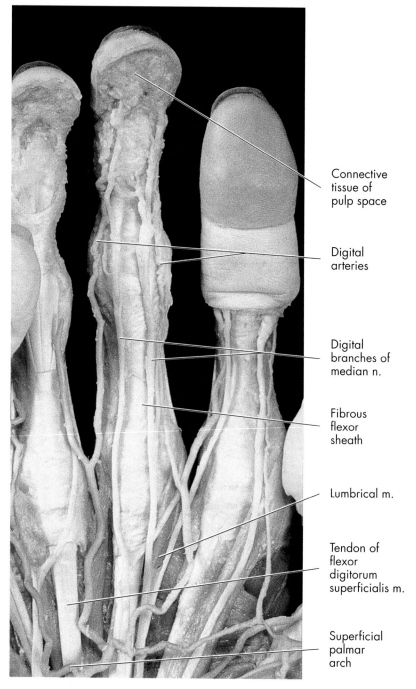

Connective
tissue of
pulp space

Digital
arteries

Digital
branches of
median n.

Fibrous
flexor
sheath

Lumbrical m.

Tendon of
flexor
digitorum
superficialis m.

Superficial
palmar
arch

Figure 3-59   Palmar digital vessels and nerves of the fingers.

See DISSECTIONS, Section 3, p. 11
See PRINCIPLES, Fig. 3-44

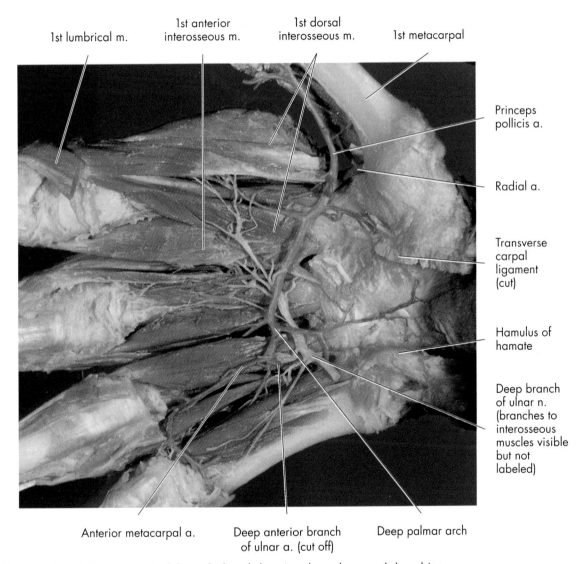

1st lumbrical m.

1st anterior
interosseous m.

1st dorsal
interosseous m.

1st metacarpal

Princeps
pollicis a.

Radial a.

Transverse
carpal
ligament
(cut)

Hamulus of
hamate

Deep branch
of ulnar n.
(branches to
interosseous
muscles visible
but not
labeled)

Anterior metacarpal a.

Deep anterior branch
of ulnar a. (cut off)

Deep palmar arch

Figure 3-60   Palmar aspect of the right hand showing the palmar and dorsal interosseous
muscles. The adductor pollicis muscle has been removed. The first dorsal interosseous
muscle has been detached from its origin on the first metacarpal bone.

See PRINCIPLES, FIG. 3-16

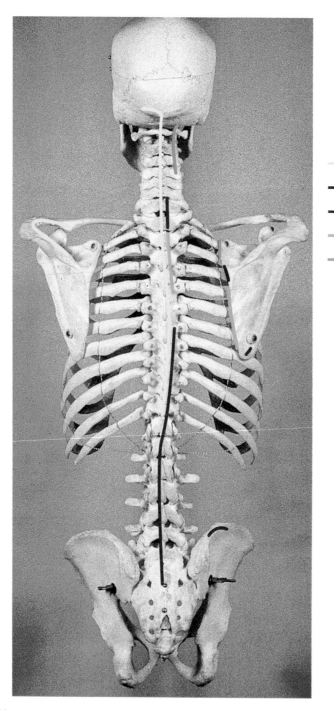

Trapezius m.
Rhomboid minor m.
Latissimus dorsi m.
Rhomboid major m.
Levator scapulae m.

Figure 3-61 Attachments of the trapezius, rhomboid major and minor, levator scapulae, and latissimus dorsi muscles. Latissimus dorsi inserts on the humerus, but, as it passes the inferior angle of the scapula, it may pick up minor attachments.

SEE DISSECTIONS, SECTION 4, P. 2
SEE PRINCIPLES, FIG. 3-16

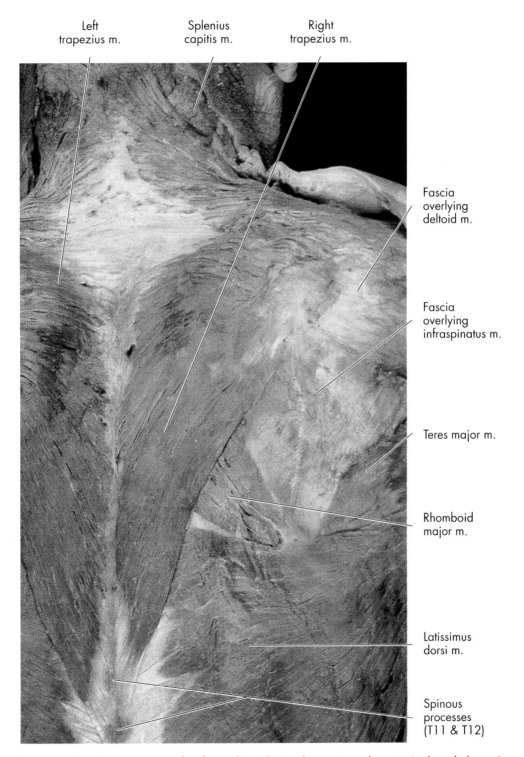

Left
trapezius m.

Splenius
capitis m.

Right
trapezius m.

Fascia
overlying
deltoid m.

Fascia
overlying
infraspinatus m.

Teres major m.

Rhomboid
major m.

Latissimus
dorsi m.

Spinous
processes
(T11 & T12)

Figure 3-62   Trapezius muscles have fascial attachments to the cervical and thoracic spinous processes and, in this dissection, are asymmetric inferiorly.

See DISSECTIONS, Section 4, p. 3
See PRINCIPLES, Fig. 3-16

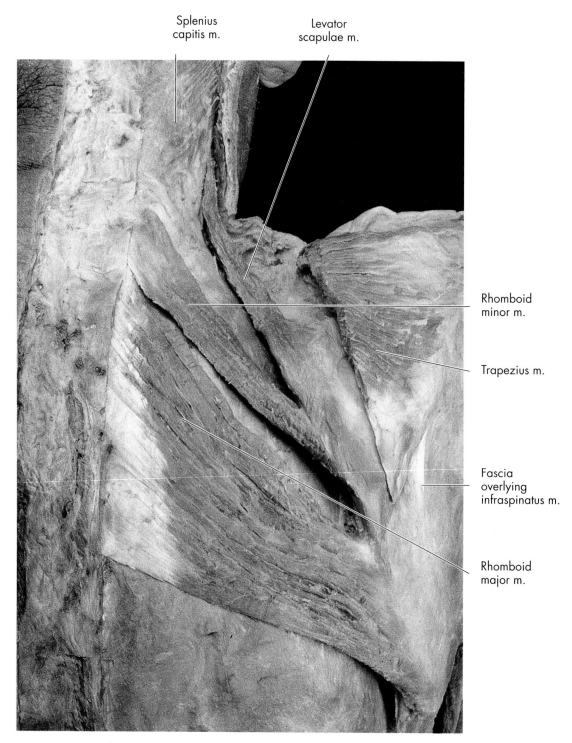

Splenius capitis m.

Levator scapulae m.

Rhomboid minor m.

Trapezius m.

Fascia overlying infraspinatus m.

Rhomboid major m.

Figure 3-63 Levator scapulae and rhomboid muscles exposed by removal of the trapezius.

See DISSECTIONS, Section 4, p. 2
See PRINCIPLES, Fig. 3-16

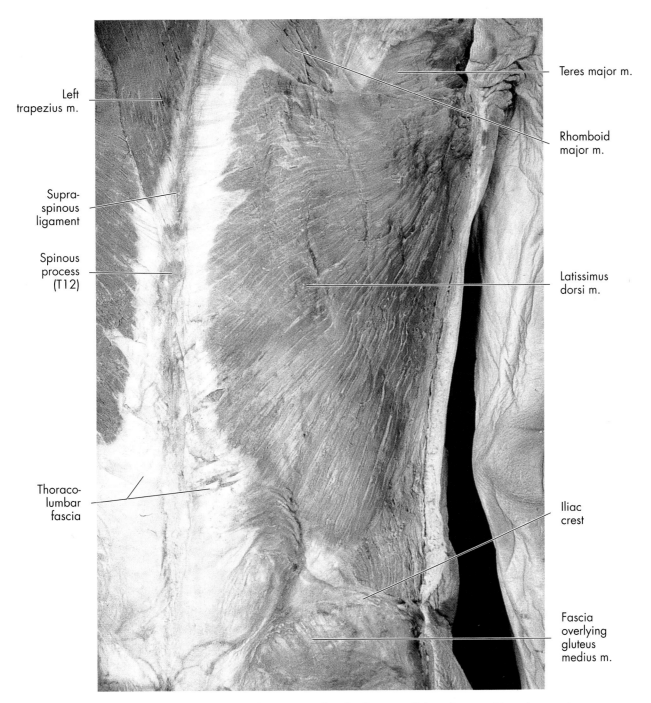

Left
trapezius m.

Supra-
spinous
ligament

Spinous
process
(T12)

Thoraco-
lumbar
fascia

Teres major m.

Rhomboid
major m.

Latissimus
dorsi m.

Iliac
crest

Fascia
overlying
gluteus
medius m.

Figure 3-64   Latissimus dorsi. The anterior border lies parallel to the cut skin edge, and the thoracic attachment has been exposed by removal of the trapezius.

SEE PRINCIPLES, FIGS. 3-3, 3-6

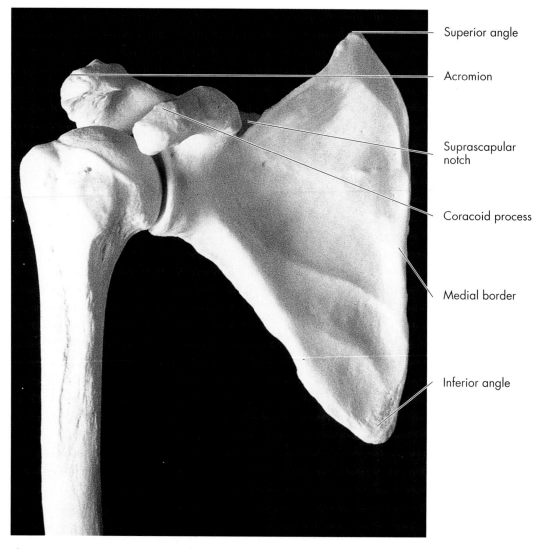

Superior angle

Acromion

Suprascapular notch

Coracoid process

Medial border

Inferior angle

Figure 3-65   Anterior aspects of the scapula with its subscapularis fossa and the proximal end of the humerus. The head of the humerus is partly obscured by the overlying coracoid process of the scapula.

See **DISSECTIONS**, Section 3, p. 2

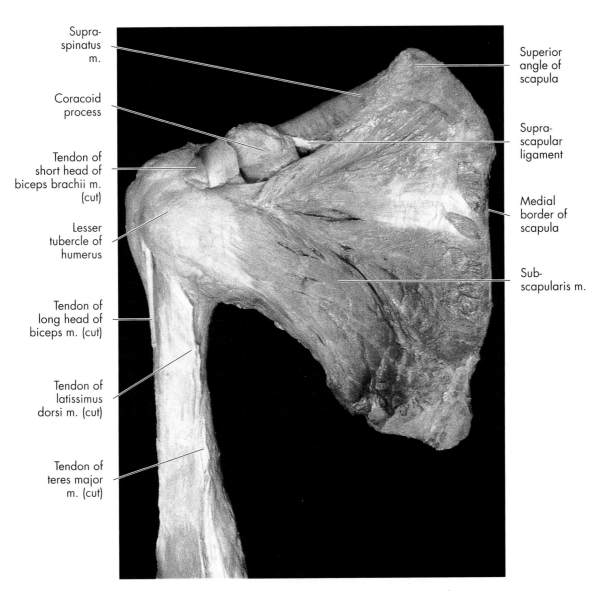

Supra-spinatus m.

Coracoid process

Tendon of short head of biceps brachii m. (cut)

Lesser tubercle of humerus

Tendon of long head of biceps m. (cut)

Tendon of latissimus dorsi m. (cut)

Tendon of teres major m. (cut)

Superior angle of scapula

Supra-scapular ligament

Medial border of scapula

Sub-scapularis m.

Figure 3-66 Anterior view of the subscapularis. The attachment of serratus anterior to the medial border of the scapula has been excised.

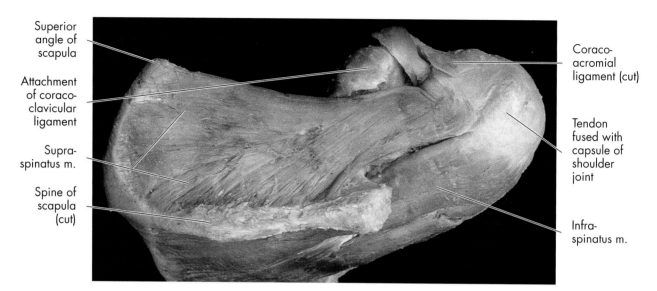

Superior angle of scapula

Attachment of coraco-clavicular ligament

Supra-spinatus m.

Spine of scapula (cut)

Coraco-acromial ligament (cut)

Tendon fused with capsule of shoulder joint

Infra-spinatus m.

Figure 3-67 Superior view of supraspinatus after removal of the acromion of the scapula.

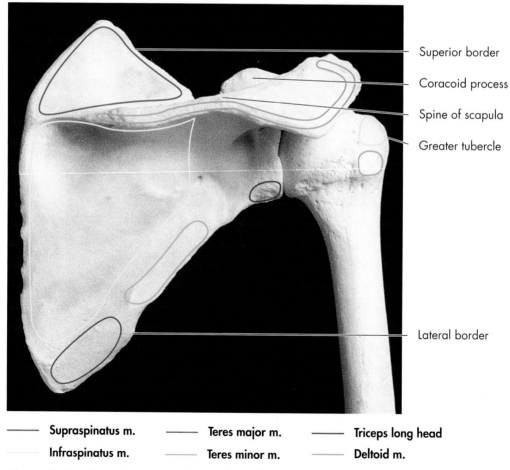

Superior border

Coracoid process

Spine of scapula

Greater tubercle

Lateral border

—— **Supraspinatus m.** —— **Teres major m.** —— **Triceps long head**

—— **Infraspinatus m.** —— **Teres minor m.** —— **Deltoid m.**

Figure 3-68 Posterior aspects of scapula and proximal end of humerus. The head of the humerus is partly obscured by the overlying acromion of the scapula.

See DISSECTIONS, Section 3, p. 2
See PRINCIPLES, Fig. 3-22

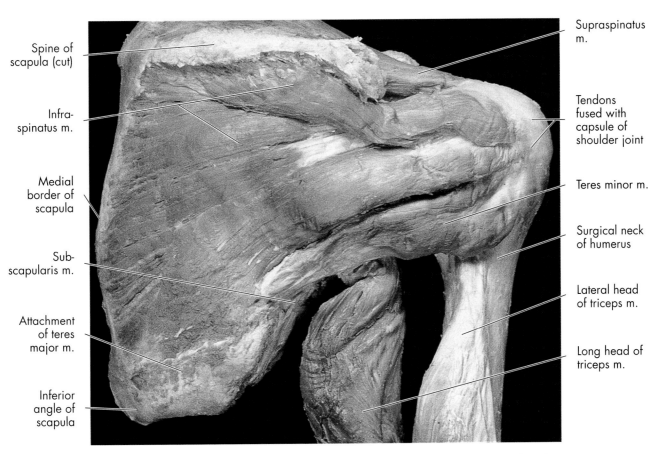

Spine of
scapula (cut)

Infra-
spinatus m.

Medial
border of
scapula

Sub-
scapularis m.

Attachment
of teres
major m.

Inferior
angle of
scapula

Supraspinatus
m.

Tendons
fused with
capsule of
shoulder joint

Teres minor m.

Surgical neck
of humerus

Lateral head
of triceps m.

Long head of
triceps m.

Figure 3-69   Posterior view of infraspinatus and teres minor. Teres major has been removed.

SEE **DISSECTIONS**, SECTION 3, P. 2

SEE **PRINCIPLES**, FIG. 3-22

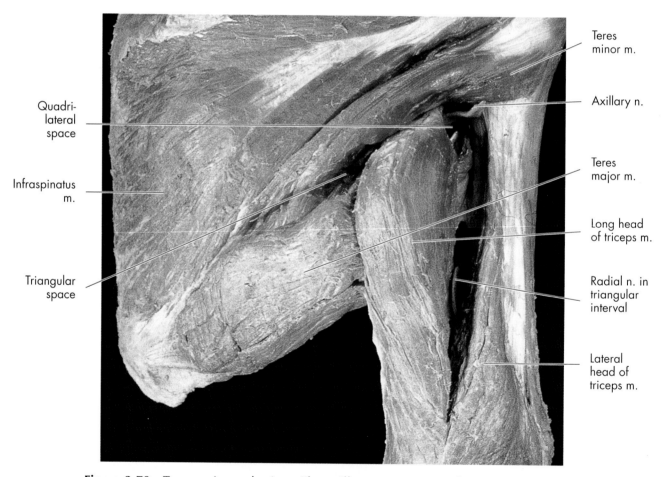

Quadri-
lateral
space

Infraspinatus
m.

Triangular
space

Teres
minor m.

Axillary n.

Teres
major m.

Long head
of triceps m.

Radial n. in
triangular
interval

Lateral
head of
triceps m.

Figure 3-70   Teres major and minor. The axillary nerve passes above the teres major while the radial nerve lies below the muscle. Both nerves pass medial to the long head of the triceps.

SEE DISSECTIONS, SECTION 3, PP. 2 AND 6

SEE PRINCIPLES, FIG. 3-22

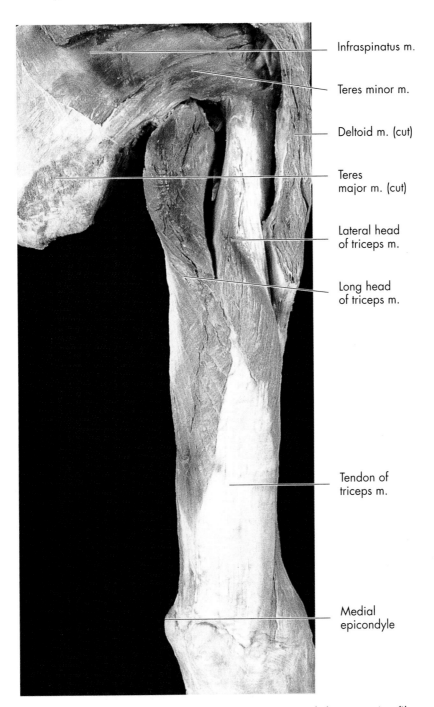

Infraspinatus m.

Teres minor m.

Deltoid m. (cut)

Teres
major m. (cut)

Lateral head
of triceps m.

Long head
of triceps m.

Tendon of
triceps m.

Medial
epicondyle

Figure 3-71 Posterior aspect of the triceps. Teres major and the posterior fibers of the deltoid have been excised.

See DISSECTIONS, Section 3, pp. 2 and 6

See PRINCIPLES, Fig. 3-27

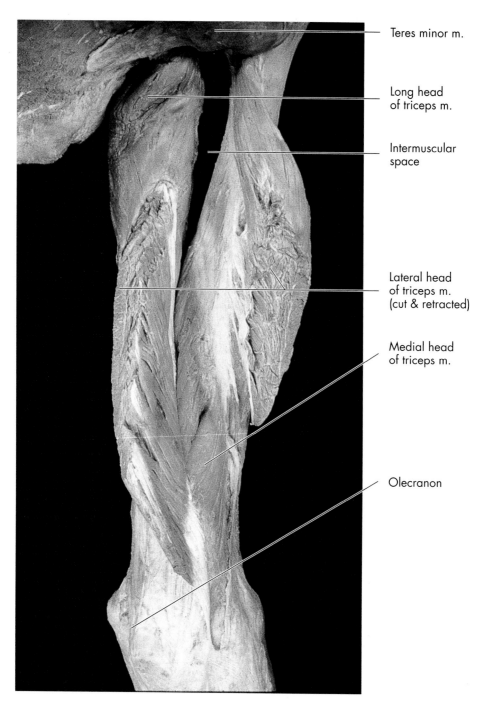

Teres minor m.

Long head
of triceps m.

Intermuscular
space

Lateral head
of triceps m.
(cut & retracted)

Medial head
of triceps m.

Olecranon

Figure 3-72   Medial head of the triceps has been exposed by removal of the deltoid muscle and division and retraction of the lateral head of the triceps.

See PRINCIPLES, Fig. 3-9

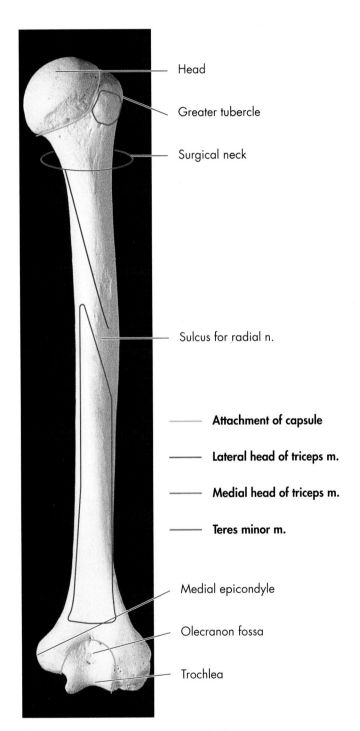

Head

Greater tubercle

Surgical neck

Sulcus for radial n.

Attachment of capsule

Lateral head of triceps m.

Medial head of triceps m.

Teres minor m.

Medial epicondyle

Olecranon fossa

Trochlea

Figure 3-73   Posterior aspect of the humerus.

SEE DISSECTIONS, SECTION 3, P. 6

SEE PRINCIPLES, FIG. 3-27

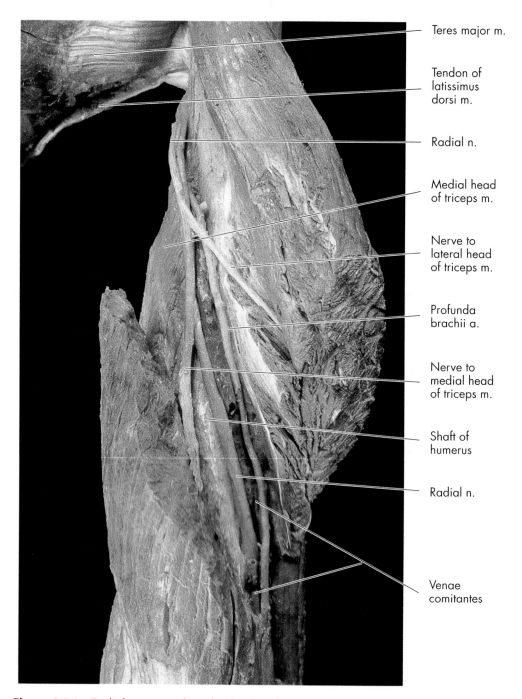

Teres major m.

Tendon of latissimus dorsi m.

Radial n.

Medial head of triceps m.

Nerve to lateral head of triceps m.

Profunda brachii a.

Nerve to medial head of triceps m.

Shaft of humerus

Radial n.

Venae comitantes

Figure 3-74   Radial nerve and profundus brachii artery in the spiral groove, seen after retraction of the cut lateral head of the triceps. The long head has been excised.

See **DISSECTIONS, Section 3, p. 8**
See **PRINCIPLES, Fig. 3-55**

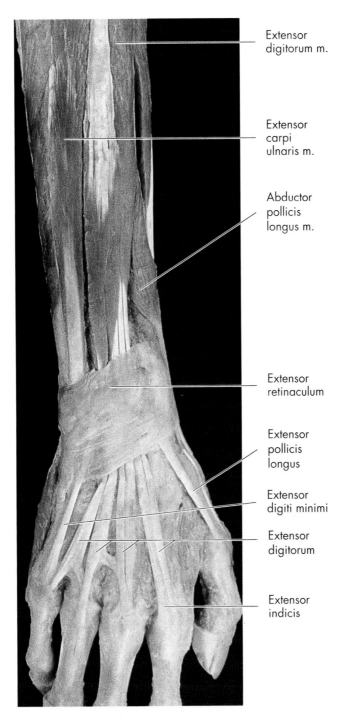

Extensor
digitorum m.

Extensor
carpi
ulnaris m.

Abductor
pollicis
longus m.

Extensor
retinaculum

Extensor
pollicis
longus

Extensor
digiti minimi

Extensor
digitorum

Extensor
indicis

Figure 3-75   Extensor retinaculum exposed by removal of superficial and deep fascia. The fibers of the retinaculum run obliquely, passing medially and inferiorly from the radius toward the hamate and pisiform bones.

See **DISSECTIONS**, Section 3, p. 8

See **PRINCIPLES**, Fig. 3-41

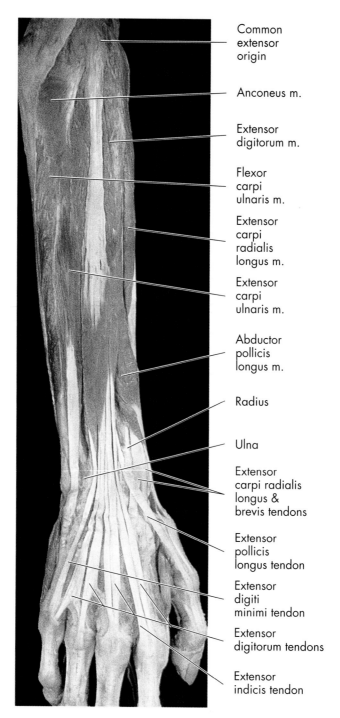

Common
extensor
origin

Anconeus m.

Extensor
digitorum m.

Flexor
carpi
ulnaris m.

Extensor
carpi
radialis
longus m.

Extensor
carpi
ulnaris m.

Abductor
pollicis
longus m.

Radius

Ulna

Extensor
carpi radialis
longus &
brevis tendons

Extensor
pollicis
longus tendon

Extensor
digiti
minimi tendon

Extensor
digitorum tendons

Extensor
indicis tendon

Figure 3-76   Superficial muscles of the posterior compartment exposed by removal of deep fascia and the extensor retinaculum. The flexor and extensor carpi ulnaris lie edge-to-edge along the subcutaneous border of the ulna.

See **DISSECTIONS**, Section 3, p. 8
See **PRINCIPLES**, Fig. 3-41

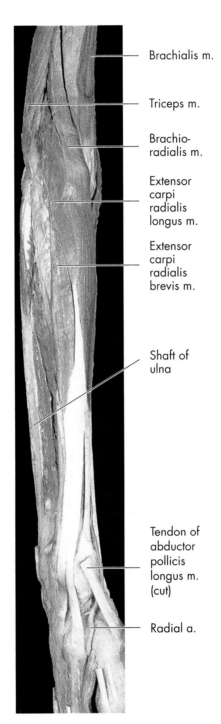

Brachialis m.

Triceps m.

Brachio-
radialis m.

Extensor
carpi
radialis
longus m.

Extensor
carpi
radialis
brevis m.

Shaft of
ulna

Tendon of
abductor
pollicis
longus m.
(cut)

Radial a.

Figure 3-77   Extensor carpi radialis longus and brevis and brachioradialis after removal of abductor pollicis longus and extensor pollicis longus and brevis.

SEE **DISSECTIONS**, SECTION 3, P. 8
SEE **PRINCIPLES**, FIG. 3-41

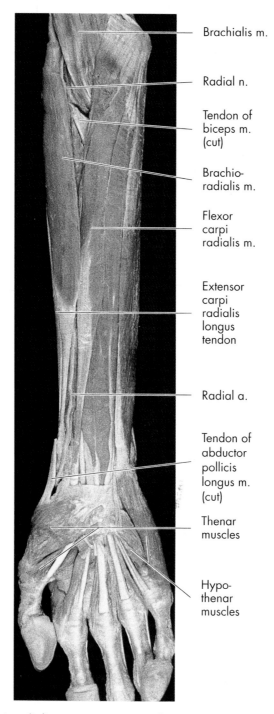

Brachialis m.

Radial n.

Tendon of
biceps m.
(cut)

Brachio-
radialis m.

Flexor
carpi
radialis m.

Extensor
carpi
radialis
longus
tendon

Radial a.

Tendon of
abductor
pollicis
longus m.
(cut)

Thenar
muscles

Hypo-
thenar
muscles

Figure 3-78   Brachioradialis, anterior aspect. The muscle forms the lateral boundary of the cubital fossa and covers the radial artery and the superficial branch of the radial nerve in the forearm.

See **PRINCIPLES,** Fig. **3-42**

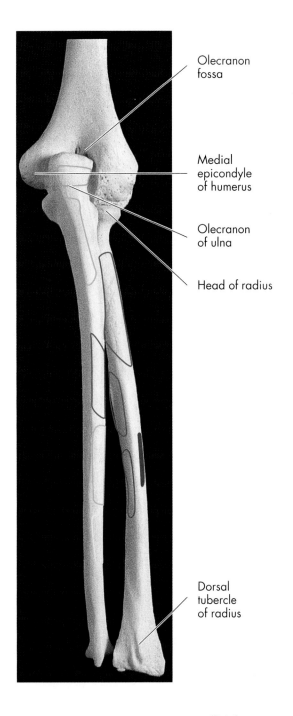

Olecranon
fossa

Medial
epicondyle
of humerus

Olecranon
of ulna

Head of radius

Dorsal
tubercle
of radius

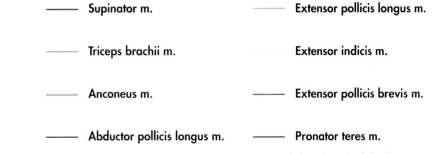

——— Supinator m.   ——— Extensor pollicis longus m.

——— Triceps brachii m.   ——— Extensor indicis m.

——— Anconeus m.   ——— Extensor pollicis brevis m.

——— Abductor pollicis longus m.   ——— Pronator teres m.

Figure 3-79   Posterior aspects of the radius, ulna, and distal end of the humerus.

See DISSECTIONS, Section 3, p. 8
See PRINCIPLES, Fig. 3-42

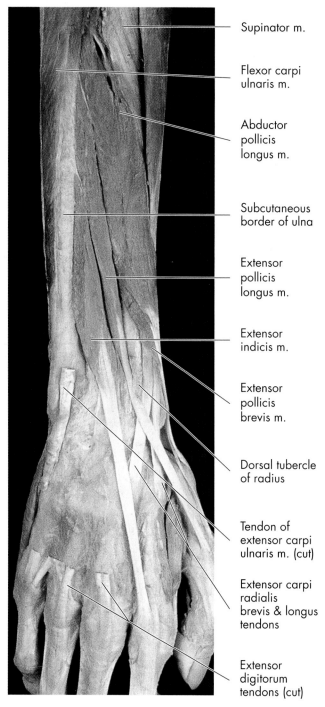

Supinator m.

Flexor carpi ulnaris m.

Abductor pollicis longus m.

Subcutaneous border of ulna

Extensor pollicis longus m.

Extensor indicis m.

Extensor pollicis brevis m.

Dorsal tubercle of radius

Tendon of extensor carpi ulnaris m. (cut)

Extensor carpi radialis brevis & longus tendons

Extensor digitorum tendons (cut)

Figure 3-80 Extensor indicis and extensor pollicis longus and brevis after division of extensor digitorum. The tendon of extensor indicis lies on the ulnar (medial) side of the index tendon of extensor digitorum.

See **DISSECTIONS**, Section 3, p. 8

See **PRINCIPLES**, p. 3-66

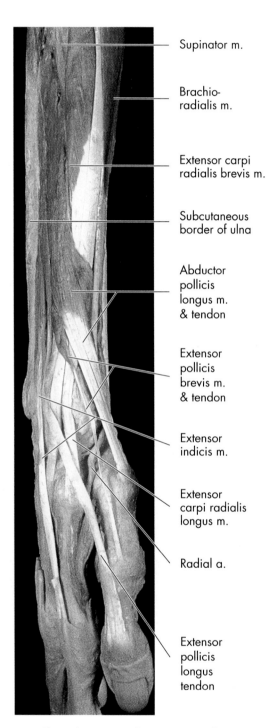

Supinator m.

Brachio-
radialis m.

Extensor carpi
radialis brevis m.

Subcutaneous
border of ulna

Abductor
pollicis
longus m.
& tendon

Extensor
pollicis
brevis m.
& tendon

Extensor
indicis m.

Extensor
carpi radialis
longus m.

Radial a.

Extensor
pollicis
longus
tendon

Figure 3-81 Abductor pollicis longus and extensor pollicis longus and brevis. At the wrist, the radial carpal extensors are crossed by the tendons of these three muscles passing to the thumb.

SEE DISSECTIONS, SECTION 3, P. 9
SEE PRINCIPLES, FIG. 3-46

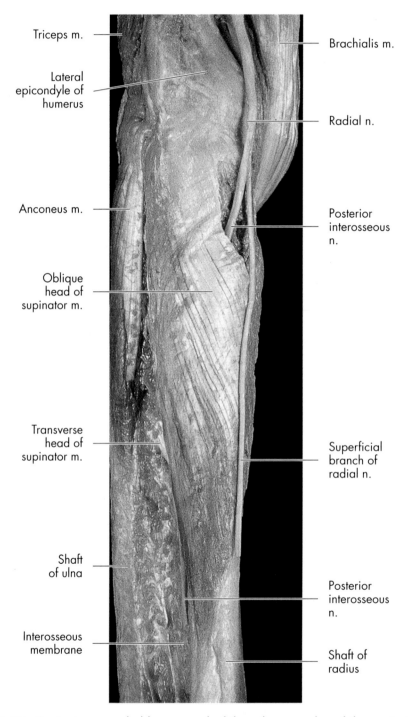

Triceps m.

Lateral epicondyle of humerus

Anconeus m.

Oblique head of supinator m.

Transverse head of supinator m.

Shaft of ulna

Interosseous membrane

Brachialis m.

Radial n.

Posterior interosseous n.

Superficial branch of radial n.

Posterior interosseous n.

Shaft of radius

Figure 3-82   Supinator, revealed by removal of the other muscles of the posterior compartment. The posterior interosseous nerve may become compressed when it passes between the transverse and oblique heads of the supinator muscle.

See **DISSECTIONS**, **Section 3**, **p. 9**
See **PRINCIPLES**, **Fig. 3-46**

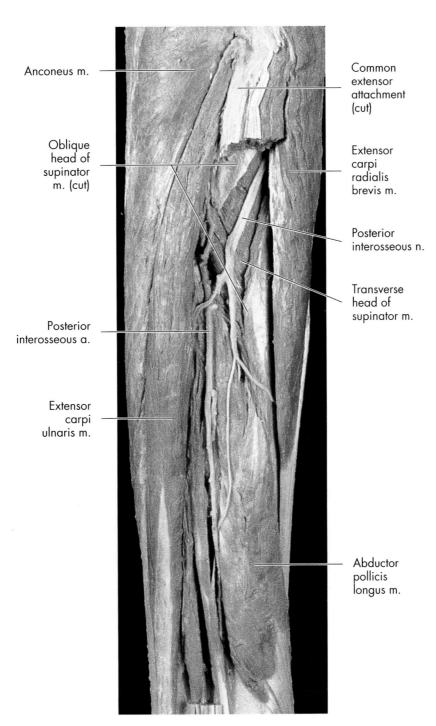

Anconeus m.

Common extensor attachment (cut)

Oblique head of supinator m. (cut)

Extensor carpi radialis brevis m.

Posterior interosseous n.

Transverse head of supinator m.

Posterior interosseous a.

Extensor carpi ulnaris m.

Abductor pollicis longus m.

Figure 3-83   Posterior interosseous artery and nerve exposed by division of the extensor digitorum and the oblique head of the supinator. The specimen is partly pronated so the radial border of the forearm faces anteriorly.

See Dissections, Section 3, p. 9

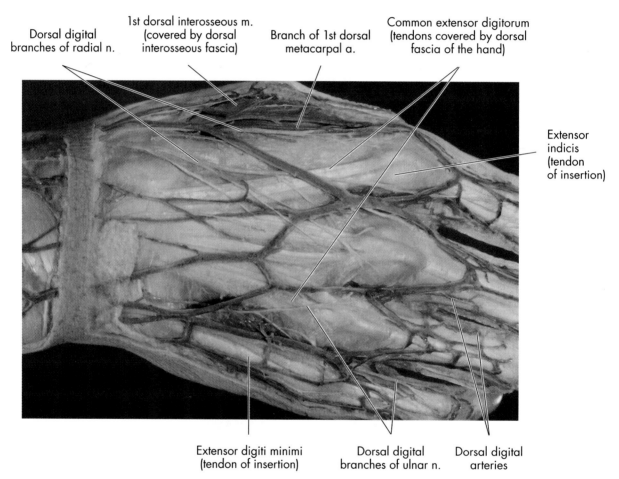

Dorsal digital
branches of radial n.

1st dorsal interosseous m.
(covered by dorsal
interosseous fascia)

Branch of 1st dorsal
metacarpal a.

Common extensor digitorum
(tendons covered by dorsal
fascia of the hand)

Extensor
indicis
(tendon
of insertion)

Extensor digiti minimi
(tendon of insertion)

Dorsal digital
branches of ulnar n.

Dorsal digital
arteries

Figure 3-84	Posterior aspect of the hand showing superficial nerves and vessels. Note the prominent network of superficial veins.

SEE DISSECTIONS, SECTION 3, P. 9

SEE PRINCIPLES, FIG. 3-48

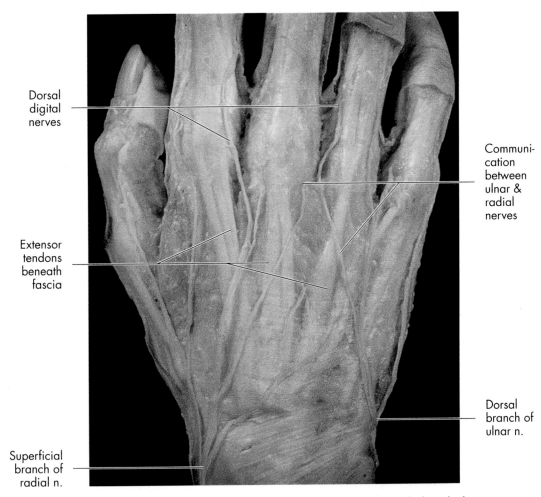

Dorsal digital nerves

Communi-cation between ulnar & radial nerves

Extensor tendons beneath fascia

Dorsal branch of ulnar n.

Superficial branch of radial n.

Figure 3-85   Cutaneous branches of the dorsal branches of the radial and ulnar nerves on the dorsum of the hand after removal of the superficial veins.

See DISSECTIONS, Section 3, p. 9
See PRINCIPLES, Fig. 3-55

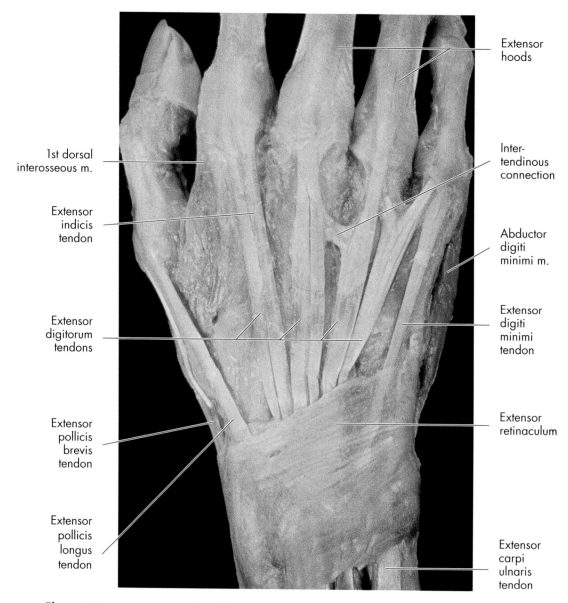

Extensor
hoods

Inter-
tendinous
connection

1st dorsal
interosseous m.

Abductor
digiti
minimi m.

Extensor
indicis
tendon

Extensor
digitorum
tendons

Extensor
digiti
minimi
tendon

Extensor
pollicis
brevis
tendon

Extensor
retinaculum

Extensor
pollicis
longus
tendon

Extensor
carpi
ulnaris
tendon

Figure 3-86   Extensor retinaculum and extensor tendons exposed by removal of the
superficial fascia. The tendons pass through fibro-osseous tunnels deep to the retinaculum and are enveloped by synovial sheaths (*here removed*) that continue beyond the
edges of the retinaculum.

See DISSECTIONS, Section 1, p. 9
See PRINCIPLES, Fig. 3-13

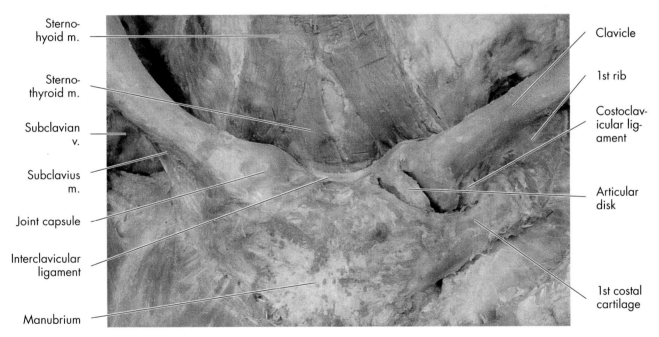

Sterno-
hyoid m.

Sterno-
thyroid m.

Subclavian
v.

Subclavius
m.

Joint capsule

Interclavicular
ligament

Manubrium

Clavicle

1st rib

Costoclav-
icular lig-
ament

Articular
disk

1st costal
cartilage

Figure 3-87   Sternoclavicular joints after removal of the sternocleidomastoid muscles. On the left, the joint capsule and subclavius have been excised to reveal the cartilaginous disk and costoclavicular ligament. Pleura is exposed in the first left intercostal space.

See PRINCIPLES, Fig. 3-8

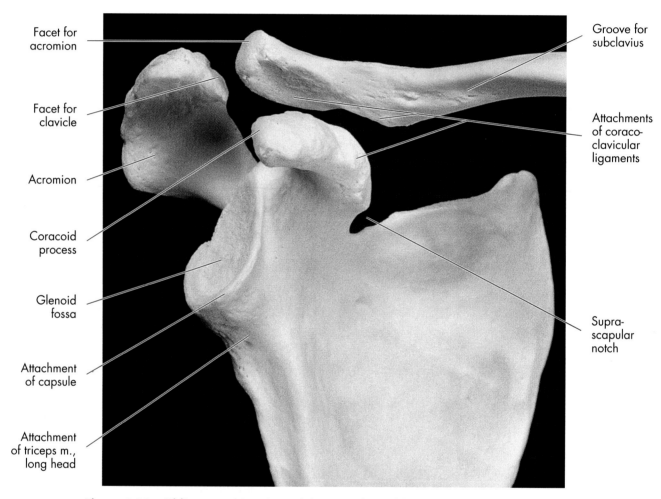

Facet for
acromion

Facet for
clavicle

Acromion

Coracoid
process

Glenoid
fossa

Attachment
of capsule

Attachment
of triceps m.,
long head

Groove for
subclavius

Attachments
of coraco-
clavicular
ligaments

Supra-
scapular
notch

Figure 3-88   Oblique anterior view of the scapula and lateral part of the clavicle. The bones have been separated to show the articular surfaces of the acromioclavicular joint and the sites of attachment of the coracoclavicular ligament.

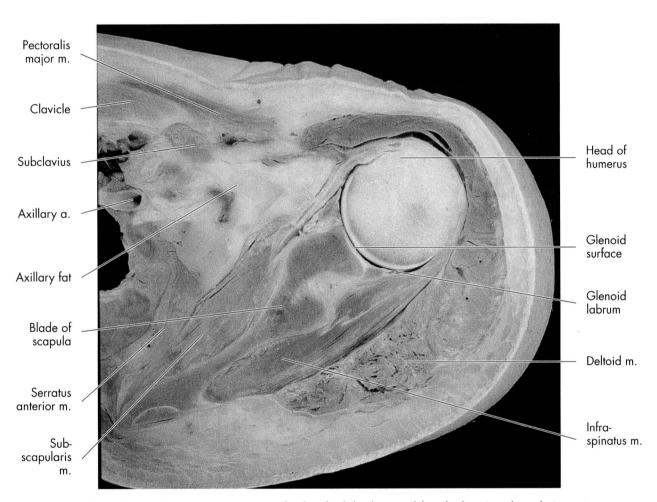

Pectoralis
major m.

Clavicle

Subclavius

Axillary a.

Axillary fat

Blade of
scapula

Serratus
anterior m.

Sub-
scapularis
m.

Head of
humerus

Glenoid
surface

Glenoid
labrum

Deltoid m.

Infra-
spinatus m.

Figure 3-89   Transverse section at the level of the humeral head, showing the relationships of the shoulder joint.

SEE DISSECTIONS, SECTION 3, P. 3
SEE PRINCIPLES, FIG. 3-10

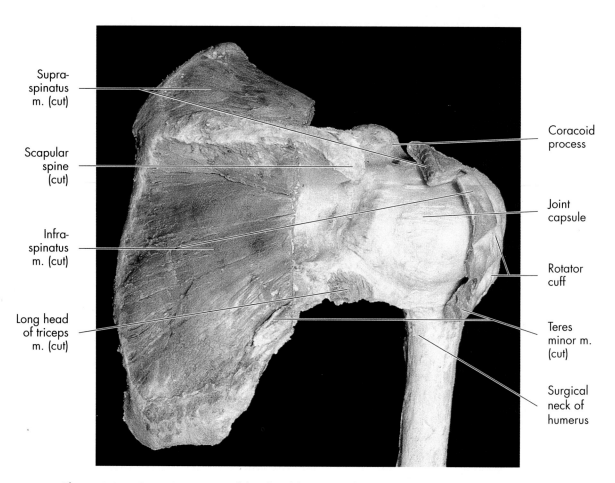

Figure 3-90   Posterior aspect of the shoulder joint. The acromion and parts of the rotator cuff muscles have been excised to reveal the joint capsule.

SEE **DISSECTIONS**, SECTION 3, P. 5
SEE **PRINCIPLES**, FIG. 3-11

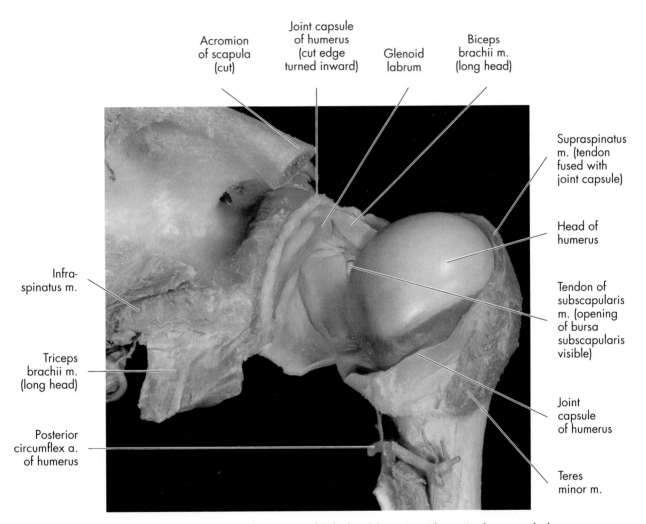

Acromion of scapula (cut)

Joint capsule of humerus (cut edge turned inward)

Glenoid labrum

Biceps brachii m. (long head)

Supraspinatus m. (tendon fused with joint capsule)

Head of humerus

Tendon of subscapularis m. (opening of bursa subscapularis visible)

Joint capsule of humerus

Teres minor m.

Infra-spinatus m.

Triceps brachii m. (long head)

Posterior circumflex a. of humerus

Figure 3-91   Posterior view of the cavity of left shoulder joint. The articular capsule has been incised vertically and the humerus retracted laterally. The head of the humerus has been rotated posteriorly.

SEE PRINCIPLES, FIG. 3-6

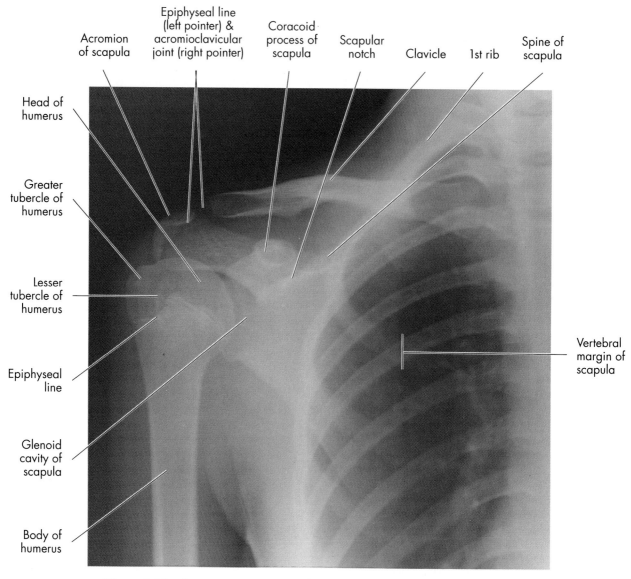

Acromion of scapula

Epiphyseal line (left pointer) & acromioclavicular joint (right pointer)

Coracoid process of scapula

Scapular notch

Clavicle

1st rib

Spine of scapula

Head of humerus

Greater tubercle of humerus

Lesser tubercle of humerus

Epiphyseal line

Glenoid cavity of scapula

Body of humerus

Vertebral margin of scapula

Figure 3-92 Anteroposterior x-ray of the right shoulder of a 16-year-old-girl.

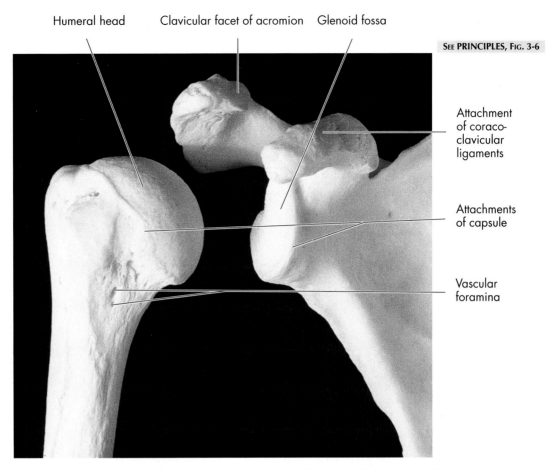

Humeral head   Clavicular facet of acromion   Glenoid fossa

Attachment
of coraco-
clavicular
ligaments

Attachments
of capsule

Vascular
foramina

Figure 3-93 Bones that form the shoulder joint separated to reveal their articular surfaces.

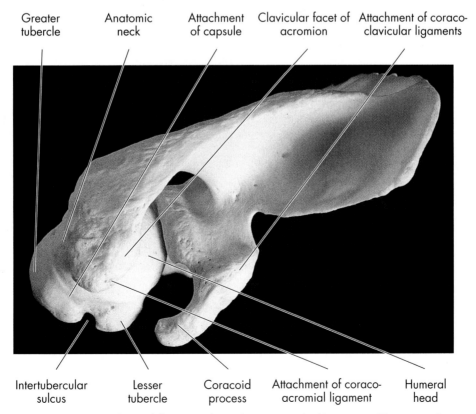

Greater
tubercle   Anatomic
neck   Attachment
of capsule   Clavicular facet of
acromion   Attachment of coraco-
clavicular ligaments

Intertubercular
sulcus   Lesser
tubercle   Coracoid
process   Attachment of coraco-
acromial ligament   Humeral
head

Figure 3-94 Superior view of the scapula and upper end of humerus. The acromion and coracoacromial ligament prevent upward displacement of the humeral head.

SEE PRINCIPLES, FIG. 3-5

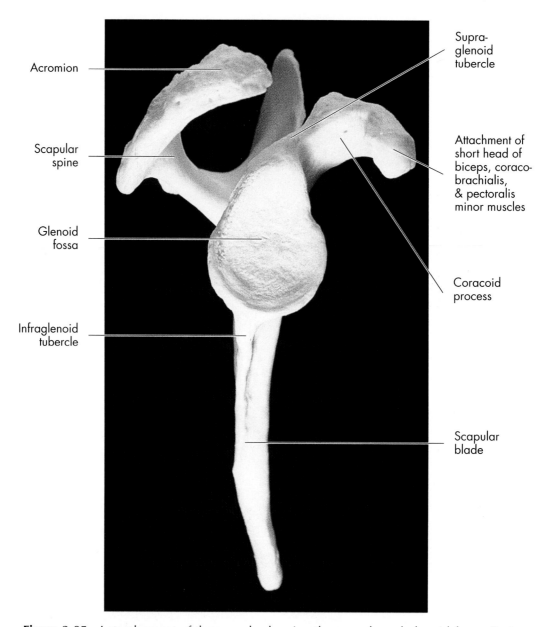

Acromion

Scapular
spine

Glenoid
fossa

Infraglenoid
tubercle

Supra-
glenoid
tubercle

Attachment of
short head of
biceps, coraco-
brachialis,
& pectoralis
minor muscles

Coracoid
process

Scapular
blade

Figure 3-95   Lateral aspect of the scapula showing the pear-shaped glenoid fossa. Positions of the supraspinous, infraspinous, and subscapular fossae can be appreciated.

See **DISSECTIONS**, Section 3, p. 5
See **PRINCIPLES**, Fig. 3-7

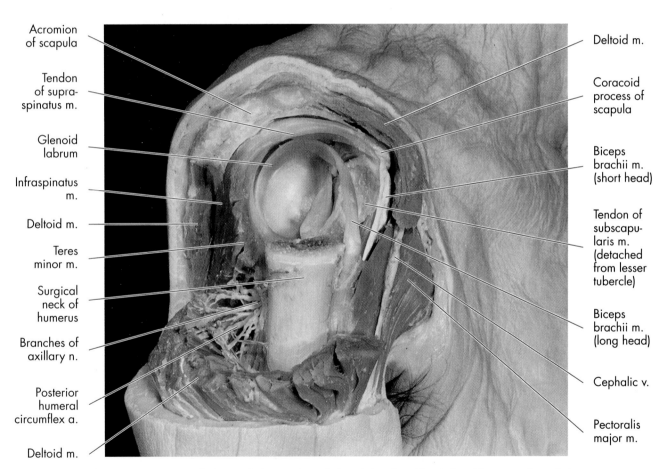

Acromion of scapula

Tendon of supraspinatus m.

Glenoid labrum

Infraspinatus m.

Deltoid m.

Teres minor m.

Surgical neck of humerus

Branches of axillary n.

Posterior humeral circumflex a.

Deltoid m.

Deltoid m.

Coracoid process of scapula

Biceps brachii m. (short head)

Tendon of subscapularis m. (detached from lesser tubercle)

Biceps brachii m. (long head)

Cephalic v.

Pectoralis major m.

Figure 3-96 Lateral view of the cavity of the right shoulder joint. The muscles of the shoulder have been resected, and the lateral part of the joint capsule has been cut away. The upper part of the humerus has been removed.

See DISSECTIONS, Section 3, p. 5
See PRINCIPLES, Fig. 3-7

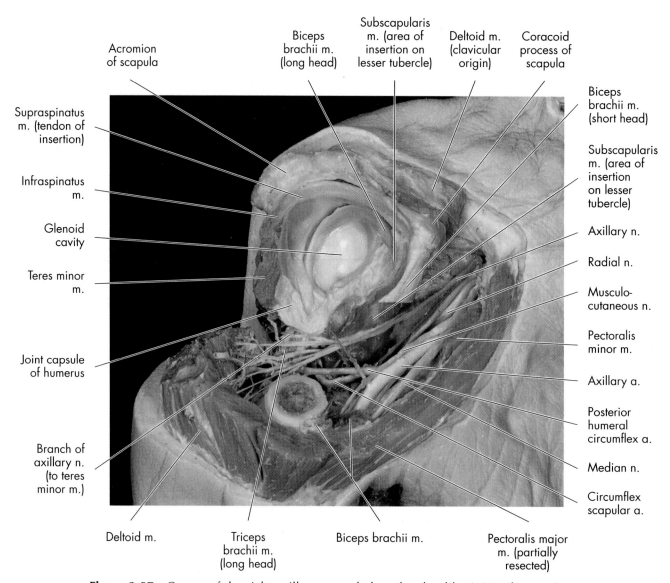

Acromion of scapula

Biceps brachii m. (long head)

Subscapularis m. (area of insertion on lesser tubercle)

Deltoid m. (clavicular origin)

Coracoid process of scapula

Supraspinatus m. (tendon of insertion)

Infraspinatus m.

Glenoid cavity

Teres minor m.

Joint capsule of humerus

Branch of axillary n. (to teres minor m.)

Biceps brachii m. (short head)

Subscapularis m. (area of insertion on lesser tubercle)

Axillary n.

Radial n.

Musculo-cutaneous n.

Pectoralis minor m.

Axillary a.

Posterior humeral circumflex a.

Median n.

Circumflex scapular a.

Deltoid m.

Triceps brachii m. (long head)

Biceps brachii m.

Pectoralis major m. (partially resected)

Figure 3-97   Course of the right axillary nerve below the shoulder joint. The specimen shown in Figure 3-96 has been dissected to illustrate the relationships of the axillary nerve. *The shallow glenoid fossa makes the shoulder joint subject to dislocation. The weak inferior capsule makes inferior dislocation common, thereby jeopardizing the axillary nerve that passes close to the joint capsule. Examination of the axillary nerve in a patient with a dislocated shoulder should include evaluation of voluntary contraction of the deltoid muscle and a check for sensory loss over the lateral aspect of the shoulder in the deltoid region before reduction of the dislocation is carried out.*

SEE **PRINCIPLES**, FIG. 3-31

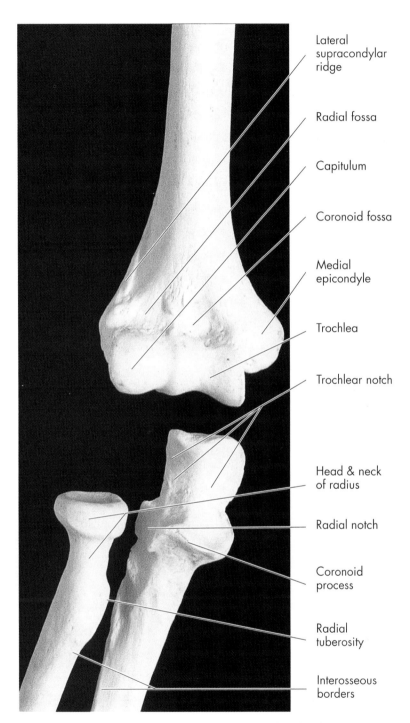

Lateral supracondylar ridge

Radial fossa

Capitulum

Coronoid fossa

Medial epicondyle

Trochlea

Trochlear notch

Head & neck of radius

Radial notch

Coronoid process

Radial tuberosity

Interosseous borders

Figure 3-98 Bones that form the elbow and proximal radioulnar joints separated to reveal their articular surfaces.

SEE **DISSECTIONS, SECTION** 3, p. 9
SEE **PRINCIPLES, FIG.** 3-31

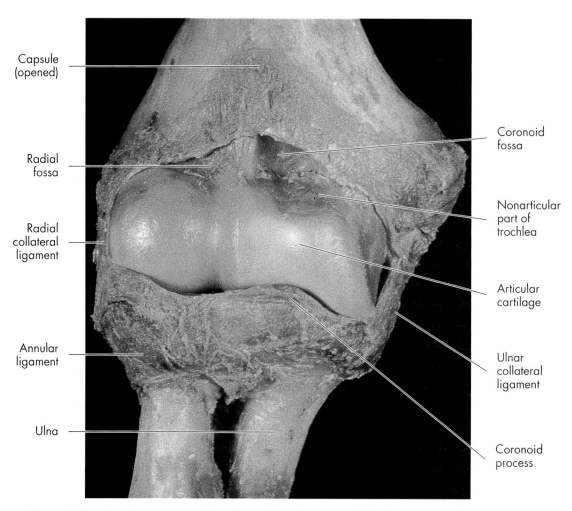

Capsule
(opened)

Radial
fossa

Radial
collateral
ligament

Annular
ligament

Ulna

Coronoid
fossa

Nonarticular
part of
trochlea

Articular
cartilage

Ulnar
collateral
ligament

Coronoid
process

Figure 3-99   Anterior aspect of the elbow joint. The capsule has been opened to expose
the interior of the joint.

See **DISSECTIONS**, Section 3, p. 9

See **PRINCIPLES**, Fig. 3-31

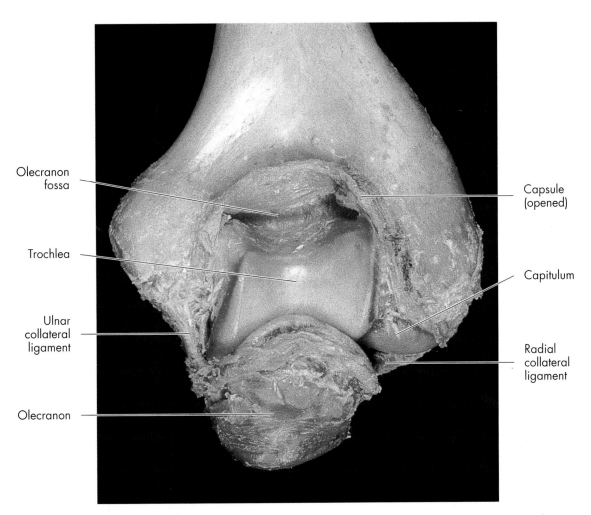

Olecranon fossa

Trochlea

Ulnar collateral ligament

Olecranon

Capsule (opened)

Capitulum

Radial collateral ligament

Figure 3-100   Posterior aspect of the flexed elbow joint. The capsule has been opened to reveal the olecranon fossa.

SEE PRINCIPLES, FIG. 3-31

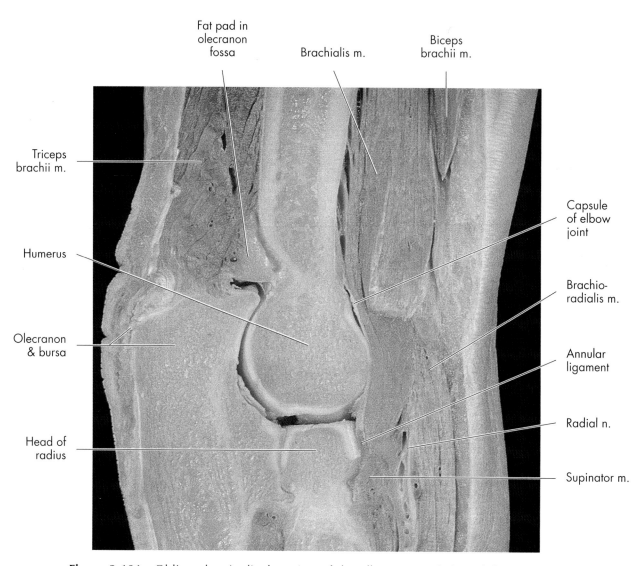

Fat pad in
olecranon
fossa

Brachialis m.

Biceps
brachii m.

Triceps
brachii m.

Humerus

Olecranon
& bursa

Head of
radius

Capsule
of elbow
joint

Brachio-
radialis m.

Annular
ligament

Radial n.

Supinator m.

Figure 3-101   Oblique longitudinal section of the elbow (extended) and the proximal radioulnar joints showing the articular surfaces and relationships of the joints.

See DISSECTIONS, Section 3, p. 9

See PRINCIPLES, Fig. 3-33

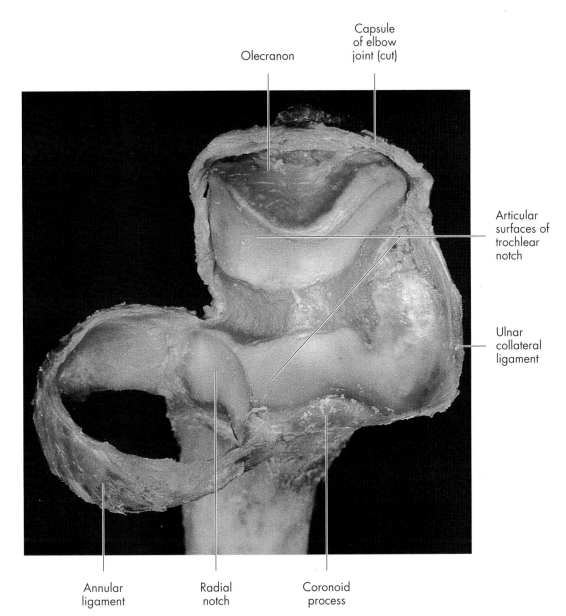

Olecranon

Capsule
of elbow
joint (cut)

Articular
surfaces of
trochlear
notch

Ulnar
collateral
ligament

Annular
ligament

Radial
notch

Coronoid
process

Figure 3-102   Anterior view of the proximal end of ulna with attached annular ligament
showing articular surfaces of the trochlear and radial notches.

See PRINCIPLES, Fig. 3-34

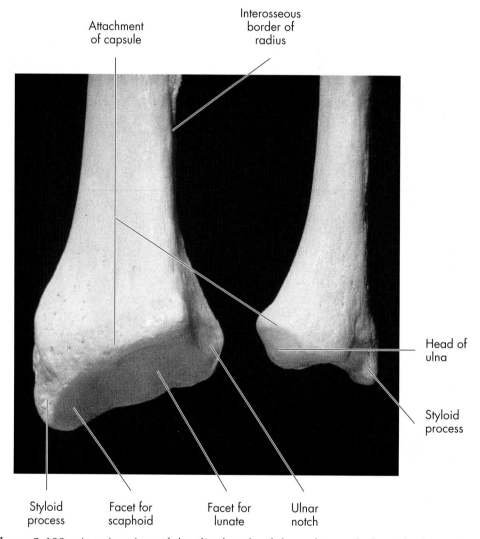

Figure 3-103   Anterior view of the distal ends of the radius and ulna. The bones have been separated to reveal the ulnar notch.

See **PRINCIPLES**, Fig. 3-53

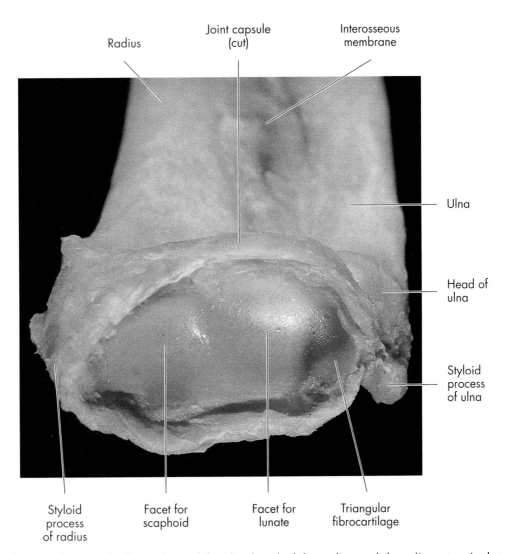

Radius

Joint capsule (cut)

Interosseous membrane

Ulna

Head of ulna

Styloid process of ulna

Styloid process of radius

Facet for scaphoid

Facet for lunate

Triangular fibrocartilage

Figure 3-104   Articular surface of the distal end of the radius and the adjacent articular disk or triangular fibrocartilage.

See PRINCIPLES, Fig. 3-49

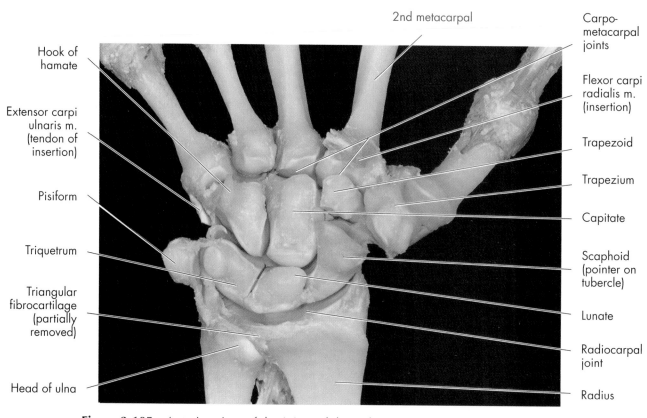

Hook of hamate

2nd metacarpal

Carpo-metacarpal joints

Extensor carpi ulnaris m. (tendon of insertion)

Flexor carpi radialis m. (insertion)

Pisiform

Trapezoid

Trapezium

Triquetrum

Capitate

Triangular fibrocartilage (partially removed)

Scaphoid (pointer on tubercle)

Lunate

Head of ulna

Radiocarpal joint

Radius

Figure 3-105 Anterior view of the joints of the right wrist and hand. The anterior ligaments have been removed and the articular capsules incised to allow the carpal and metacarpal bones to be separated. The interosseous ligaments of the bases of the metacarpals have been incised. The head of the ulna is separated from the carpals by the triangular fibrocartilage or articular disk.

See **PRINCIPLES**, Fig. 3-53

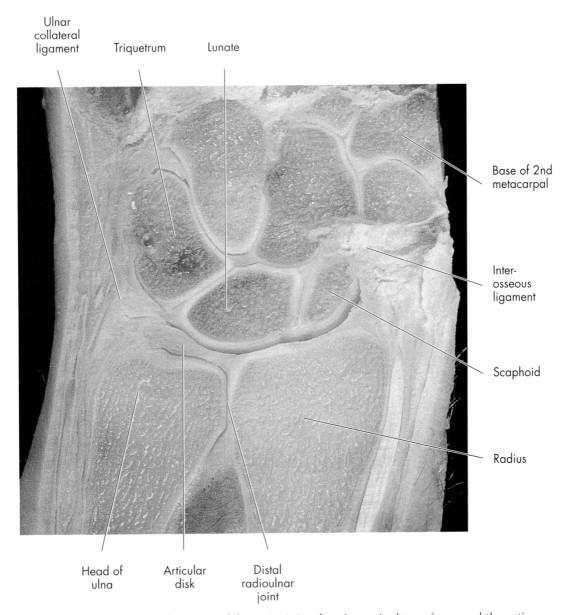

Figure 3-106 Coronal section of the wrist joint showing articular surfaces and the articular disk or triangular fibrocartilage.

See PRINCIPLES, Fig. 3-53

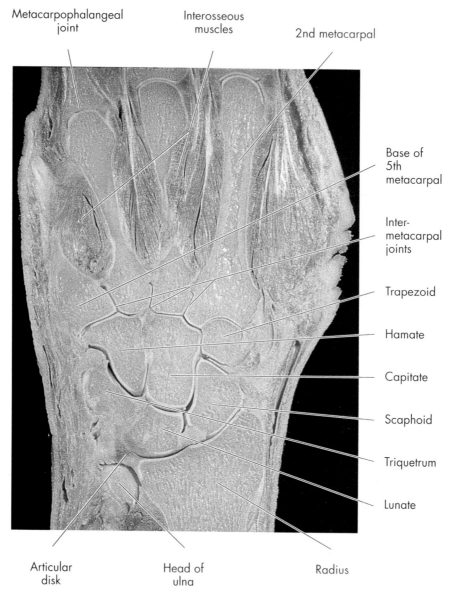

Metacarpophalangeal joint

Interosseous muscles

2nd metacarpal

Base of 5th metacarpal

Inter-metacarpal joints

Trapezoid

Hamate

Capitate

Scaphoid

Triquetrum

Lunate

Articular disk

Head of ulna

Radius

Figure 3-107   Coronal section of the hand showing the joints of the carpal region. The thumb and little finger lie anterior to the plane of section. The triangular fibrocartilage or articular disk can be seen separating the ulnar head from the carpals, lunate, and triquetrum.

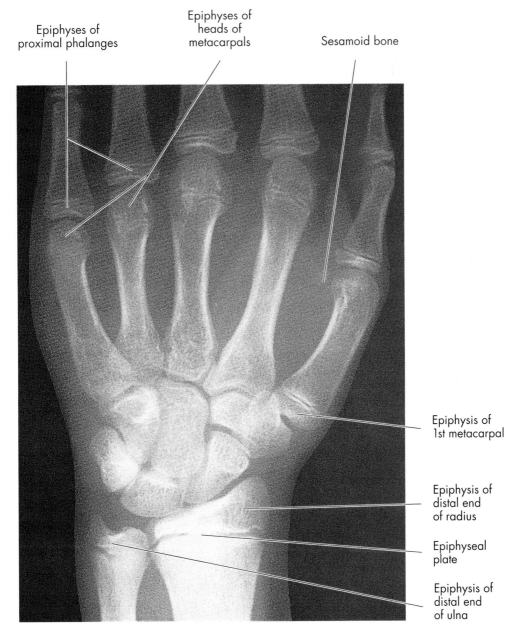

Epiphyses of
proximal phalanges

Epiphyses of
heads of
metacarpals

Sesamoid bone

Epiphysis of
1st metacarpal

Epiphysis of
distal end
of radius

Epiphyseal
plate

Epiphysis of
distal end
of ulna

Figure 3-108   Radiograph of the hand of an adolescent showing metacarpal and carpal bones. Epiphyseal plates are present as dark, radiolucent lines (cartilage) separating the epiphyses from the diaphyses.

SEE **DISSECTIONS**, SECTION 3, P. 11
SEE **PRINCIPLES**, FIG. 3-54

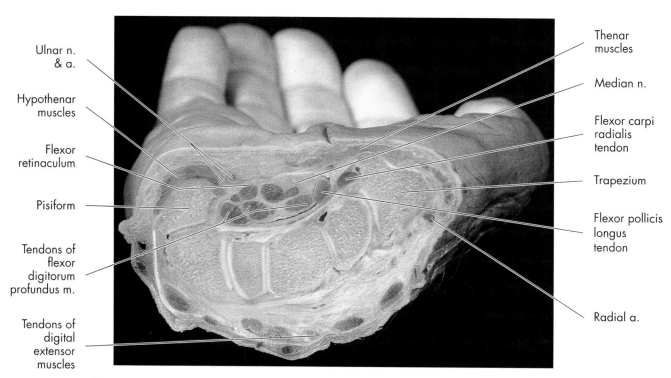

Ulnar n. & a.

Hypothenar muscles

Flexor retinaculum

Pisiform

Tendons of flexor digitorum profundus m.

Tendons of digital extensor muscles

Thenar muscles

Median n.

Flexor carpi radialis tendon

Trapezium

Flexor pollicis longus tendon

Radial a.

Figure 3-109   Transverse section through the carpus showing the carpal tunnel and its contents. The flexor digitorum superficialis tendons (unlabeled) lie palmar to the profundi with ring and long finger tendons palmar to the index and little finger tendons.

See DISSECTIONS, Section 3, p. 11
See PRINCIPLES, Fig. 3-54

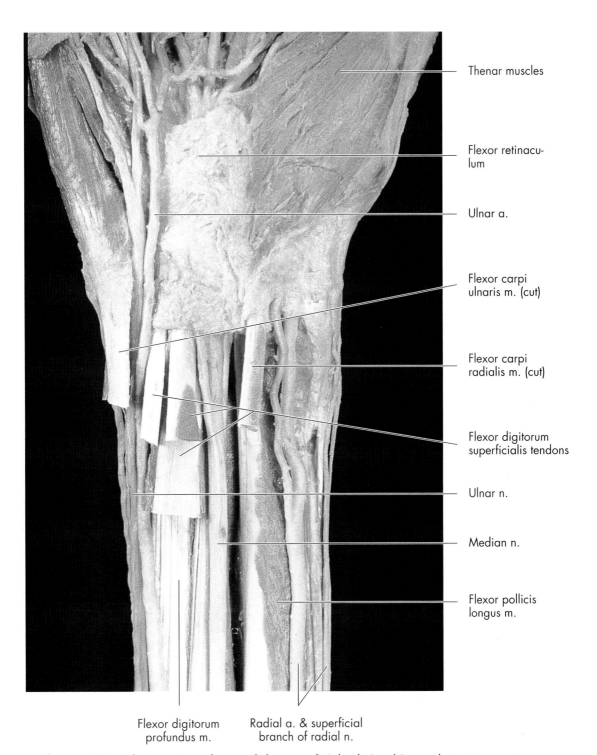

Thenar muscles

Flexor retinaculum

Ulnar a.

Flexor carpi ulnaris m. (cut)

Flexor carpi radialis m. (cut)

Flexor digitorum superficialis tendons

Ulnar n.

Median n.

Flexor pollicis longus m.

Flexor digitorum profundus m.

Radial a. & superficial branch of radial n.

Figure 3-110   Flexor retinaculum and the superficial relationships and structures entering the carpal tunnel.

SEE PRINCIPLES, FIG. 3-51

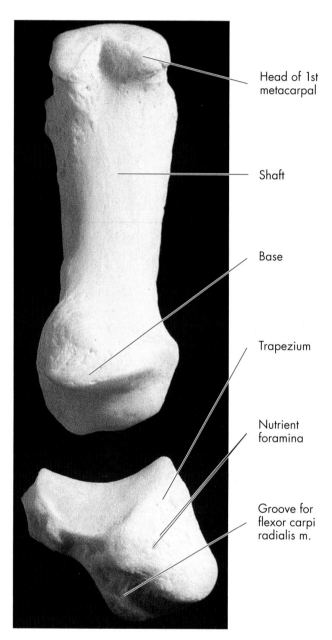

Head of 1st
metacarpal

Shaft

Base

Trapezium

Nutrient
foramina

Groove for
flexor carpi
radialis m.

Figure 3-111   Trapezium and metacarpal of the thumb separated to show the double saddle-shaped articular surfaces of the metacarpotrapezial joint.

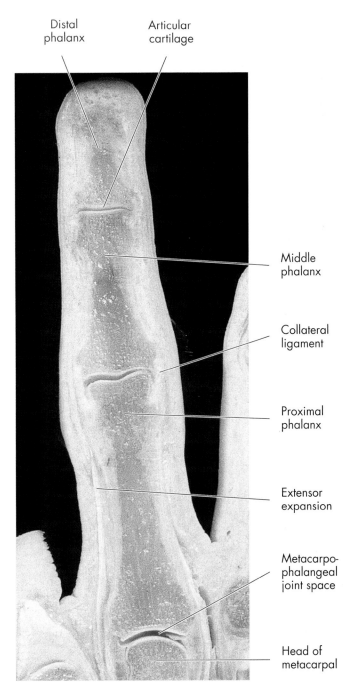

Distal
phalanx

Articular
cartilage

Middle
phalanx

Collateral
ligament

Proximal
phalanx

Extensor
expansion

Metacarpo-
phalangeal
joint space

Head of
metacarpal

Figure 3-112   Coronal section of a finger. The joint spaces have been exaggerated by hyperextension of the specimen.

SEE **PRINCIPLES**, FIG. 3-65

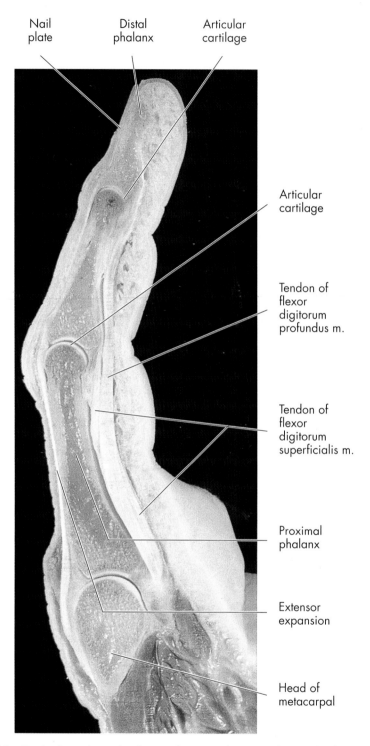

Nail plate

Distal phalanx

Articular cartilage

Articular cartilage

Tendon of flexor digitorum profundus m.

Tendon of flexor digitorum superficialis m.

Proximal phalanx

Extensor expansion

Head of metacarpal

Figure 3-113   Sagittal section of a finger showing the capsules and relationships of the joints.

SECTION FOUR

Back and Spinal Cord

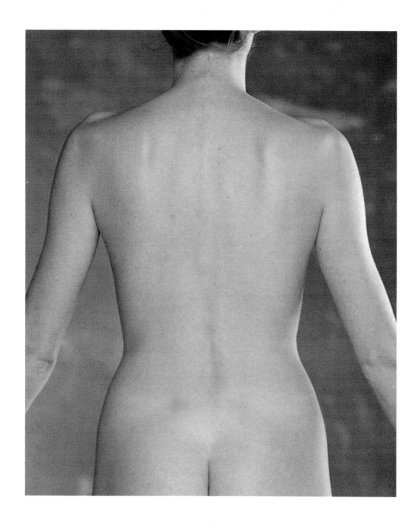

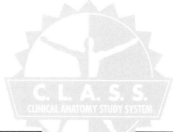

SEE PRINCIPLES, FIG. 4-31

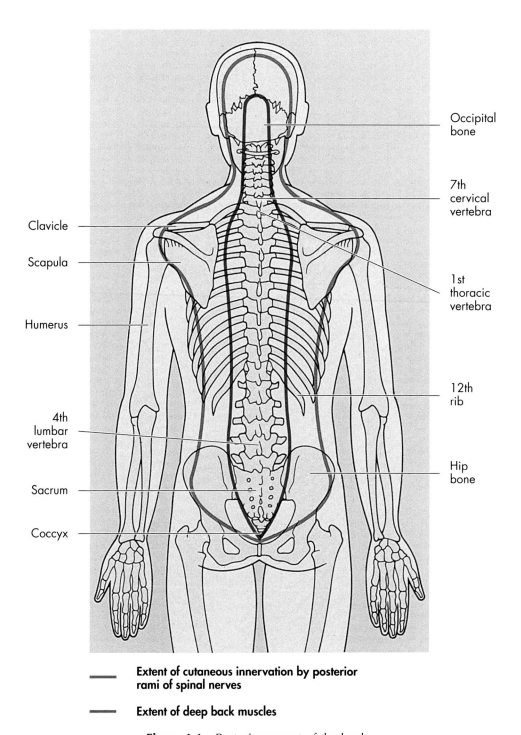

Occipital
bone

7th
cervical
vertebra

Clavicle

Scapula

1st
thoracic
vertebra

Humerus

12th
rib

4th
lumbar
vertebra

Hip
bone

Sacrum

Coccyx

——— **Extent of cutaneous innervation by posterior
rami of spinal nerves**

——— **Extent of deep back muscles**

Figure 4-1   Posterior aspect of the back.

SEE **PRINCIPLES,** FIG. 4-1

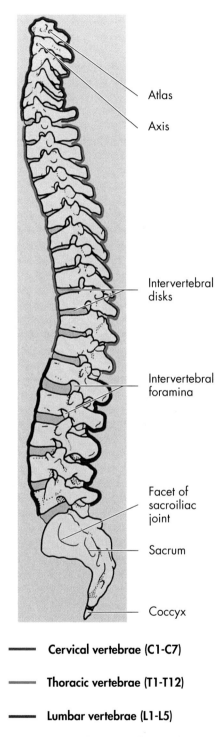

Atlas

Axis

Intervertebral
disks

Intervertebral
foramina

Facet of
sacroiliac
joint

Sacrum

Coccyx

—— **Cervical vertebrae (C1-C7)**

—— **Thoracic vertebrae (T1-T12)**

—— **Lumbar vertebrae (L1-L5)**

Figure 4-2   Lateral view of the vertebral column.

See **PRINCIPLES**, Fig. 4-2

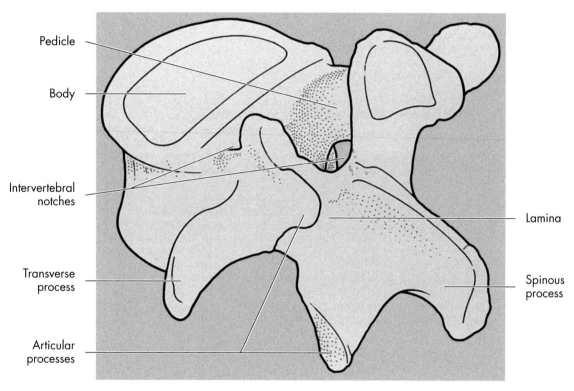

Pedicle

Body

Intervertebral
notches

Transverse
process

Articular
processes

Lamina

Spinous
process

Figure 4-3   Oblique view of a lumbar vertebra showing its processes, vertebral foramen, and intervertebral notches.

Rib   Transverse process   Transversospinalis m.   Erector spinae m.

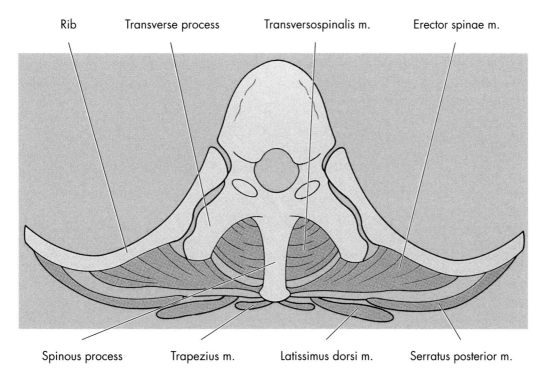

Spinous process   Trapezius m.   Latissimus dorsi m.   Serratus posterior m.

Figure 4-4 Superior view of a thoracic vertebra showing the arrangement of the main groups of back muscles.

See **PRINCIPLES**, Figs. 4-31, 4-36

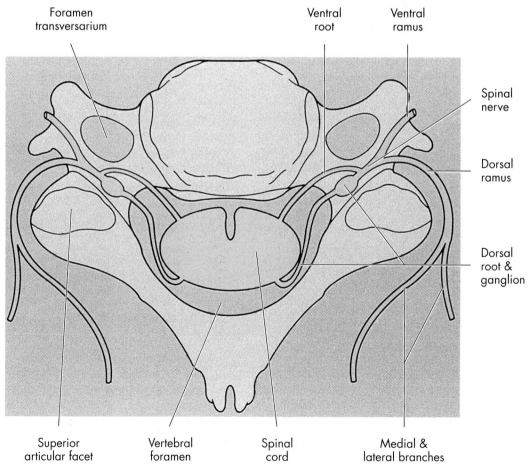

Foramen
transversarium

Ventral
root

Ventral
ramus

Spinal
nerve

Dorsal
ramus

Dorsal
root &
ganglion

Superior
articular facet

Vertebral
foramen

Spinal
cord

Medial &
lateral branches

Figure 4-5 Superior view of a cervical vertebra, the spinal cord, and a pair of spinal nerves.

See PRINCIPLES, Fig. 4-5

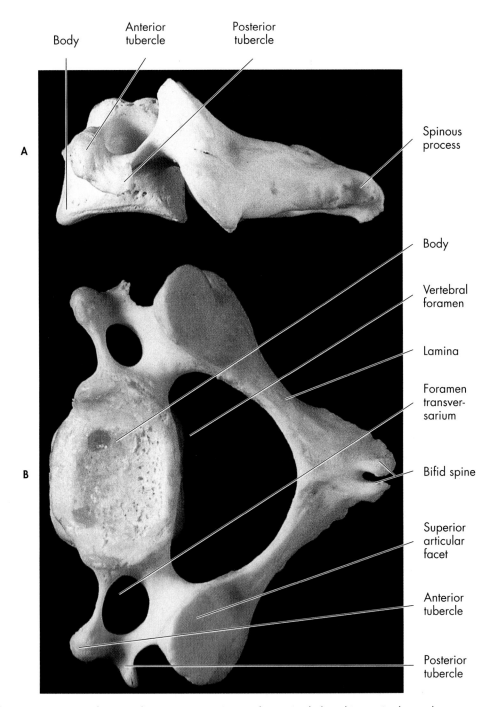

Figure 4-6   Lateral (**A**) and superior (**B**) views of a typical (fourth) cervical vertebra.

SEE **PRINCIPLES**, FIG. 4-5

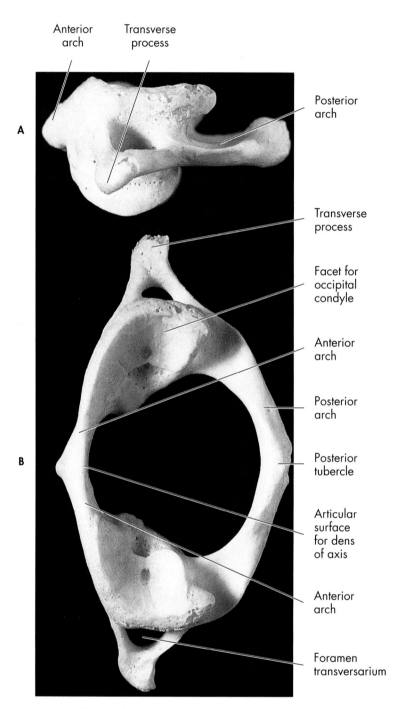

Anterior arch

Transverse process

Posterior arch

A

Transverse process

Facet for occipital condyle

Anterior arch

Posterior arch

Posterior tubercle

Articular surface for dens of axis

B

Anterior arch

Foramen transversarium

Figure 4-7   Lateral (**A**) and superior (**B**) views of the first cervical vertebra, the atlas.

See **PRINCIPLES**, Fig. 4-5

Dens   Body   Transverse
                            process

A

Spinous
process

Foramen
transversarium

B

Articular facets
for atlas

Bifid spinous
process

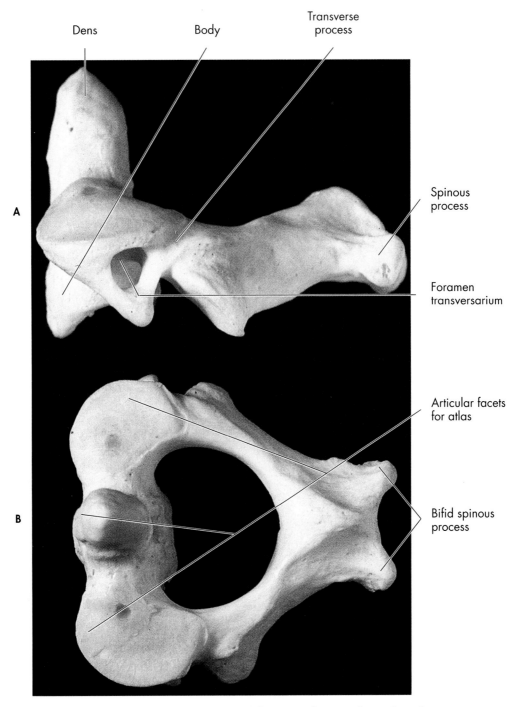

Figure 4-8   Lateral (**A**) and superior (**B**) views of the second cervical vertebra, the axis.

See PRINCIPLES, Fig. 4-6

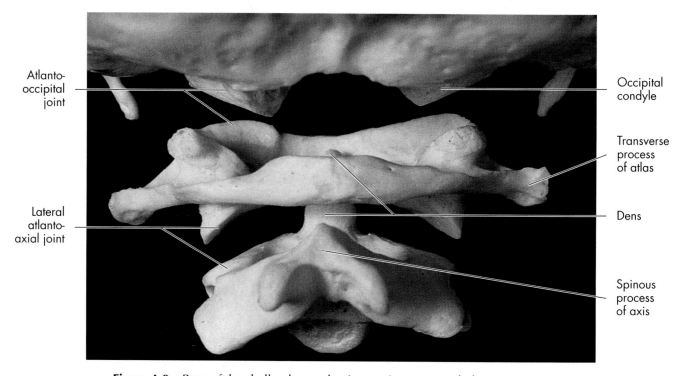

Atlanto-
occipital
joint

Occipital
condyle

Transverse
process
of atlas

Lateral
atlanto-
axial joint

Dens

Spinous
process
of axis

Figure 4-9   Base of the skull, atlas, and axis seen in an expanded posterior view.

SEE **PRINCIPLES, FIG. 4-7**

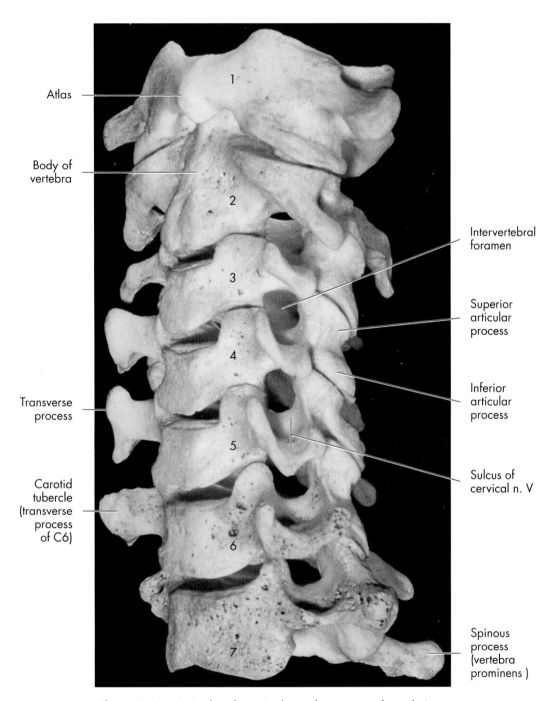

Atlas

Body of
vertebra

Transverse
process

Carotid
tubercle
(transverse
process
of C6)

Intervertebral
foramen

Superior
articular
process

Inferior
articular
process

Sulcus of
cervical n. V

Spinous
process
(vertebra
prominens)

Figure 4-10   Articulated cervical vertebrae, anterolateral view.

SEE PRINCIPLES, FIG. 4-15

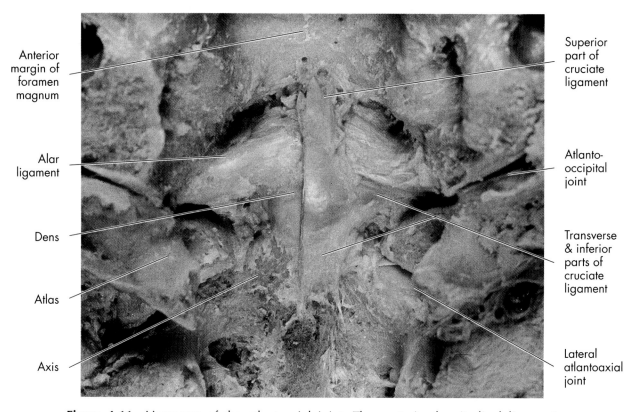

Anterior margin of foramen magnum

Alar ligament

Dens

Atlas

Axis

Superior part of cruciate ligament

Atlanto-occipital joint

Transverse & inferior parts of cruciate ligament

Lateral atlantoaxial joint

Figure 4-11　Ligaments of the atlantoaxial joint. The posterior longitudinal ligament, spinal cord and meninges, vertebral arches, and the posterior part of the skull have been removed. On the left side, part of the cruciate ligament has been excised.

See PRINCIPLES, Fig. 4-8

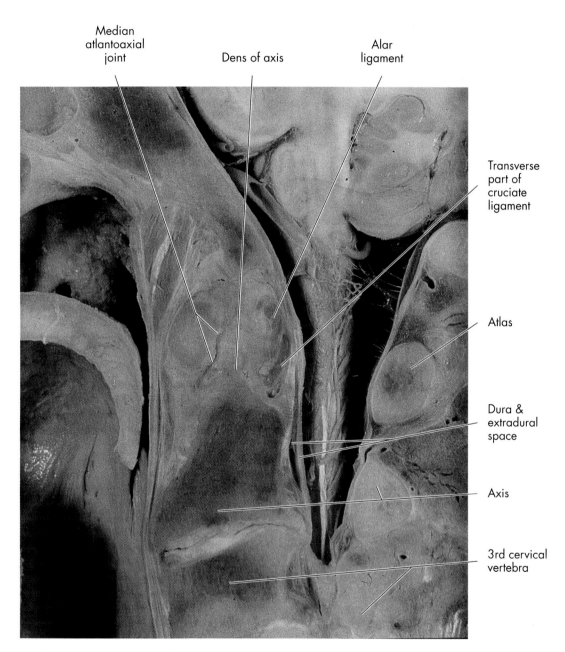

Figure 4-12   Near sagittal section through the median atlantoaxial joint.

SEE **PRINCIPLES**, FIG. 4-5

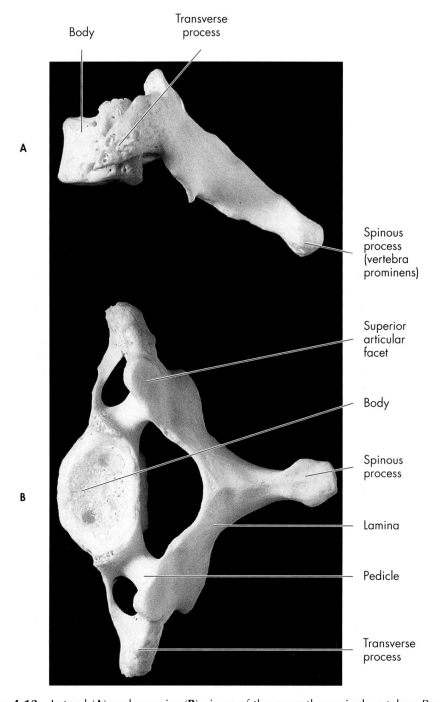

Body

Transverse process

A

Spinous process (vertebra prominens)

Superior articular facet

Body

Spinous process

B

Lamina

Pedicle

Transverse process

Figure 4-13   Lateral (**A**) and superior (**B**) views of the seventh cervical vertebra. Because of its prominent and easily palpable spinous process, it is called the *vertebra prominens*.

Sterno-   Levator   Longus   Pharyngeal   Scalene
mastoid m.   scapulae m.   colli m.   wall   muscles

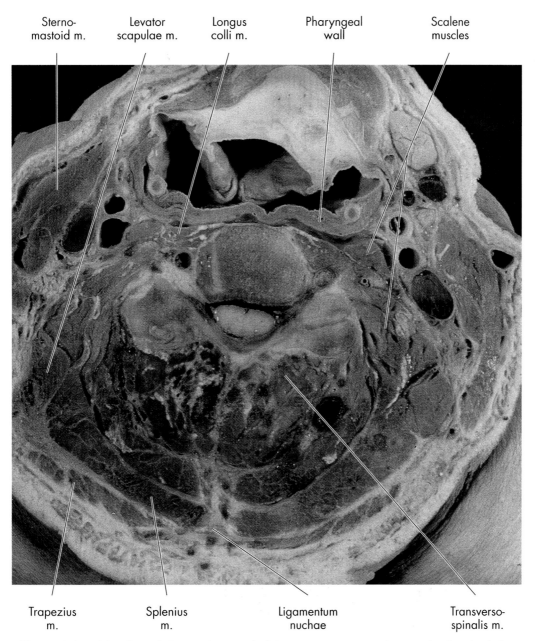

Trapezius   Splenius   Ligamentum   Transverso-
m.   m.   nuchae   spinalis m.

Figure 4-14   Muscles of the neck revealed in a transverse section at the level of the fourth cervical vertebra.

SEE **PRINCIPLES, FIG. 4-9**

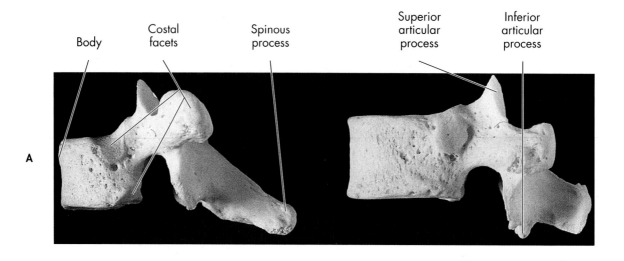

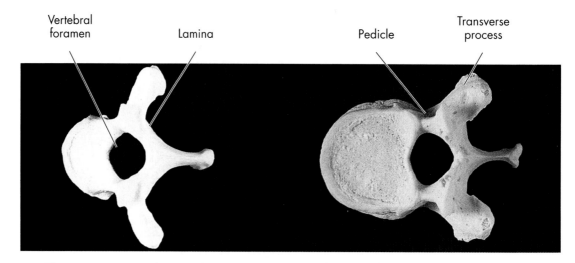

Figure 4-15   Lateral (**A**) and superior (**B**) views of the second and tenth thoracic vertebrae.

SEE **PRINCIPLES**, FIGS. 4-2, 4-11

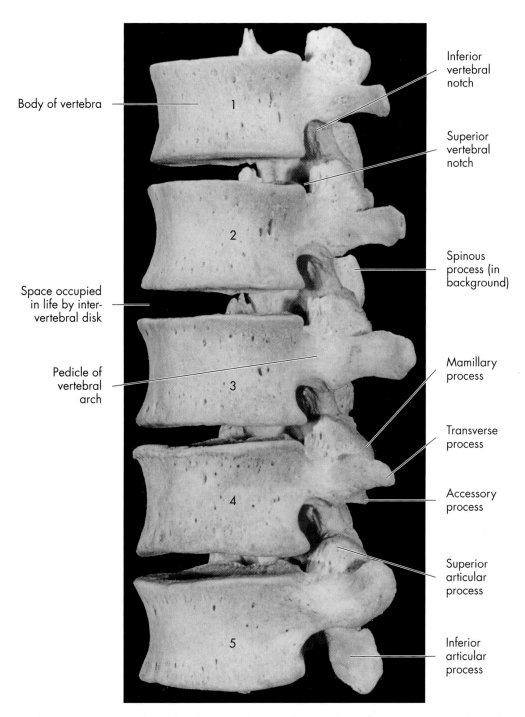

Figure 4-16 Articulated lumbar vertebrae, left anterolateral view. Together the inferior and superior vertebral notches form each of the intervertebral foramina.

See PRINCIPLES, Fig. 4-17

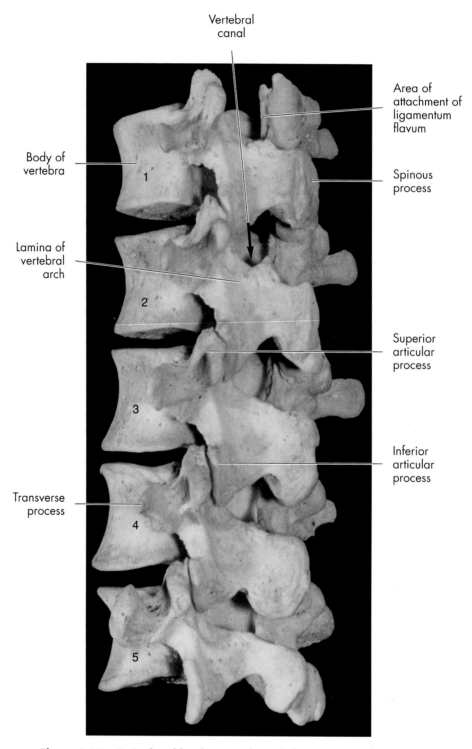

Vertebral
canal

Area of
attachment of
ligamentum
flavum

Body of
vertebra

Spinous
process

Lamina of
vertebral
arch

Superior
articular
process

Inferior
articular
process

Transverse
process

Figure 4-17   Articulated lumbar vertebrae, left posteroanterior view.

SEE **PRINCIPLES,** FIG. **4-2**

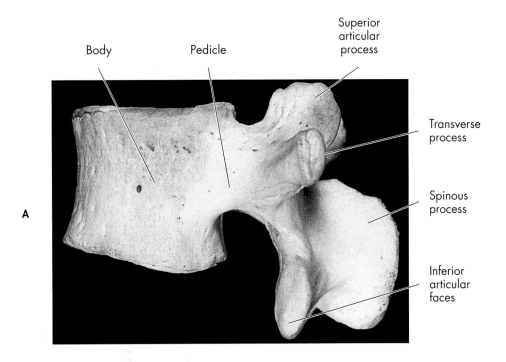

Body   Pedicle   Superior articular process

Transverse process

Spinous process

Inferior articular faces

A

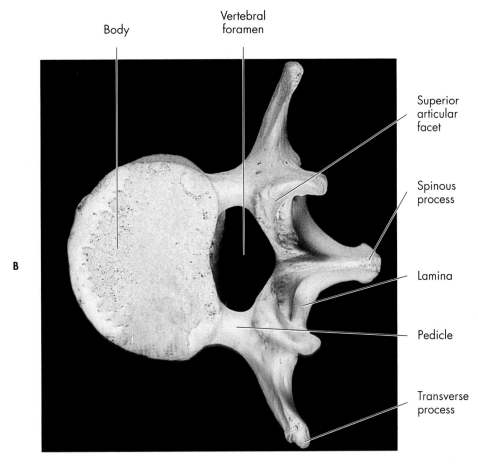

Body   Vertebral foramen

Superior articular facet

Spinous process

Lamina

Pedicle

Transverse process

B

Figure 4-18   Lateral (**A**) and superior (**B**) views of a typical (third) lumbar vertebra.

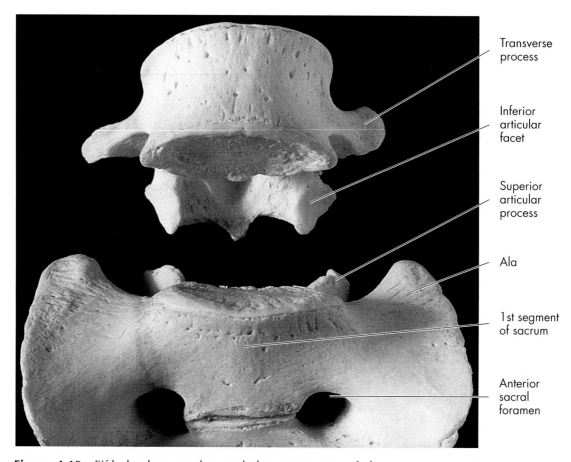

Transverse
process

Inferior
articular
facet

Superior
articular
process

Ala

1st segment
of sacrum

Anterior
sacral
foramen

Figure 4-19 Fifth lumbar vertebra and the upper part of the sacrum, seen in an expanded anterior view.

SEE PRINCIPLES, FIG. 4-13

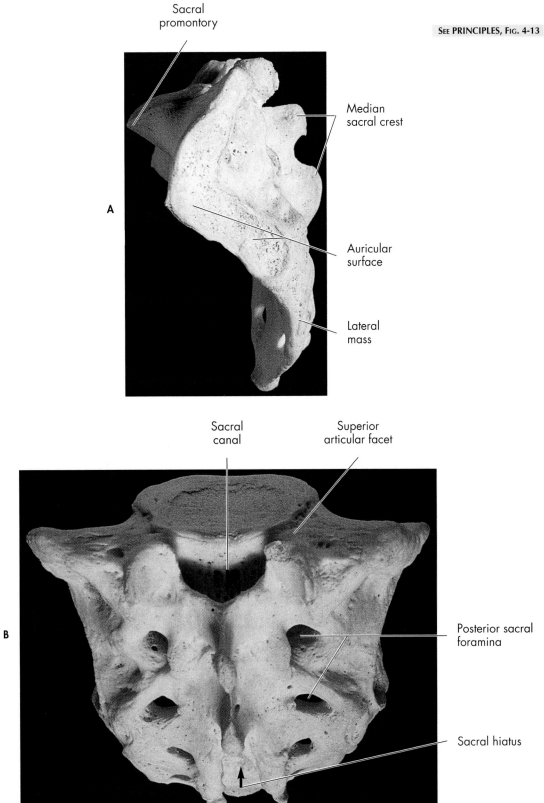

Sacral
promontory

Median
sacral crest

A

Auricular
surface

Lateral
mass

Sacral
canal

Superior
articular facet

B

Posterior sacral
foramina

Sacral hiatus

Figure 4-20 Lateral (**A**) and posterosuperior (**B**) views of the sacrum. *A sacral epidural injection of local anesthetic (caudal block) results in anesthesia of the perineal area including the vagina, anorectal region, scrotal skin, and vulva. The needle insertion is through the sacral hiatus into the epidural fat. The dural sac generally ends at the level of S2; thus the injection is made outside the sac (extradural) and bathes the sacral nerve roots. It is used in obstetric deliveries, some pediatric procedures, and for chronic pain control.*

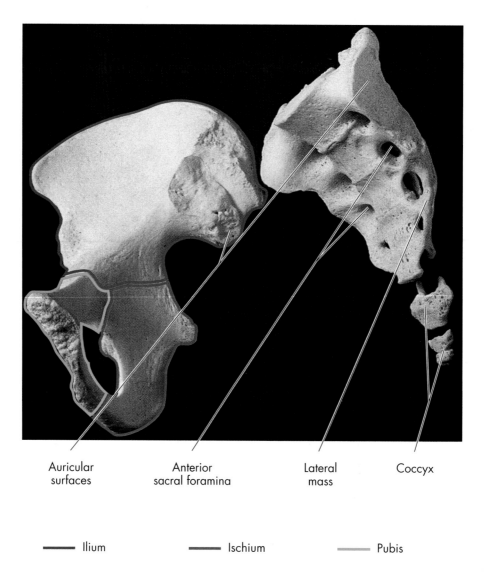

Auricular
surfaces

Anterior
sacral foramina

Lateral
mass

Coccyx

━━━ Ilium   ━━━ Ischium   ━━━ Pubis

Figure 4-21   Oblique view of the sacrum, coccyx, and the right hip bone.

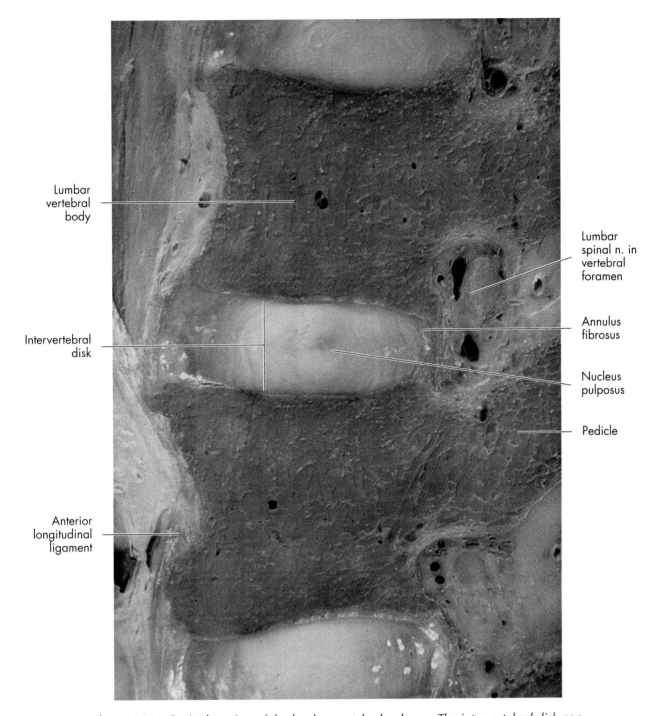

Lumbar
vertebral
body

Lumbar
spinal n. in
vertebral
foramen

Annulus
fibrosus

Intervertebral
disk

Nucleus
pulposus

Pedicle

Anterior
longitudinal
ligament

Figure 4-22 Sagittal section of the lumbar vertebral column. *The intervertebral disk consists of a peripheral annulus fibrosus and a central gelatinous nucleus pulposus. The tough annulus fibrosis degenerates with age and wear and tear, particularly in areas of greatest motion: the cervical and lumbar spines. Disk degeneration may lead to a break in continuity of the annulus fibrosus and a protrusion of part of the nucleus pulposus. Anatomically, such a posterolateral protrusion impinges on the nerve roots or spinal nerves, resulting in pain or numbness and muscle weakness or paralysis in the affected segment. Rest and traction may reverse the problem. If not, surgical removal of the protruding nucleus pulposus may be necessary.*

SEE DISSECTIONS, SECTION 6, PP. 11 AND 12

Anterior
sacroiliac
ligament

Anterior
longitudinal
ligament

Lumbosacral
disk

Erector
spinae m.

Anterior rami of
S1, S2, & S3
(cut)

Piriformis

Sacrospinous
ligament

Sacrotuberous
ligament

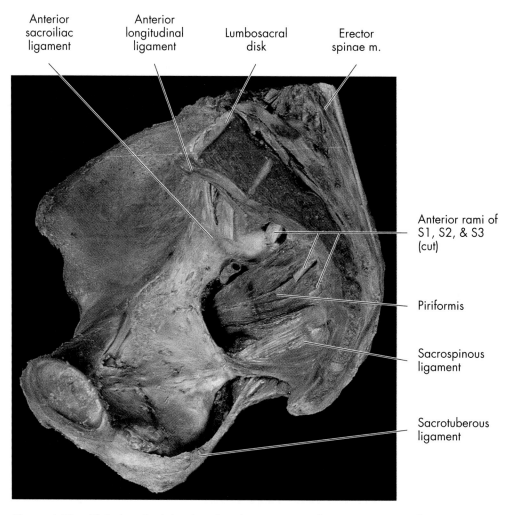

Figure 4-23   Right hemipelvis, showing the sacrum and coccyx in sagittal section.

SEE PRINCIPLES, FIGS. 4-17, 4-18

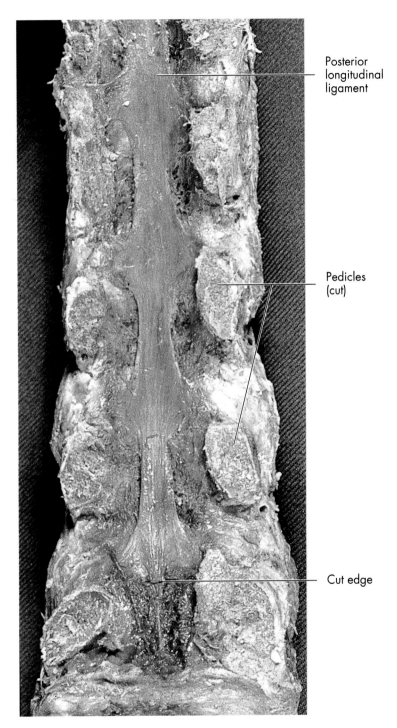

Posterior
longitudinal
ligament

Pedicles
(cut)

Cut edge

Figure 4-24   Posterior longitudinal ligament exposed by removal of the vertebral arches, meninges, and spinal cord.

See PRINCIPLES, Figs. 4-17, 4-18

Anterior
longitudinal
ligament

Interverte-
bral disks

4th lumbar
vertebral
body

Cut edge

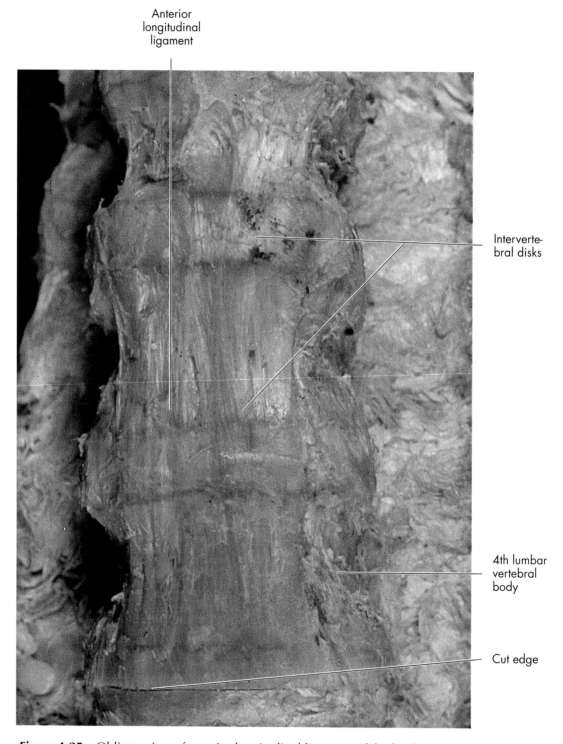

Figure 4-25   Oblique view of anterior longitudinal ligament of the lumbar spine.

See PRINCIPLES, Fig. 4-20

Nucleus
pulposus

Spinous
process of L3
vertebra

Erector
spinae m.

Thoraco-
lumbar fascia

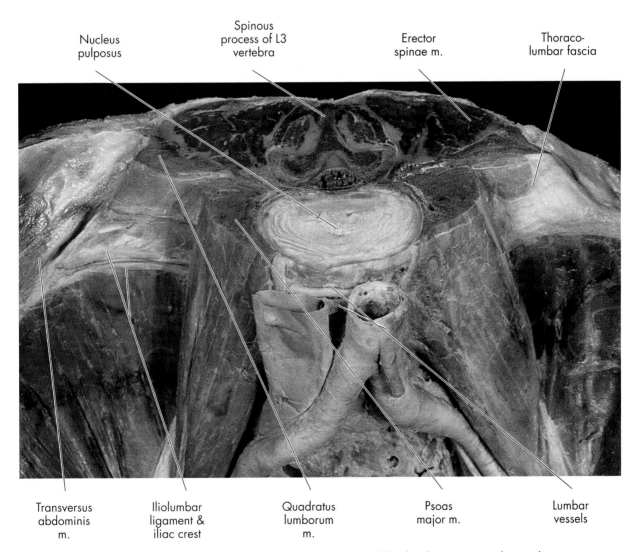

Transversus
abdominis
m.

Iliolumbar
ligament &
iliac crest

Quadratus
lumborum
m.

Psoas
major m.

Lumbar
vessels

Figure 4-26   Oblique view of a transverse section of the lumbar spine and muscles at
the level of the disk between the third and fourth lumbar vertebrae.

See PRINCIPLES, Fig. 4-23

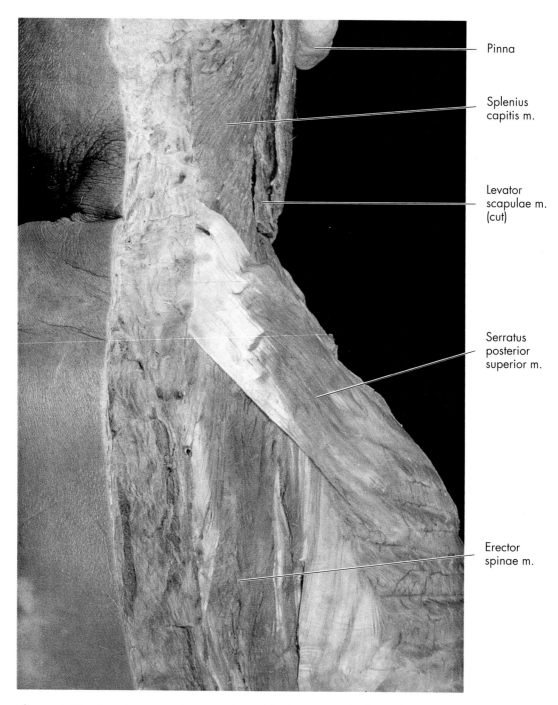

Pinna

Splenius
capitis m.

Levator
scapulae m.
(cut)

Serratus
posterior
superior m.

Erector
spinae m.

Figure 4-27   Serratus posterior superior with the upper limb girdle and its muscles removed.

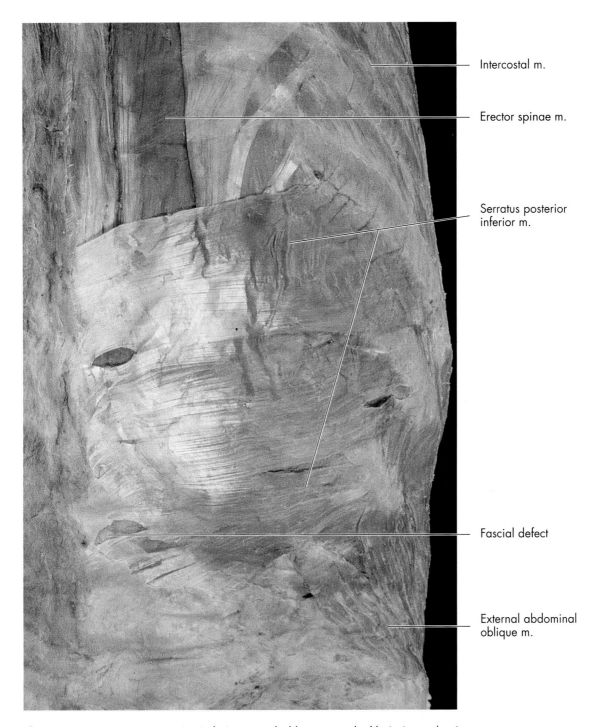

Intercostal m.

Erector spinae m.

Serratus posterior
inferior m.

Fascial defect

External abdominal
oblique m.

Figure 4-28   Serratus posterior inferior revealed by removal of latissimus dorsi.

See DISSECTIONS, Section 4, p. 4

See PRINCIPLES, Fig. 4-23

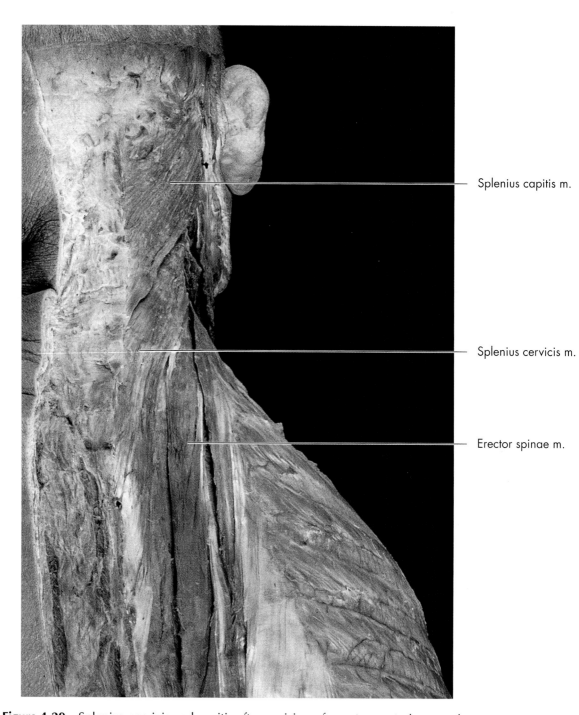

Splenius capitis m.

Splenius cervicis m.

Erector spinae m.

Figure 4-29   Splenius cervicis and capitis after excision of serratus posterior superior.

See PRINCIPLES, Fig. 4-31

Extradural
space

Thoracic
spinal cord

Anterior
longitudinal
ligament

Descending
aorta

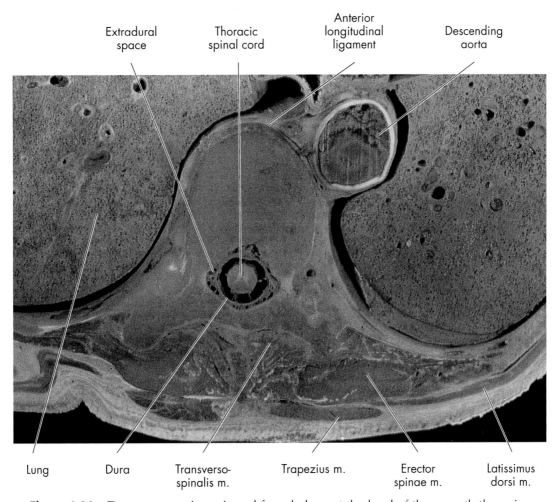

Lung   Dura   Transverso-   Trapezius m.   Erector   Latissimus
                            spinalis m.   spinae m.   dorsi m.

Figure 4-30   Transverse section, viewed from below, at the level of the seventh thoracic
vertebra showing the back muscles and the contents of the vertebral foramen.

324   **Clinical Anatomy Atlas**

SEE DISSECTIONS, SECTION 4, P. 4

SEE PRINCIPLES, FIG. 4-24

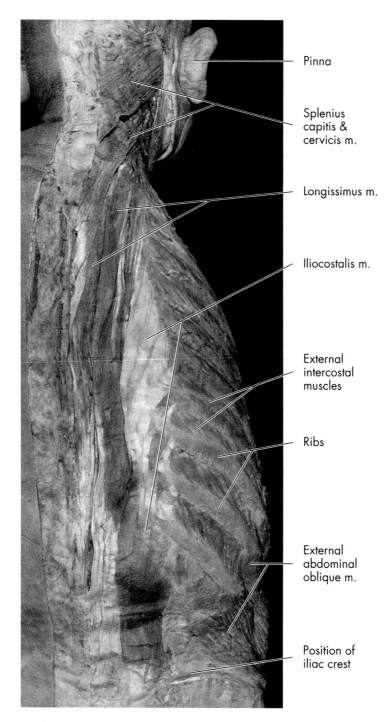

Pinna

Splenius
capitis &
cervicis m.

Longissimus m.

Iliocostalis m.

External
intercostal
muscles

Ribs

External
abdominal
oblique m.

Position of
iliac crest

Figure 4-31   Splenius and erector spinae exposed by removal of overlying muscles and
fasciae.

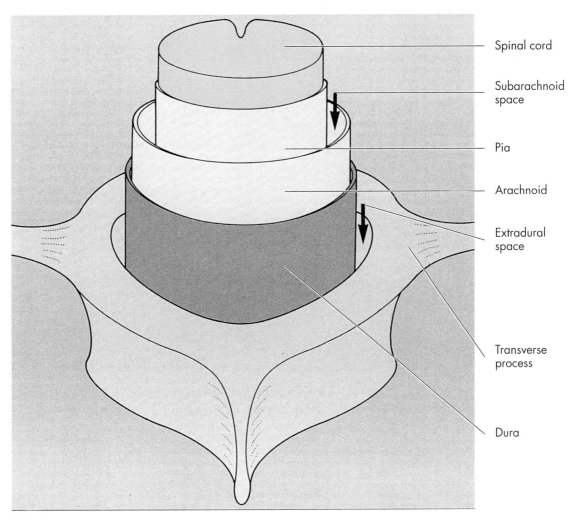

- Spinal cord
- Subarachnoid space
- Pia
- Arachnoid
- Extradural space
- Transverse process
- Dura

Figure 4-32   Spinal meninges.

See DISSECTIONS, Section 4, p. 4
See PRINCIPLES, Fig. 4-23

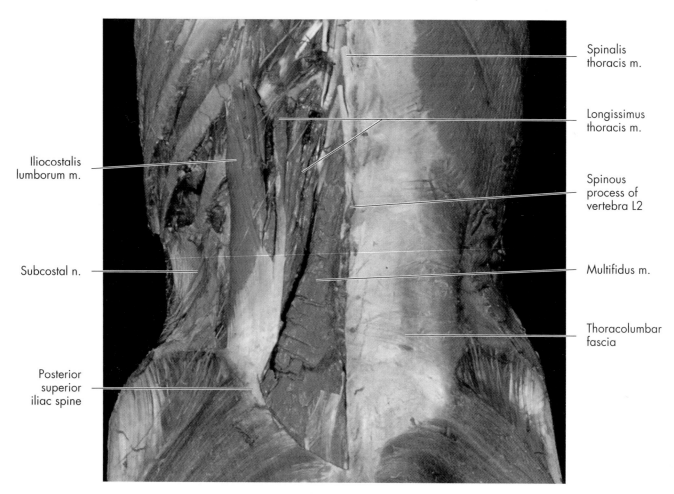

Spinalis
thoracis m.

Longissimus
thoracis m.

Spinous
process of
vertebra L2

Multifidus m.

Thoracolumbar
fascia

Iliocostalis
lumborum m.

Subcostal n.

Posterior
superior
iliac spine

Figure 4-33 Thoracic and lumbosacral regions of the back. Posterior view shows the iliocostalis lumborum, longissimus thoracis, and multifidus muscles. The longissimus inserts into the ribs, the transverse processes, and the lumbar vertebrae.

See DISSECTIONS, Section 4, p. 4

See PRINCIPLES, Fig. 4-25

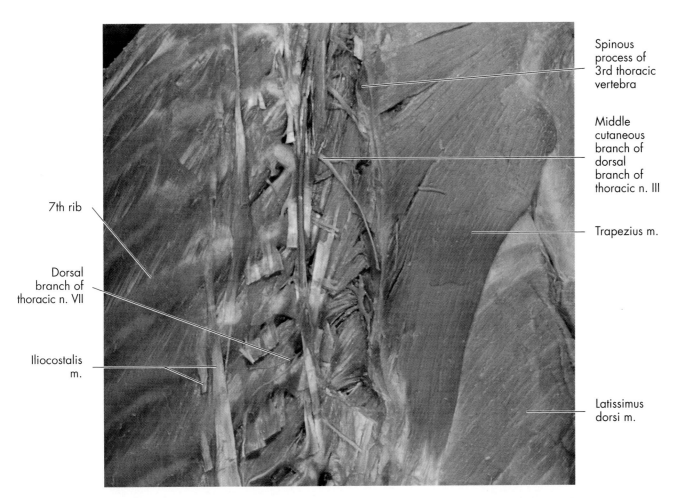

Spinous
process of
3rd thoracic
vertebra

Middle
cutaneous
branch of
dorsal
branch of
thoracic n. III

Trapezius m.

7th rib

Dorsal
branch of
thoracic n. VII

Iliocostalis
m.

Latissimus
dorsi m.

Figure 4-34   Thoracic and lumbosacral regions of the back. Posterior view shows multifidus and rotator muscles in the midthoracic region. Parts of the semispinalis have been
cut away to expose the more deeply placed multifidus and rotator muscles.

See DISSECTIONS, Section 4, p. 4

See PRINCIPLES, Fig. 4-25

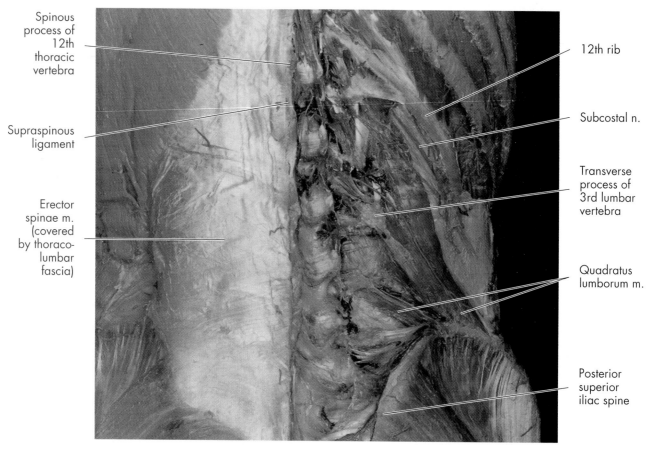

Spinous process of 12th thoracic vertebra

Supraspinous ligament

Erector spinae m. (covered by thoraco-lumbar fascia)

12th rib

Subcostal n.

Transverse process of 3rd lumbar vertebra

Quadratus lumborum m.

Posterior superior iliac spine

Figure 4-35   Thoracic and lumbosacral regions of the back. Posterior view shows the quadratus lumborum muscle. The middle layer of the thoracolumbar fascia has been removed from the posterior surface of the quadratus lumborum muscle.

See **DISSECTIONS**, Section 4, p. 4

See **PRINCIPLES**, Fig. 4-38

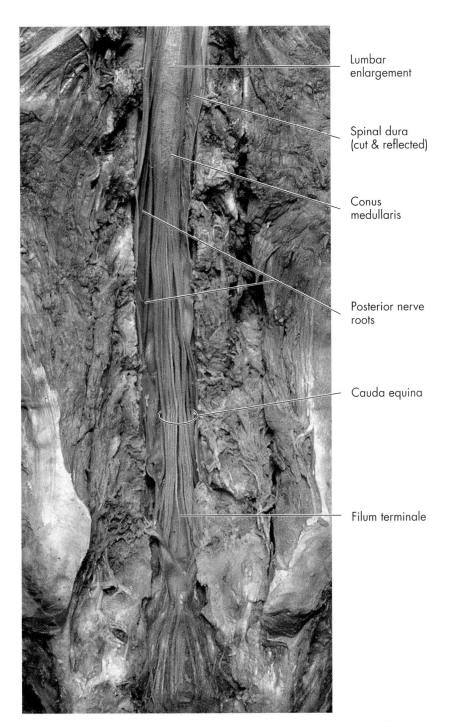

Lumbar
enlargement

Spinal dura
(cut & reflected)

Conus
medullaris

Posterior nerve
roots

Cauda equina

Filum terminale

Figure 4-36   Spinal dura and arachnoid opened posteriorly and reflected laterally,
exposing the lumbar enlargement, conus medullaris, and cauda equina.

See DISSECTIONS, Section 4, p. 4

See PRINCIPLES, Fig. 4-36

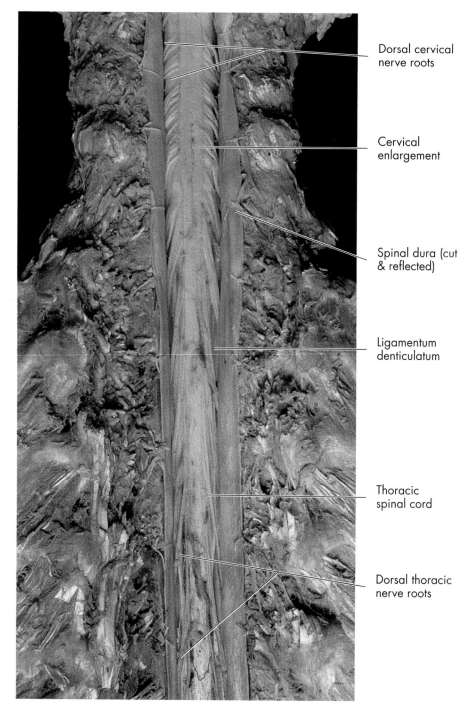

Dorsal cervical
nerve roots

Cervical
enlargement

Spinal dura (cut
& reflected)

Ligamentum
denticulatum

Thoracic
spinal cord

Dorsal thoracic
nerve roots

Figure 4-37   Cervical spinal cord and dorsal nerve roots. The spinal dura has been reflected laterally.

See DISSECTIONS, Section 4, p. 4

See PRINCIPLES, Fig. 4-35

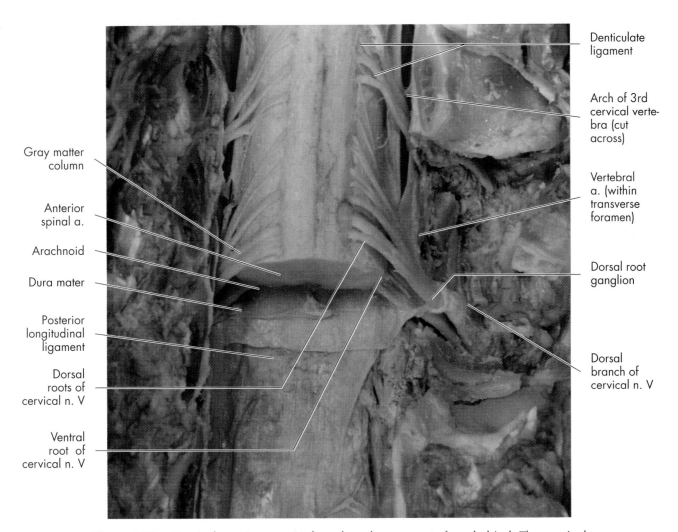

Denticulate
ligament

Arch of 3rd
cervical verte-
bra (cut
across)

Vertebral
a. (within
transverse
foramen)

Dorsal root
ganglion

Dorsal
branch of
cervical n. V

Gray matter
column

Anterior
spinal a.

Arachnoid

Dura mater

Posterior
longitudinal
ligament

Dorsal
roots of
cervical n. V

Ventral
root of
cervical n. V

Figure 4-38   Cervical meninges, spinal cord, and nerve roots from behind. The cervical
spinal cord and nerve roots are shown in relation to the meninges. The spinal cord has
been divided between the roots of the V and VI cervical nerves. Note the dura fuses to
nerve roots medial to the ganglion.

Psoas
major m.

Kidney

Quadratus
lumborum
m.

Spinous
process

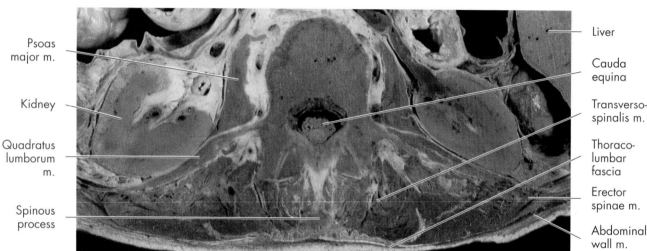

Liver

Cauda
equina

Transverso-
spinalis m.

Thoraco-
lumbar
fascia

Erector
spinae m.

Abdominal
wall m.

Figure 4-39 Transverse section, looking from above, at the level of the second lumbar vertebra showing back muscles and contents of the vertebral foramen. *Lumbar puncture or spinal tap is a frequently performed diagnostic procedure and is also used to administer intrathecal (intradural or subarachnoid) regional anesthesia. The lumbar area below L2 is ideal for needle insertion into the subarachnoid space. The spinal cord ends in the conus medullaris at the level of L1, thus injury to the cord is avoided. The lumbar spinous processes protrude posteriorly, and flexion of the trunk widens the space between processes and opens the interlaminar space to afford access for a needle. Anesthetic fluid injected into this space bathes nerve roots and results in loss of sensibility and motor paralysis below the level of injection.*

Abdomen

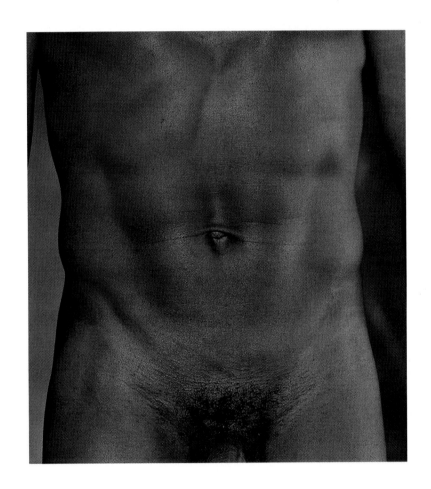

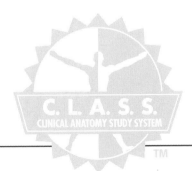

See PRINCIPLES, FIG. 5-6

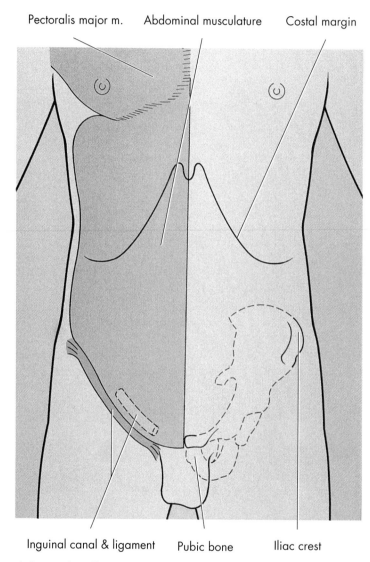

Pectoralis major m.   Abdominal musculature   Costal margin

Inguinal canal & ligament   Pubic bone   Iliac crest

Figure 5-1   Abdominal wall showing position of the inguinal canal and the way some of the abdominal muscles overlap the rib cage.

SEE PRINCIPLES, FIG. 5-7

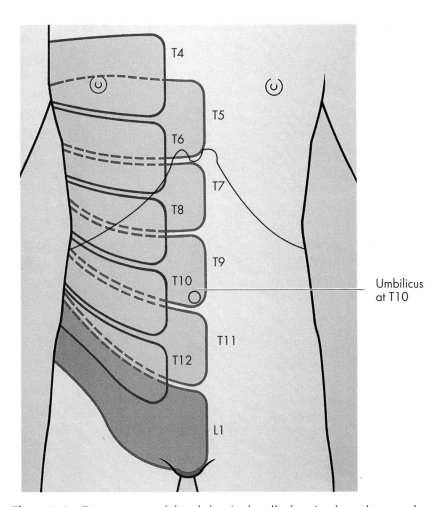

Figure 5-2   Dermatomes of the abdominal wall, showing how they overlap.

See **PRINCIPLES**, Figs. 5-25, 5-29

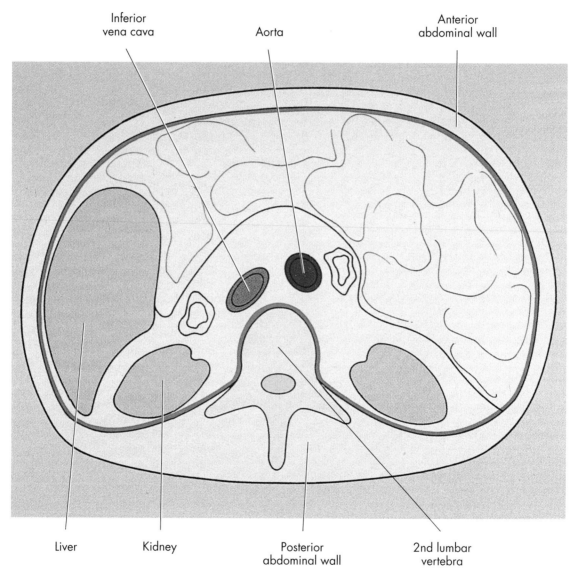

Figure 5-3   Transverse section through the abdomen looking from inferior to superior, demonstrating the shape of the abdominal cavity.

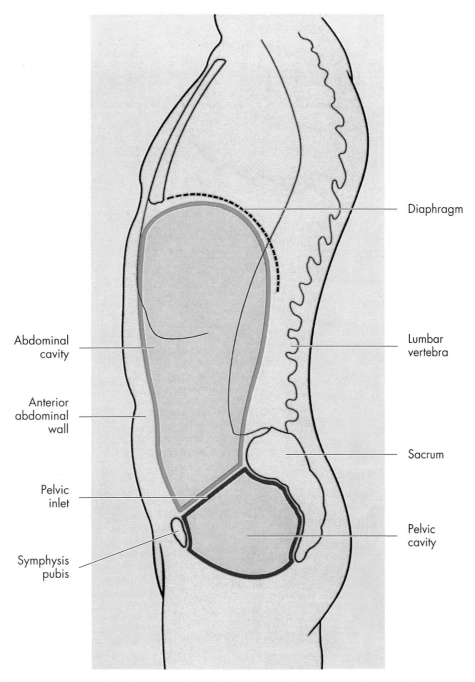

Figure 5-4   Longitudinal section through abdomen showing its shape and superior and inferior boundaries.

SEE PRINCIPLES, FIG. 5-48

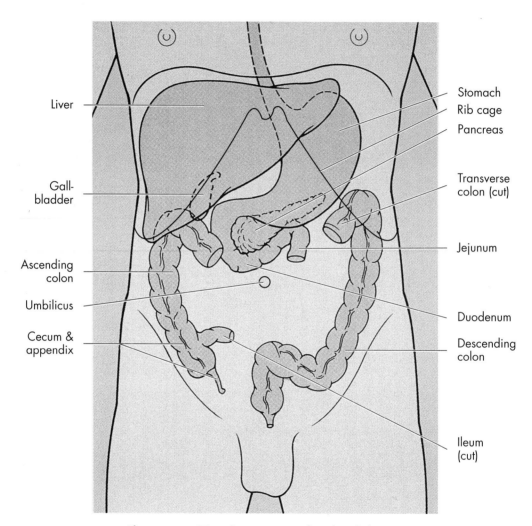

Liver

Gall-
bladder

Ascending
colon

Umbilicus

Cecum &
appendix

Stomach
Rib cage
Pancreas

Transverse
colon (cut)

Jejunum

Duodenum

Descending
colon

Ileum
(cut)

Figure 5-5   Digestive organs within the abdomen.

See **PRINCIPLES**, Fig. 5-33

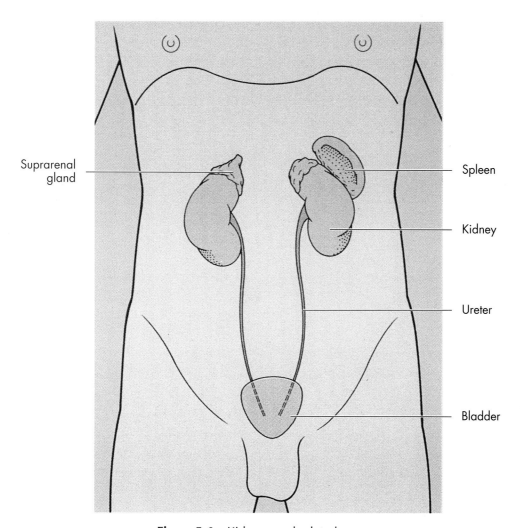

Figure 5-6   Kidneys and related organs.

SEE PRINCIPLES, FIG. 5-17

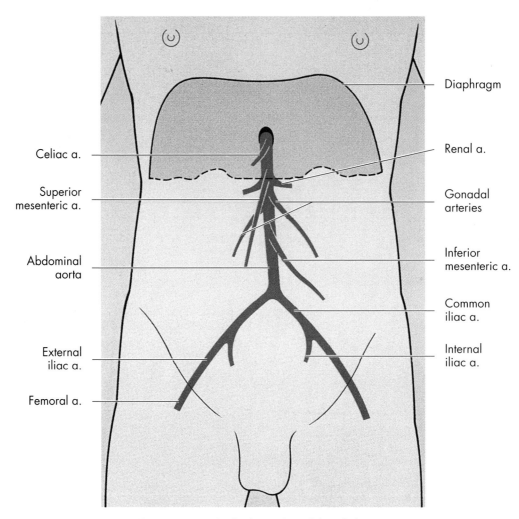

Celiac a.

Superior
mesenteric a.

Abdominal
aorta

External
iliac a.

Femoral a.

Diaphragm

Renal a.

Gonadal
arteries

Inferior
mesenteric a.

Common
iliac a.

Internal
iliac a.

Figure 5-7   Principal arteries of the abdomen.

SEE PRINCIPLES, FIG. 5-60

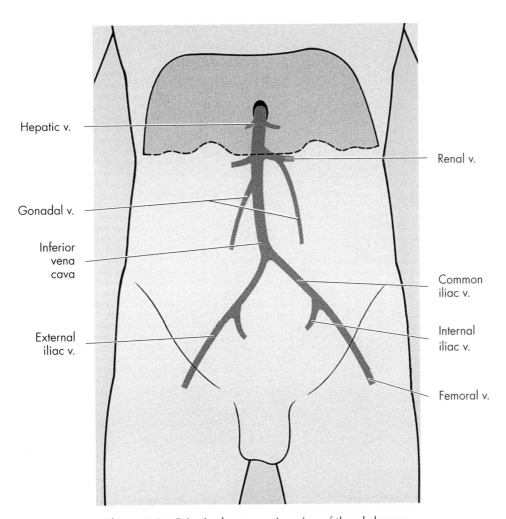

Hepatic v.

Renal v.

Gonadal v.

Inferior
vena
cava

Common
iliac v.

Internal
iliac v.

External
iliac v.

Femoral v.

Figure 5-8   Principal systematic veins of the abdomen.

SEE PRINCIPLES, FIG. 5-19

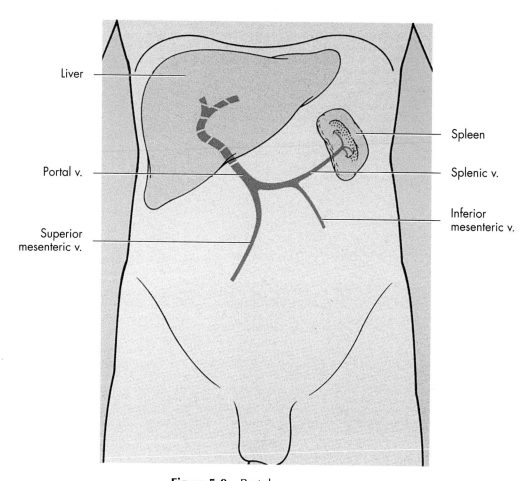

Liver

Portal v.

Superior
mesenteric v.

Spleen

Splenic v.

Inferior
mesenteric v.

Figure 5-9   Portal venous system.

See **DISSECTIONS, Section 5, p. 2**

See **PRINCIPLES, Fig. 5-1**

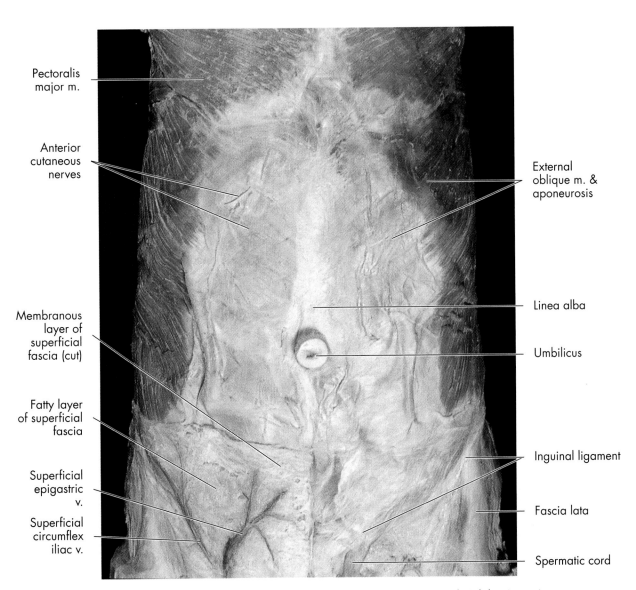

Pectoralis
major m.

Anterior
cutaneous
nerves

Membranous
layer of
superficial
fascia (cut)

Fatty layer
of superficial
fascia

Superficial
epigastric
v.

Superficial
circumflex
iliac v.

External
oblique m. &
aponeurosis

Linea alba

Umbilicus

Inguinal ligament

Fascia lata

Spermatic cord

Figure 5-10   External oblique muscles and aponeuroses. Some superficial fascia, veins, and cutaneous nerves have been preserved on the right side.

SEE DISSECTIONS, SECTION 5, P. 2
SEE PRINCIPLES, FIG. 5-5

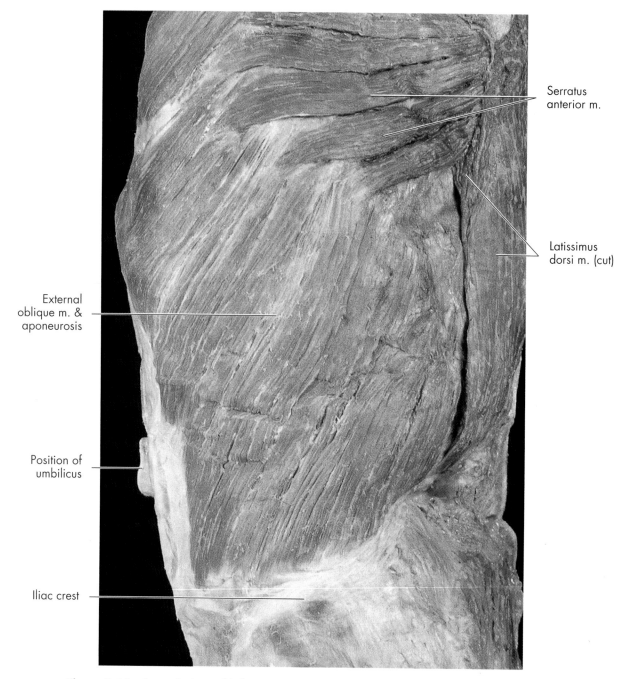

Serratus
anterior m.

Latissimus
dorsi m. (cut)

External
oblique m. &
aponeurosis

Position of
umbilicus

Iliac crest

Figure 5-11   Lateral view of left external oblique muscle showing its attachments to the lower ribs and the iliac crest.

See **DISSECTIONS, Section 5, pp. 2 AND 3**

See **PRINCIPLES, Fig. 5-5**

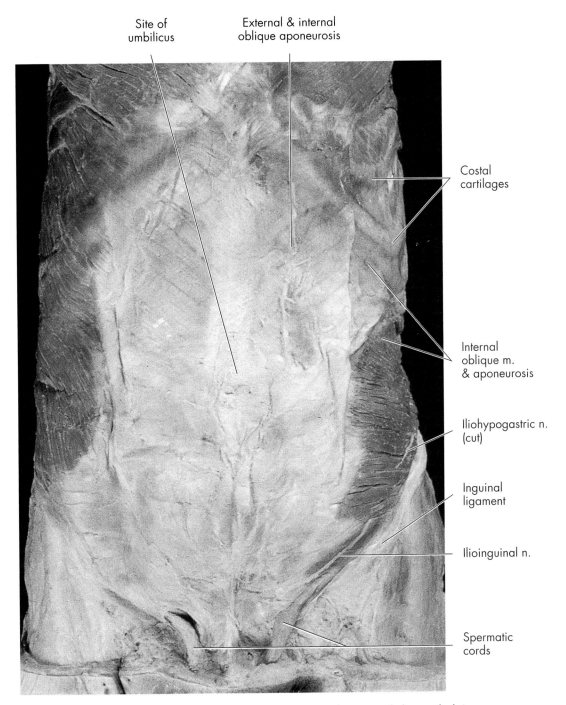

Site of
umbilicus

External & internal
oblique aponeurosis

Costal
cartilages

Internal
oblique m.
& aponeurosis

Iliohypogastric n.
(cut)

Inguinal
ligament

Ilioinguinal n.

Spermatic
cords

Figure 5-12   Most of the left external oblique muscle excised to reveal the underlying
internal oblique.

SEE DISSECTIONS, SECTION 5, P. 3

SEE PRINCIPLES, FIG. 5-5

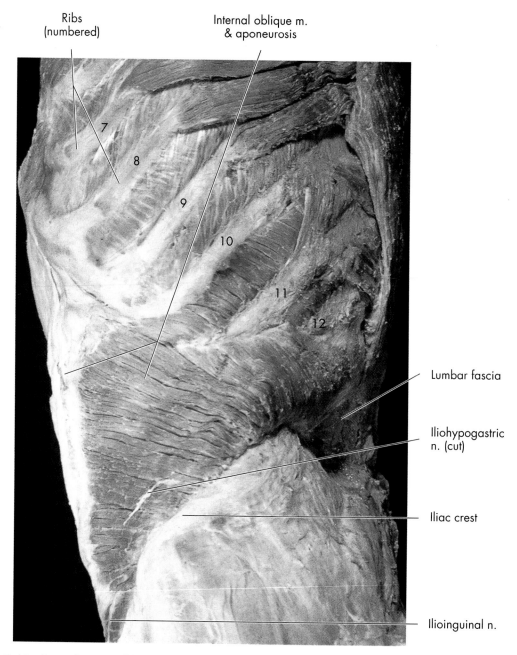

Ribs
(numbered)

Internal oblique m.
& aponeurosis

7

8

9

10

11

12

Lumbar fascia

Iliohypogastric
n. (cut)

Iliac crest

Ilioinguinal n.

Figure 5-13 Lateral view of left internal oblique muscle and attachments revealed by removal of the external oblique muscle. In this specimen the costal attachments of the serratus anterior include the ninth rib.

See **DISSECTIONS, Section 5, p. 4**
See **PRINCIPLES, Fig. 5-5**

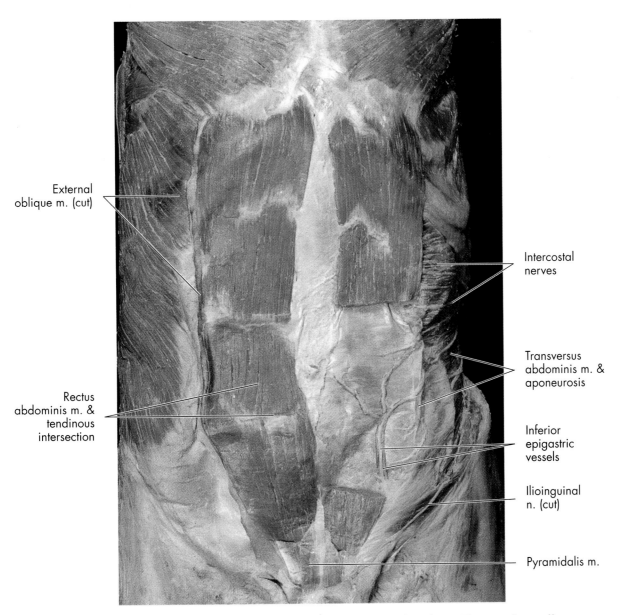

External
oblique m. (cut)

Intercostal
nerves

Transversus
abdominis m. &
aponeurosis

Rectus
abdominis m. &
tendinous
intersection

Inferior
epigastric
vessels

Ilioinguinal
n. (cut)

Pyramidalis m.

Figure 5-14 Rectus abdominis muscles and the neurovascular plane. The anterior walls of both rectus sheaths, the left oblique muscles, and part of the left rectus abdominis have been removed.

SEE DISSECTIONS, SECTION 5, P. 4

SEE PRINCIPLES, FIG. 5-5

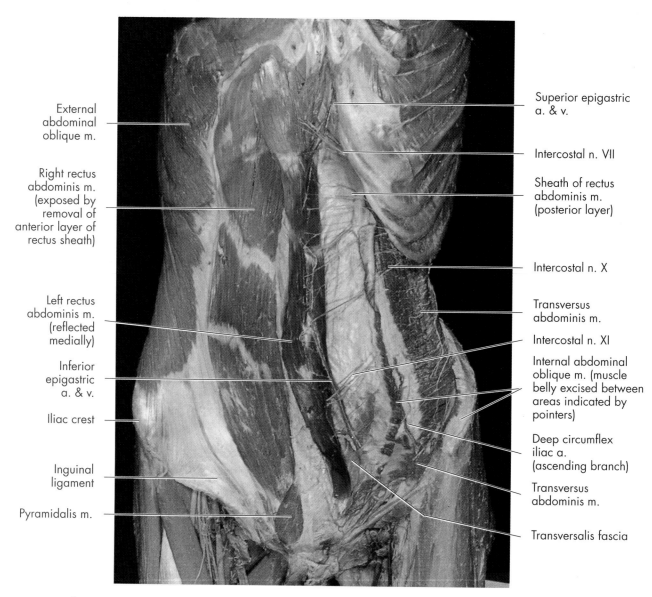

External abdominal oblique m.

Right rectus abdominis m. (exposed by removal of anterior layer of rectus sheath)

Left rectus abdominis m. (reflected medially)

Inferior epigastric a. & v.

Iliac crest

Inguinal ligament

Pyramidalis m.

Superior epigastric a. & v.

Intercostal n. VII

Sheath of rectus abdominis m. (posterior layer)

Intercostal n. X

Transversus abdominis m.

Intercostal n. XI

Internal abdominal oblique m. (muscle belly excised between areas indicated by pointers)

Deep circumflex iliac a. (ascending branch)

Transversus abdominis m.

Transversalis fascia

Figure 5-15   Both rectus muscles exposed within their sheaths. The left rectus has been reflected medially to expose its posterior surface. *A vertical surgical incision lateral to the rectus abdominis muscle will divide some of the intercostal nerves, resulting in partial paralysis of the rectus abdominis. The robust anastomoses between the inferior and superior epigastric arteries allows the surgeon to carry tissues such as skin, fat, and fascia from the lower abdominal wall to the chest wall for breast reconstruction. Sternal defects can be repaired using the rectus abdominis with an intact superior epigastric artery as a vascular pedicle.*

SEE **DISSECTIONS**, SECTION 5, P. 4

SEE **PRINCIPLES**, FIG. 5-5

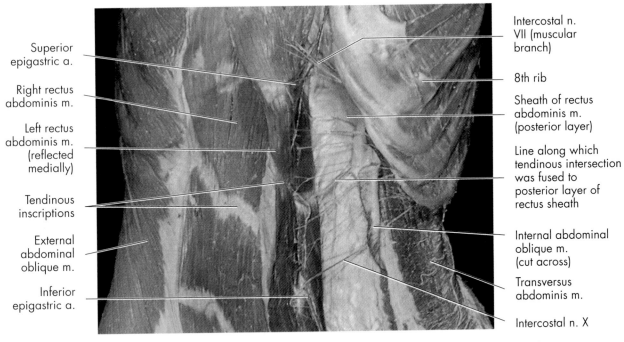

Superior
epigastric a.

Right rectus
abdominis m.

Left rectus
abdominis m.
(reflected
medially)

Tendinous
inscriptions

External
abdominal
oblique m.

Inferior
epigastric a.

Intercostal n.
VII (muscular
branch)

8th rib

Sheath of rectus
abdominis m.
(posterior layer)

Line along which
tendinous intersection
was fused to
posterior layer of
rectus sheath

Internal abdominal
oblique m.
(cut across)

Transversus
abdominis m.

Intercostal n. X

Figure 5-16   Close-up view of the midportion of the rectus abdominis muscles. The left
rectus is reflected medially to show its innervation, epigastric arteries, and posterior rectus sheath.

SEE DISSECTIONS, SECTION 5, P. 4

SEE PRINCIPLES, FIG. 5-5

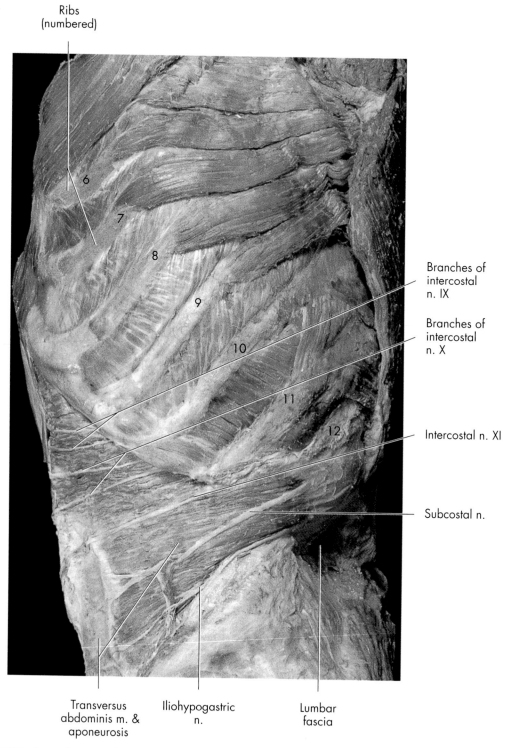

Ribs
(numbered)

6

7

8

9

10

11

12

Branches of
intercostal
n. IX

Branches of
intercostal
n. X

Intercostal n. XI

Subcostal n.

Transversus
abdominis m. &
aponeurosis

Iliohypogastric
n.

Lumbar
fascia

Figure 5-17   Lateral view of thorax. Removal of the external and internal oblique muscles reveals the transversus abdominis muscle and aponeurosis. Running across its surface are the lower intercostal, subcostal, and iliohypogastric nerves.

See DISSECTIONS, Section 5, p. 4
See PRINCIPLES, Fig. 5-5

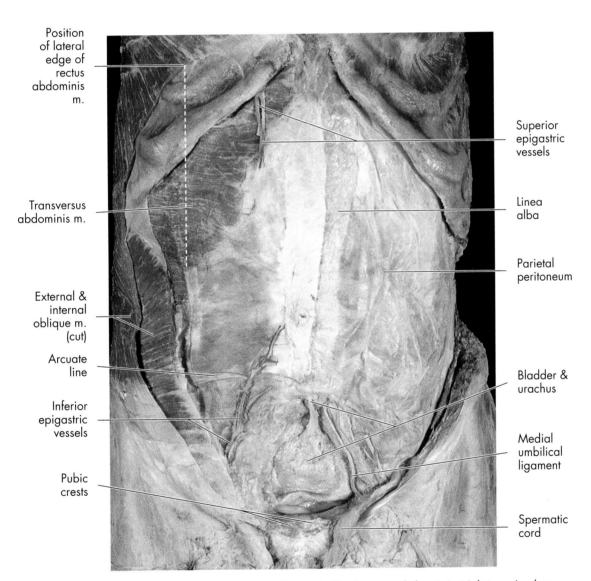

Position of lateral edge of rectus abdominis m.

Transversus abdominis m.

External & internal oblique m. (cut)

Arcuate line

Inferior epigastric vessels

Pubic crests

Superior epigastric vessels

Linea alba

Parietal peritoneum

Bladder & urachus

Medial umbilical ligament

Spermatic cord

Figure 5-18 Most of the oblique muscles and all of rectus abdominis (right) excised to reveal the posterior wall of the rectus sheath. All the muscles (left) removed to show the parietal peritoneum. The bladder is enlarged.

See PRINCIPLES, Fig. 5-5

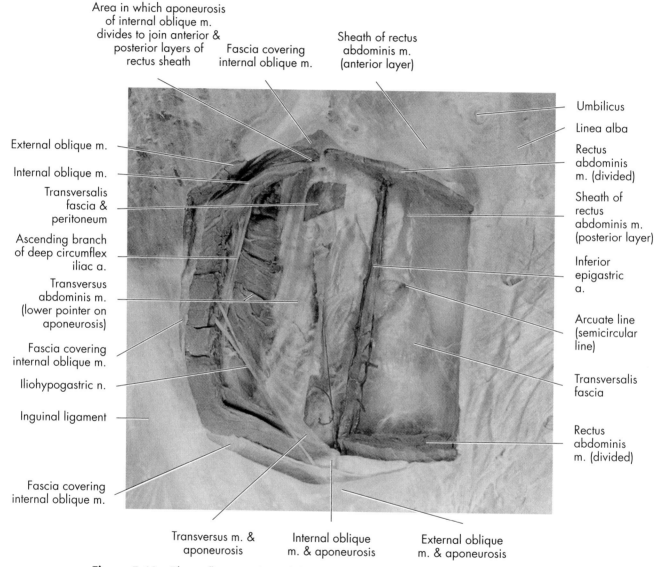

Area in which aponeurosis of internal oblique m. divides to join anterior & posterior layers of rectus sheath

Fascia covering internal oblique m.

Sheath of rectus abdominis m. (anterior layer)

External oblique m.

Internal oblique m.

Transversalis fascia & peritoneum

Ascending branch of deep circumflex iliac a.

Transversus abdominis m. (lower pointer on aponeurosis)

Fascia covering internal oblique m.

Iliohypogastric n.

Inguinal ligament

Fascia covering internal oblique m.

Umbilicus

Linea alba

Rectus abdominis m. (divided)

Sheath of rectus abdominis m. (posterior layer)

Inferior epigastric a.

Arcuate line (semicircular line)

Transversalis fascia

Rectus abdominis m. (divided)

Transversus m. & aponeurosis

Internal oblique m. & aponeurosis

External oblique m. & aponeurosis

Figure 5-19 Three flat muscles of the abdominal wall dissected on the right side to demonstrate the contribution of their aponeuroses to the formation of the sheath of the rectus muscle.

SEE **PRINCIPLES**, FIG. 5-8

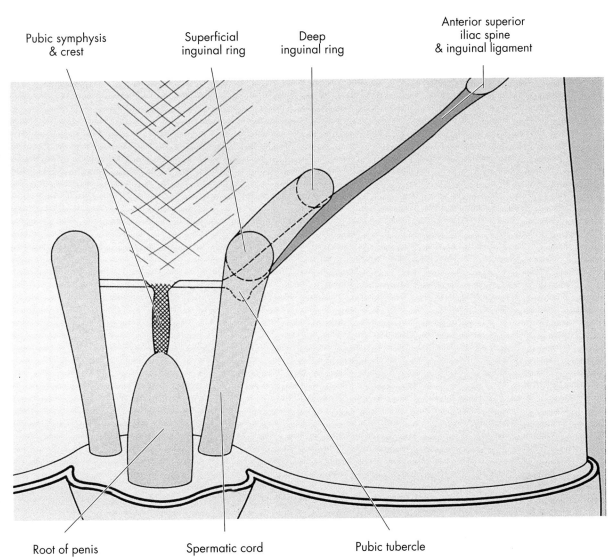

Figure 5-20 Position of the inguinal canal, superficial inguinal ring, and deep inguinal ring in relation to the inguinal ligament, the pubic bone, and the iliac crest.

See **DISSECTIONS, SECTION 5, P. 5**

See **PRINCIPLES, FIG. 5-8**

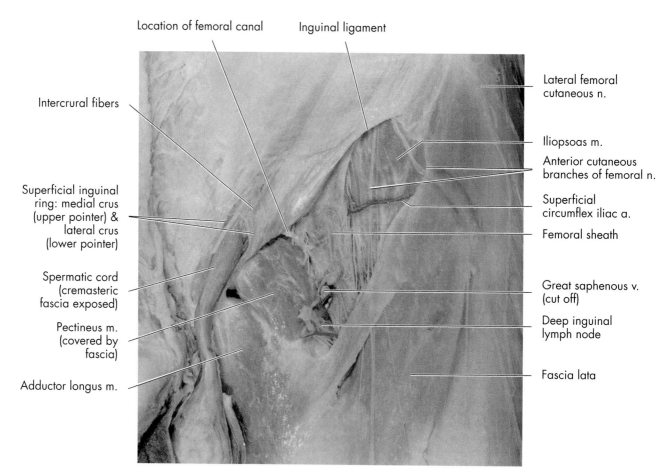

Figure 5-21   The superficial inguinal ring, a thickened rim of the external oblique aponeurosis, seen surrounding the spermatic cord. Below the inguinal ligament, the femoral sheath has been exposed by removing the superficial inguinal lymph nodes, the cribriform fascia, and part of the fascia lata, which bounds the saphenous opening. Note lymphatic vessels penetrating the femoral sheath near the femoral canal.

SEE DISSECTIONS, SECTION 5, P. 6
SEE PRINCIPLES, FIG. 5-8

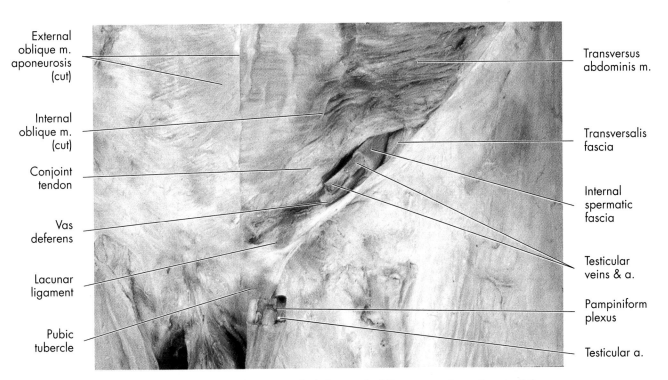

External oblique m. aponeurosis (cut)

Internal oblique m. (cut)

Conjoint tendon

Vas deferens

Lacunar ligament

Pubic tubercle

Transversus abdominis m.

Transversalis fascia

Internal spermatic fascia

Testicular veins & a.

Pampiniform plexus

Testicular a.

Figure 5-22   Lower part of the internal abdominal oblique muscle and part of the spermatic cord excised to reveal the posterior wall and floor of the canalis inguinalis.

356   **Clinical Anatomy Atlas**

See **DISSECTIONS**, Section 5, p. 5

See **PRINCIPLES**, Fig. 5-8

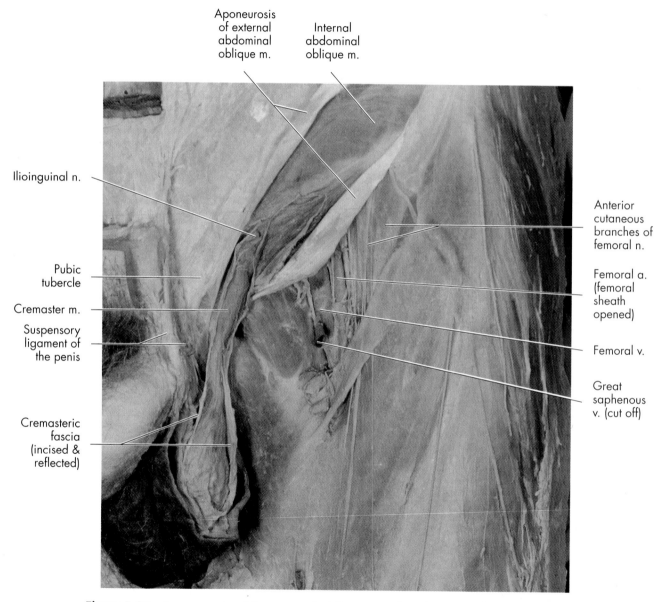

Aponeurosis of external abdominal oblique m.

Internal abdominal oblique m.

Ilioinguinal n.

Pubic tubercle

Cremaster m.

Suspensory ligament of the penis

Cremasteric fascia (incised & reflected)

Anterior cutaneous branches of femoral n.

Femoral a. (femoral sheath opened)

Femoral v.

Great saphenous v. (cut off)

Figure 5-23   Aponeurosis of the external oblique muscle split in a direction parallel to the inguinal ligament. The margins have been reflected to reveal the underlying fascia of the internal oblique, which continues into the spermatic cord as the cremasteric fascia. The cremaster muscle is displayed by division of the cremasteric fascia.

See **DISSECTIONS**, Section 5, p. 7

See **PRINCIPLES**, Fig. 5-8

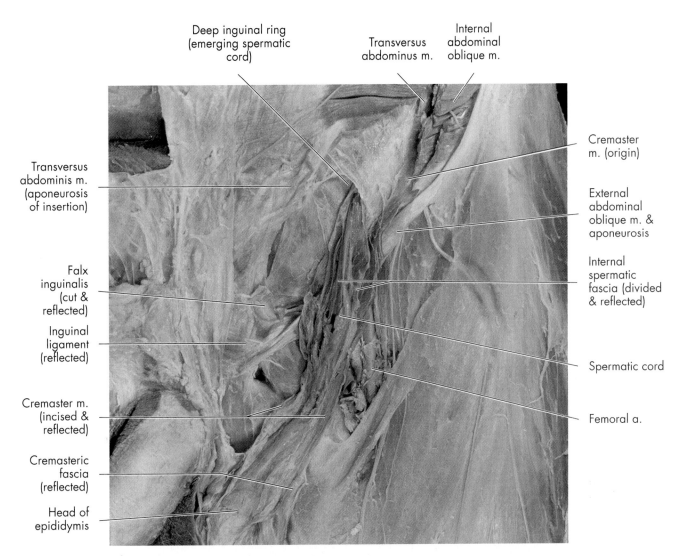

Figure 5-24   Internal oblique and transversus abdominis muscles divided close to their origins and insertions. The transversalis fascia is exposed in the area behind the inguinal canal. The internal spermatic fascia has been split longitudinally, and its margins have been retracted. *Inguinal hernias are a common consequence of bipedalism and weakness of support in the dependent inguinal region. More common in males than females, inguinal hernias are classified as direct or indirect. An indirect inguinal hernia results in ballooning forward of a finger of peritoneum along the course of the ordinarily obliterated processus vaginalis. Thus, like the core structures of the spermatic cord, it enters the inguinal canal at the internal ring lateral to the inferior epigastric vessels. A direct inguinal hernia bulges forward into the inguinal area medial to the course of the inferior epigastric vessels through the conjoined tendon in the so-called triangle of Hasselbach. This triangle is bounded by the inferior epigastric vessels laterally, the lateral border of the rectus sheath medially, and the inguinal ligament inferiorly. Both types of hernia pass through the superficial inguinal ring above the level of the pubic tubercle.*

Transversalis fascia   Inferior epigastric a. (cut)   Testicular a. entering deep inguinal ring   Lacunar ligament   Bladder

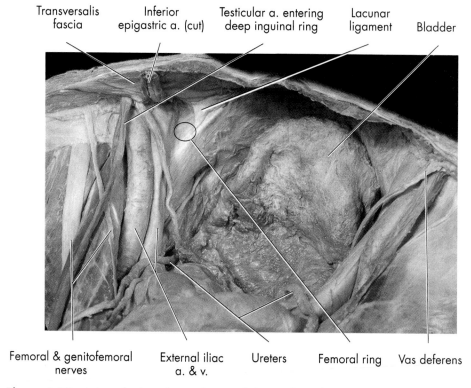

Femoral & genitofemoral nerves   External iliac a. & v.   Ureters   Femoral ring   Vas deferens

Figure 5-25 Internal view from above of the male pelvis showing the deep inguinal ring, the femoral ring, and the lacunar ligament.

Superficial inguinal ring   External oblique m. & aponeurosis (cut)   Fibers of internal oblique m.   Inguinal ligament

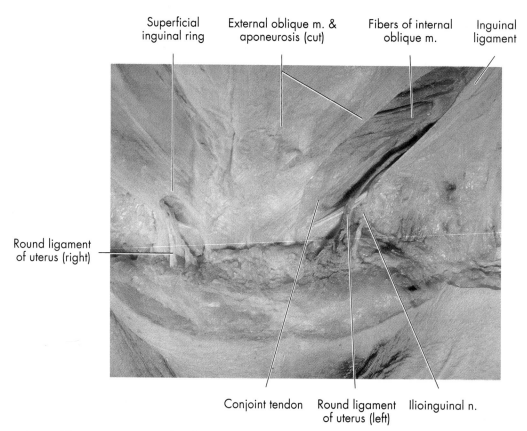

Round ligament of uterus (right)

Conjoint tendon   Round ligament of uterus (left)   Ilioinguinal n.

Figure 5-26 Superficial ring and inguinal canal in the female showing the round ligaments of the uterus.

See DISSECTIONS, Section 5, p. 6
See PRINCIPLES, Fig. 5-9

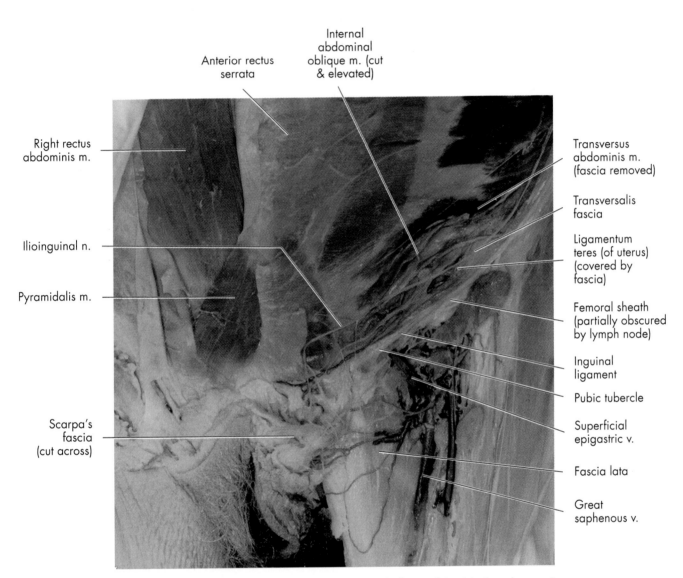

Anterior rectus
serrata

Internal
abdominal
oblique m. (cut
& elevated)

Right rectus
abdominis m.

Ilioinguinal n.

Pyramidalis m.

Scarpa's
fascia
(cut across)

Transversus
abdominis m.
(fascia removed)

Transversalis
fascia

Ligamentum
teres (of uterus)
(covered by
fascia)

Femoral sheath
(partially obscured
by lymph node)

Inguinal
ligament

Pubic tubercle

Superficial
epigastric v.

Fascia lata

Great
saphenous v.

Figure 5-27 Internal oblique muscle cut across and elevated in this female specimen. The round ligament of the uterus is exposed in the upper part of the inguinal canal. The canal is partially covered by the transversus abdominis muscle.

Inferior
epigastric
a.

Round ligament
of uterus

Transversus
abdominis
m.

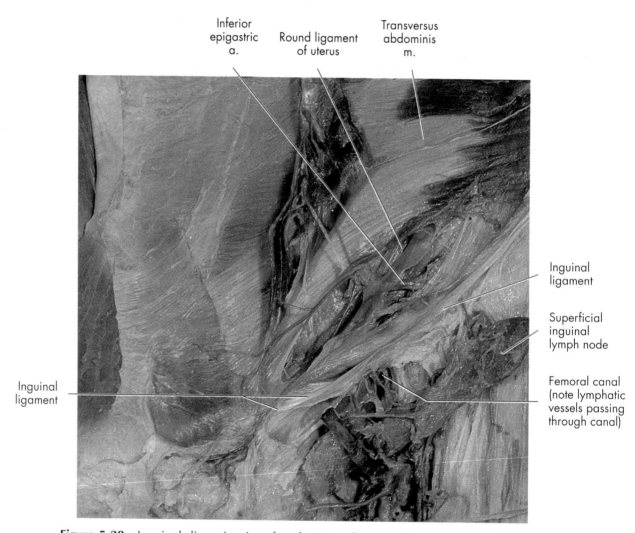

Inguinal
ligament

Superficial
inguinal
lymph node

Femoral canal
(note lymphatic
vessels passing
through canal)

Inguinal
ligament

Figure 5-28 Inguinal dissection in a female. Note the round ligament lifted away from the posterior wall of the inguinal canal. The transversus abdominis muscle has been elevated along its lower border. Note the lymphatic vessels passing through the femoral canal.

See **DISSECTIONS,** Section 5, p. 6

See **PRINCIPLES,** Fig. 5-9

Transversalis fascia   Deep inguinal ring

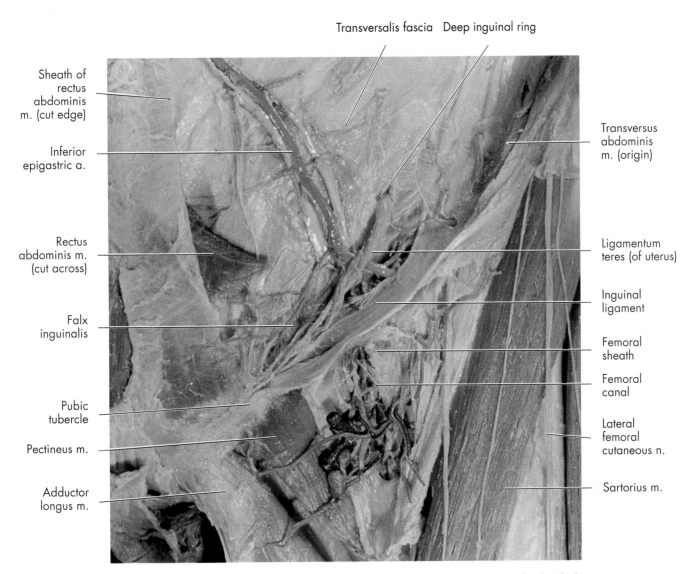

Sheath of
rectus
abdominis
m. (cut edge)

Inferior
epigastric a.

Rectus
abdominis m.
(cut across)

Falx
inguinalis

Pubic
tubercle

Pectineus m.

Adductor
longus m.

Transversus
abdominis
m. (origin)

Ligamentum
teres (of uterus)

Inguinal
ligament

Femoral
sheath

Femoral
canal

Lateral
femoral
cutaneous n.

Sartorius m.

Figure 5-29 Transversus abdominis muscle removed and the rectus muscle divided in
this dissection of the female inguinal canal.

SEE DISSECTIONS, SECTION 5, P. 7
SEE PRINCIPLES, FIGS. 5-11, 5-13

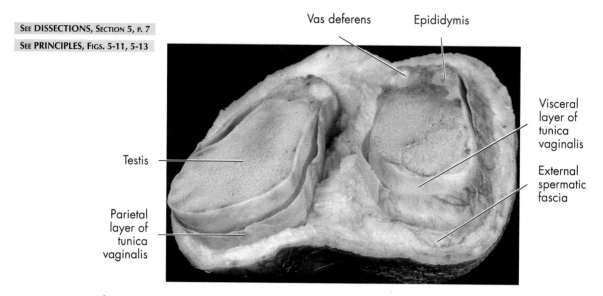

Vas deferens   Epididymis

Visceral
layer of
tunica
vaginalis

External
spermatic
fascia

Testis

Parietal
layer of
tunica
vaginalis

Figure 5-30   Transverse section through the scrotum. The spermatic fasciae are trimmed flush with the superficial fascia.

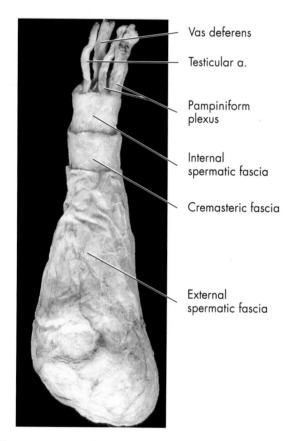

Vas deferens

Testicular a.

Pampiniform
plexus

Internal
spermatic fascia

Cremasteric fascia

External
spermatic fascia

Figure 5-31   Left testis and spermatic cord within their fascial sleeves. The internal spermatic fascia is derived from the transversalis fascia, the cremasteric from the transversus and internal oblique, and the external from the external oblique.

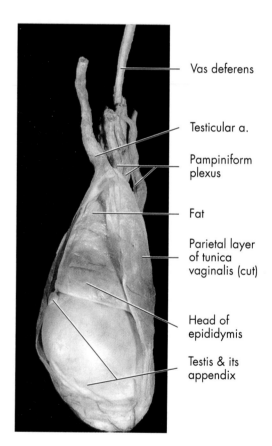

Vas deferens

Testicular a.

Pampiniform
plexus

Fat

Parietal layer
of tunica
vaginalis (cut)

Head of
epididymis

Testis & its
appendix

Figure 5-32   Anterolateral part of the parietal layer of the tunica vaginalis removed to reveal the testis and head of the epididymis. This testis bears a vestigial tag, the appendix of the testis. *Excess fluid collection and resulting distension of the tunica vaginalis creates a mass in the scrotum known as a hydrocele. A similar fluid-filled mass may occur along the ordinarily obliterated processus vaginalis and be manifested as a swelling on the spermatic cord. Such a mass is known as a hydrocele of the cord. Because hydroceles are filled with clear fluid, they ordinarily can be transilluminated using a bright flashlight in a darkened examining room.*

SEE DISSECTIONS, SECTION 5, P. 7
SEE PRINCIPLES, FIGS. 5-12, 5-13

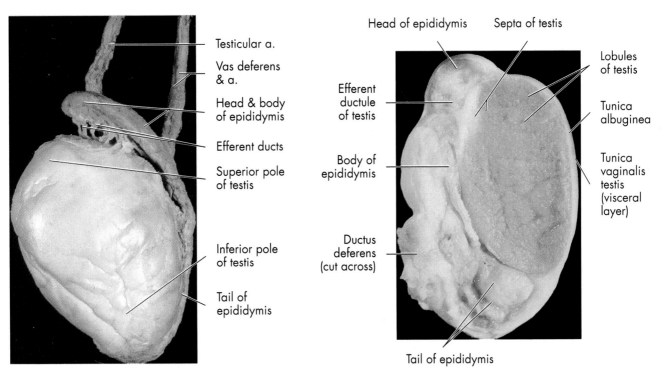

Figure 5-33 Lateral aspect of testis and epididymis after removal of the tunica vaginalis and pampiniform plexus. The head of the epididymis has been lifted to display the efferent ducts.

Figure 5-34 Testis cut in a sagittal plane. The section does not include the entire length of the epididymis since the body of the epididymis curves out of the plane of section. One or two other efferent ductules are indistinctly visible. Note the thick muscular tunic, thin mucosal tunic, and small lumen of the ductus deferens.

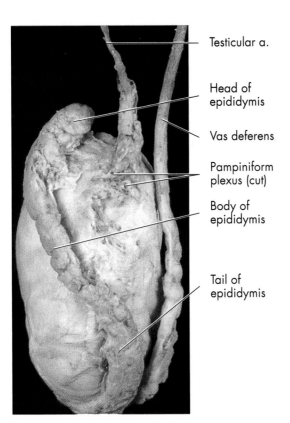

Figure 5-35 Posterior view of testis, epididymis, and vas deferens. *Inflammation of the epididymis results in swelling and acute pain, discomfort, and tenderness of the easily palpable epididymis. A testicular neoplasm is generally less tender and palpably separate from the epididymis.*

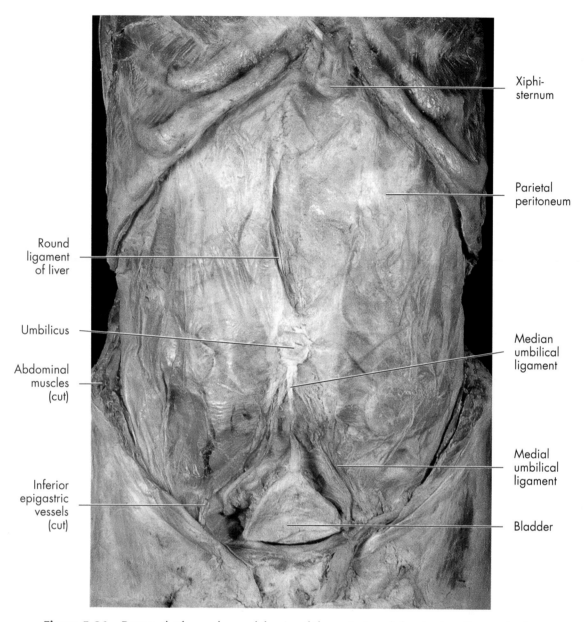

Xiphi-sternum

Parietal peritoneum

Round ligament of liver

Umbilicus

Abdominal muscles (cut)

Median umbilical ligament

Medial umbilical ligament

Inferior epigastric vessels (cut)

Bladder

Figure 5-36   Removal of muscles and fascia of the anterior abdominal wall reveals the parietal peritoneum and extraperitoneal structures. *Ordinarily the urachal connection between bladder and umbilicus is obliterated to remain as the median umbilical liga-ment in the midline of the anterior abdominal wall. The urachus sometimes remains open after birth, resulting in fluid discharge from the umbilicus (patent urachus). Partial but incomplete obliteration of the urachus results in formation of a cystic mass along the midline in the medial umbilical ligament (urachal cyst).*

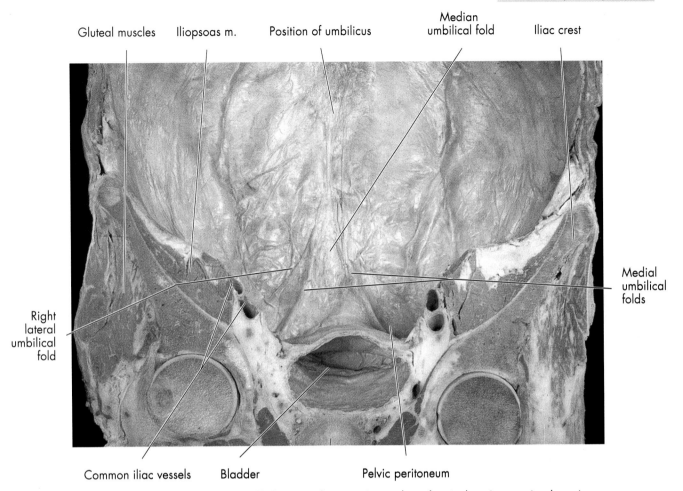

Gluteal muscles   Iliopsoas m.   Position of umbilicus   Median umbilical fold   Iliac crest

Median umbilical fold

Medial umbilical folds

Right lateral umbilical fold

Common iliac vessels   Bladder   Pelvic peritoneum

Figure 5-37   Abdominal wall from within (peritoneal surface) showing parietal peritoneum and folds.

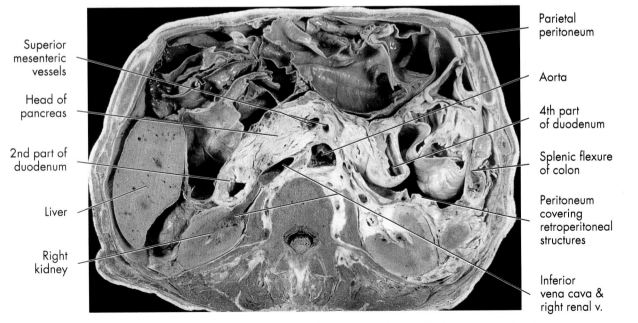

Superior mesenteric vessels

Head of pancreas

2nd part of duodenum

Liver

Right kidney

Parietal peritoneum

Aorta

4th part of duodenum

Splenic flexure of colon

Peritoneum covering retroperitoneal structures

Inferior vena cava & right renal v.

Figure 5-38   Transverse section through the abdomen at the level of the second lumbar vertebra looking upward from below showing the relationship of the peritoneum to retroperitoneal structures.

See **DISSECTIONS**, Section 5, p. 8

See **PRINCIPLES**, Figs. 5-20, 5-36, 5-37

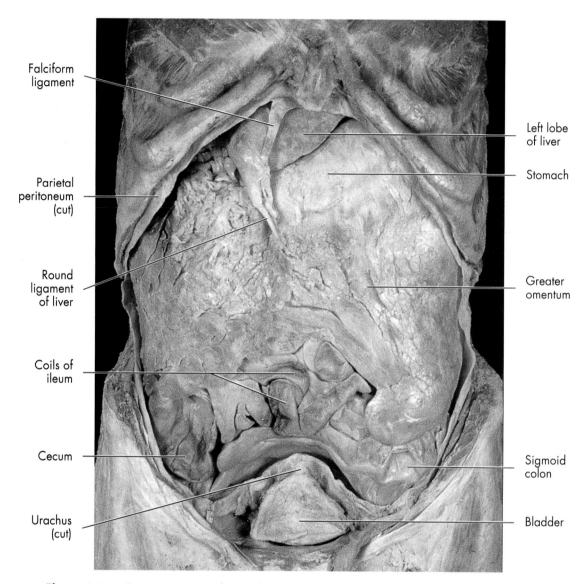

Falciform ligament

Parietal peritoneum (cut)

Round ligament of liver

Coils of ileum

Cecum

Urachus (cut)

Left lobe of liver

Stomach

Greater omentum

Sigmoid colon

Bladder

Figure 5-39 Greater peritoneal sac after removal of most of the parietal peritoneum. In this specimen, the greater omentum is adherent to the right side of the diaphragm, concealing the right lobe of the liver and the gallbladder. *The round ligament of the liver (ligamentum teres) represents the obliterated umbilical vein. Although this vein becomes obliterated, the vein remains open for several hours after birth and is often used as a means to obtain blood samples or as a site for intravenous blood transfusion.*

See DISSECTIONS, Section 5, p. 8
See PRINCIPLES, Figs. 5-37, 5-38

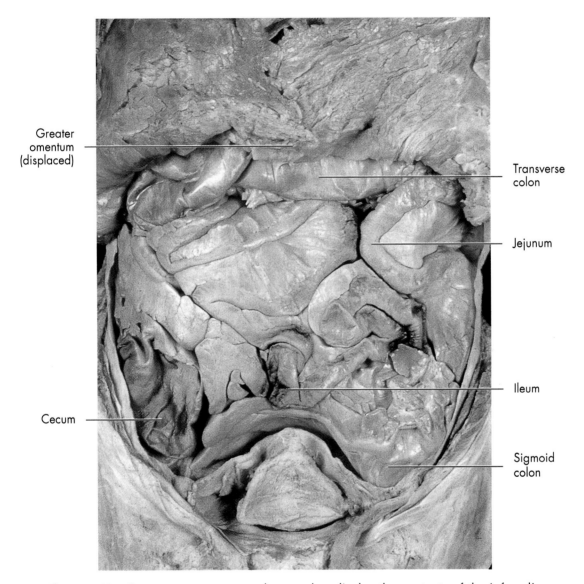

Greater omentum (displaced)

Transverse colon

Jejunum

Ileum

Cecum

Sigmoid colon

Figure 5-40 Greater omentum turned upward to display the contents of the infracolic compartment of the greater peritoneal sac.

See DISSECTIONS, Section 5, p. 9
See PRINCIPLES, Fig. 5-18

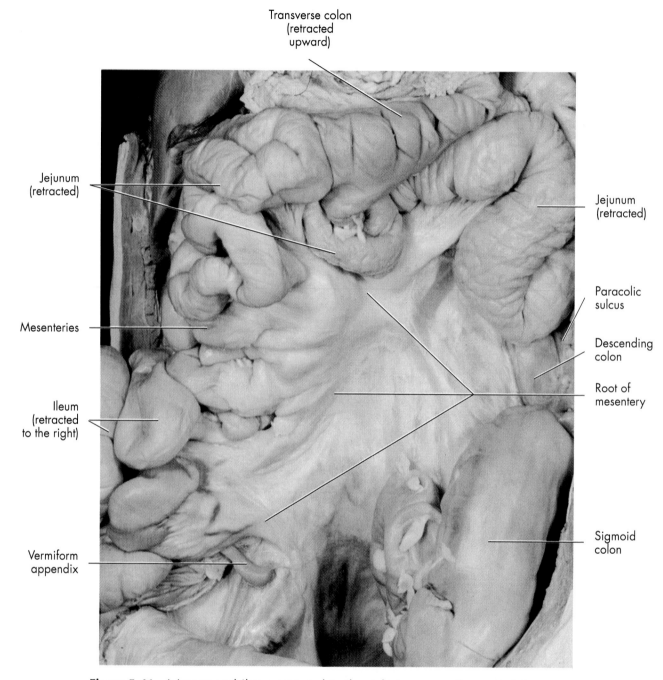

Transverse colon
(retracted
upward)

Jejunum
(retracted)

Jejunum
(retracted)

Paracolic
sulcus

Mesenteries

Descending
colon

Root of
mesentery

Ileum
(retracted
to the right)

Vermiform
appendix

Sigmoid
colon

Figure 5-41   Jejunum and ileum retracted to the right to expose the root of the mesentery and to demonstrate the posterior part of the peritoneal cavity to the left of the mesentery. *The mesentery is laden with lymphatics and lymph nodes. Acute inflammatory disorders of the bowel sometimes result in hyperplasia and enlargement of these nodes. The symptoms and signs are like those of acute appendicitis and often the surgeon operating for "acute appendicitis" will find a normal appendix but abnormal enlarged mesenteric lymph nodes (mesenteric adenitis).*

SEE DISSECTIONS, SECTION 5, P. 9
SEE PRINCIPLES, FIG. 5-18

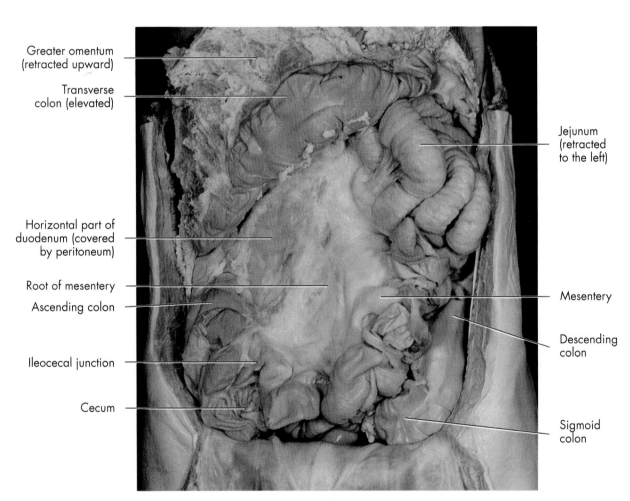

Greater omentum
(retracted upward)

Transverse
colon (elevated)

Jejunum
(retracted
to the left)

Horizontal part of
duodenum (covered
by peritoneum)

Root of mesentery

Ascending colon

Mesentery

Descending
colon

Ileocecal junction

Cecum

Sigmoid
colon

Figure 5-42 Greater omentum and transverse colon retracted upward to expose the infraomental part of the peritoneal cavity. Loops of the jejunum and ileum have been arranged to display the right side of the mesentery.

SEE DISSECTIONS, SECTION 5, P. 14
SEE PRINCIPLES, FIG. 5-18

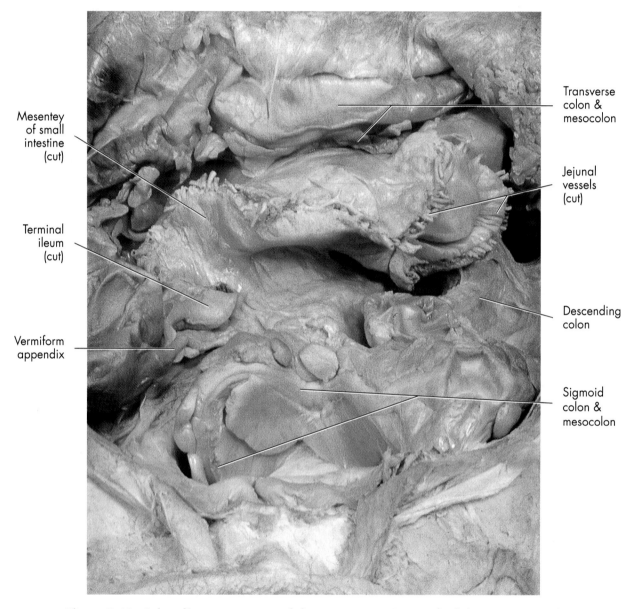

Mesentey
of small
intestine
(cut)

Terminal
ileum
(cut)

Vermiform
appendix

Transverse
colon &
mesocolon

Jejunal
vessels
(cut)

Descending
colon

Sigmoid
colon &
mesocolon

Figure 5-43 Infracolic compartment of the greater sac. Removal of the jejunum and ileum reveals their cut mesenteries. The descending colon is more medially placed than usual.

See DISSECTIONS, Section 5, p. 12

See PRINCIPLES, Fig. 5-21

Diaphragm
(cut)

Right & left
lobes of
liver

Subphrenic
spaces

Fibrous
pericardium

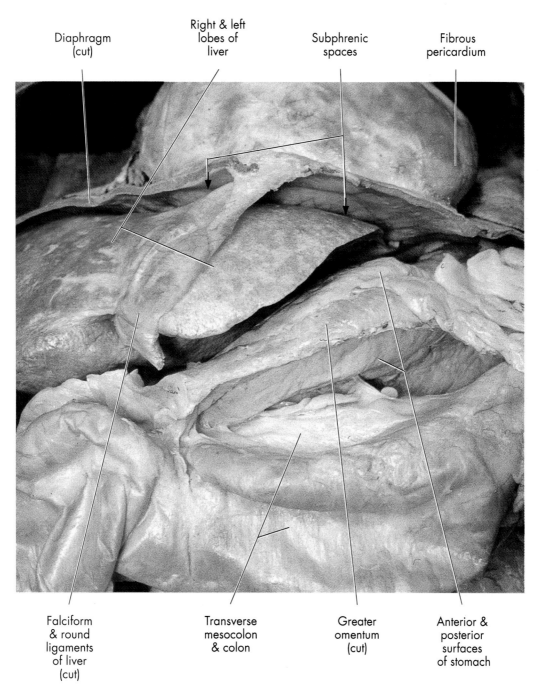

Falciform
& round
ligaments
of liver
(cut)

Transverse
mesocolon
& colon

Greater
omentum
(cut)

Anterior &
posterior
surfaces
of stomach

Figure 5-44   Supracolic compartment of the greater sac. After removal of most of the greater omentum, the greater curve of the stomach has been displaced upward to show the position of the lesser sac.

See DISSECTIONS, Section 5, pp. 10 and 12
See PRINCIPLES, Figs. 5-20, 5-37

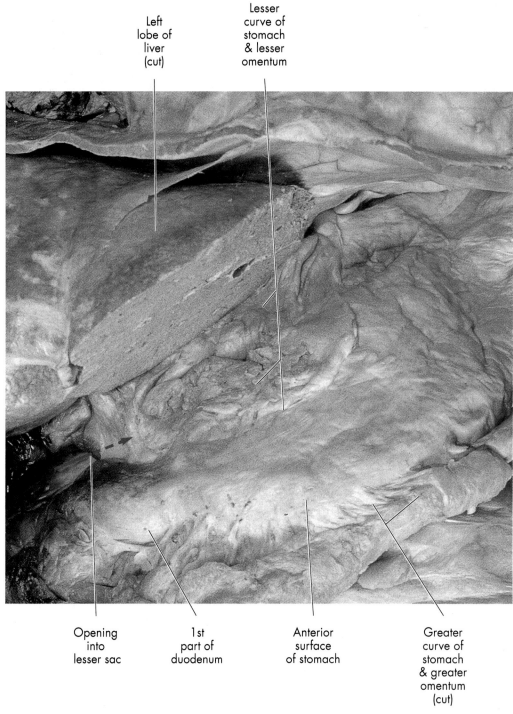

Left
lobe of
liver
(cut)

Lesser
curve of
stomach
& lesser
omentum

Opening
into
lesser sac

1st
part of
duodenum

Anterior
surface
of stomach

Greater
curve of
stomach
& greater
omentum
(cut)

Figure 5-45 Lesser omentum and opening into the lesser sac (epiploic foramen of Winslow) after removal of part of the left lobe of the liver.

SEE DISSECTIONS, SECTION 5, P. 10
SEE PRINCIPLES, FIGS. 5-25, 5-37

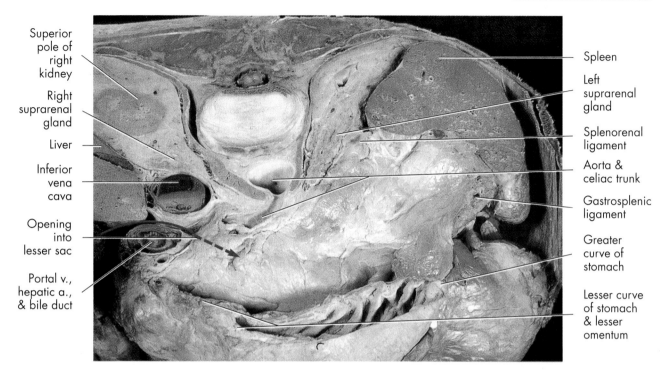

Superior pole of right kidney

Right suprarenal gland

Liver

Inferior vena cava

Opening into lesser sac

Portal v., hepatic a., & bile duct

Spleen

Left suprarenal gland

Splenorenal ligament

Aorta & celiac trunk

Gastrosplenic ligament

Greater curve of stomach

Lesser curve of stomach & lesser omentum

Figure 5-46 Transverse section at the level of the disk between the twelfth thoracic and first lumbar vertebra. This section is cut through the stomach showing the lesser sac and its opening. In this specimen, the left kidney lies lower than usual. *An ulcer on the posterior wall of the stomach or first part of the duodenum may perforate through the wall. The gastric contents leak into the lesser sac and only reach the general peritoneal cavity by passing through the epiploic foramen (of Winslow) indicated by the arrow. This contrasts with ulcers located anteriorly, which perforate directly into the general peritoneal cavity.*

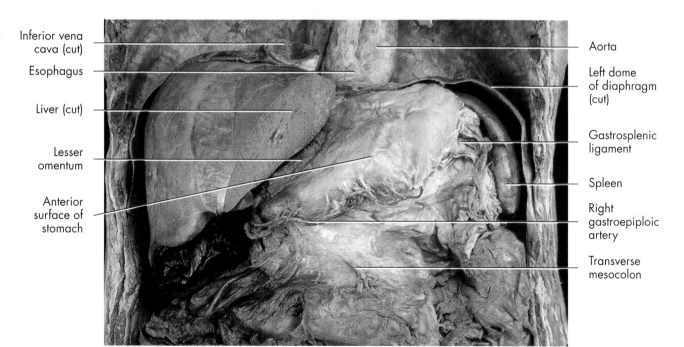

Inferior vena cava (cut)

Esophagus

Liver (cut)

Lesser omentum

Anterior surface of stomach

Aorta

Left dome of diaphragm (cut)

Gastrosplenic ligament

Spleen

Right gastroepiploic artery

Transverse mesocolon

Figure 5-47 Stomach and some of its relationships seen after removal of the anterior half of the diaphragm and left lobe of the liver and dissection of the greater omentum.

See DISSECTIONS, Section 5, p. 11
See PRINCIPLES, Fig. 5-19

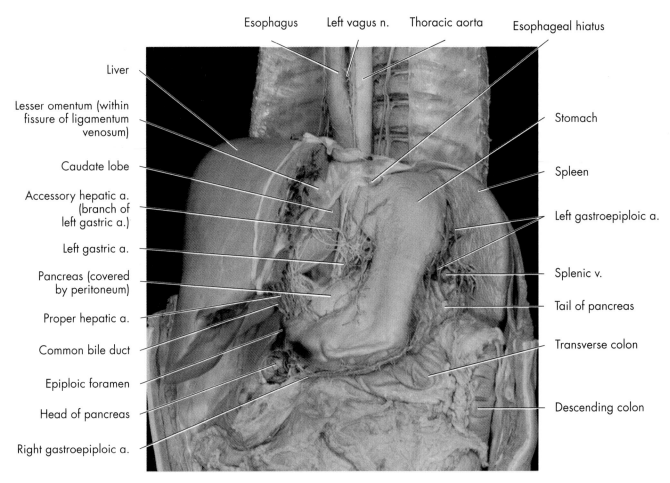

Esophagus   Left vagus n.   Thoracic aorta   Esophageal hiatus

Liver

Lesser omentum (within fissure of ligamentum venosum)

Caudate lobe

Accessory hepatic a. (branch of left gastric a.)

Left gastric a.

Pancreas (covered by peritoneum)

Proper hepatic a.

Common bile duct

Epiploic foramen

Head of pancreas

Right gastroepiploic a.

Stomach

Spleen

Left gastroepiploic a.

Splenic v.

Tail of pancreas

Transverse colon

Descending colon

Figure 5-48 Stomach dissected to show relationships to the liver, spleen, transverse colon, pancreas, and half of the left diaphragm. In this view, lymphatic vessels and nodes have been removed to display blood vessels and nerves that reach the stomach.

See DISSECTIONS, Section 5, p. 11

See PRINCIPLES, Fig. 5-19

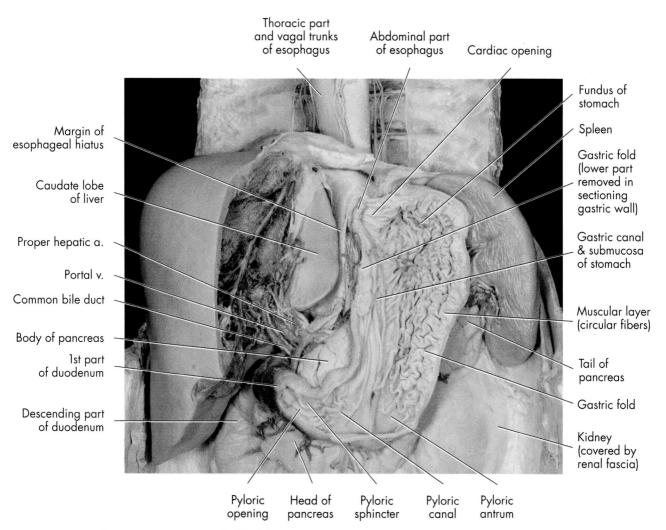

Thoracic part
and vagal trunks
of esophagus

Abdominal part
of esophagus

Cardiac opening

Margin of
esophageal hiatus

Caudate lobe
of liver

Proper hepatic a.

Portal v.

Common bile duct

Body of pancreas

1st part
of duodenum

Descending part
of duodenum

Fundus of
stomach

Spleen

Gastric fold
(lower part
removed in
sectioning
gastric wall)

Gastric canal
& submucosa
of stomach

Muscular layer
(circular fibers)

Tail of
pancreas

Gastric fold

Kidney
(covered by
renal fascia)

Pyloric
opening

Head of
pancreas

Pyloric
sphincter

Pyloric
canal

Pyloric
antrum

Figure 5-49   Anterior half of the stomach removed to show the configuration of the gastric mucosal folds and pyloric sphincter. Note the hepatic plexus of nerves accompanying the proper hepatic artery. *Since the vagus nerves (parasympathetic) stimulate acid secretion in the stomach, various surgical procedures have been developed to cut this nerve supply. A truncal vagotomy divides the vagal trunks at the level of the diaphragm. This eliminates all parasympathetic nerve supply to the foregut, midgut, and their associated structures. Thus gastric peristalsis diminishes, and the pyloric sphincter contracts so that the stomach fails to empty. With a truncal vagotomy, therefore, a procedure must be done to enhance emptying of the stomach (a pyloroplasty or a gastrojejunostomy). A highly selective vagotomy is intended to divide only those vagal branches that supply gastric secretory cells.*

See PRINCIPLES, Fig. 5-32

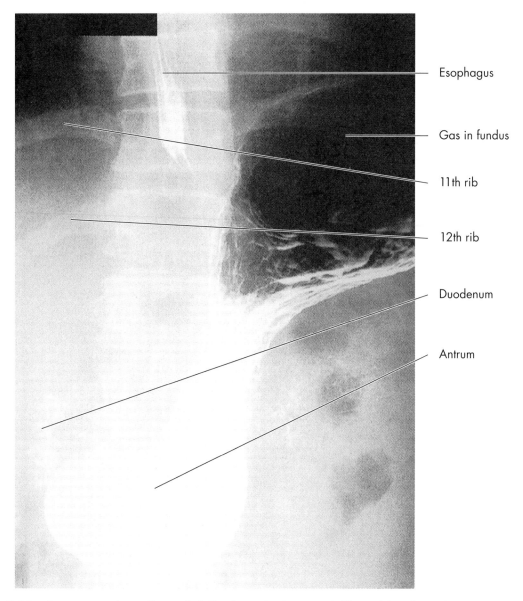

Esophagus

Gas in fundus

11th rib

12th rib

Duodenum

Antrum

Figure 5-50   Anteroposterior radiograph following a barium meal. The subject is supine and most of the barium has pooled into the antrum of the stomach.

See **PRINCIPLES**, Fig. 5-32

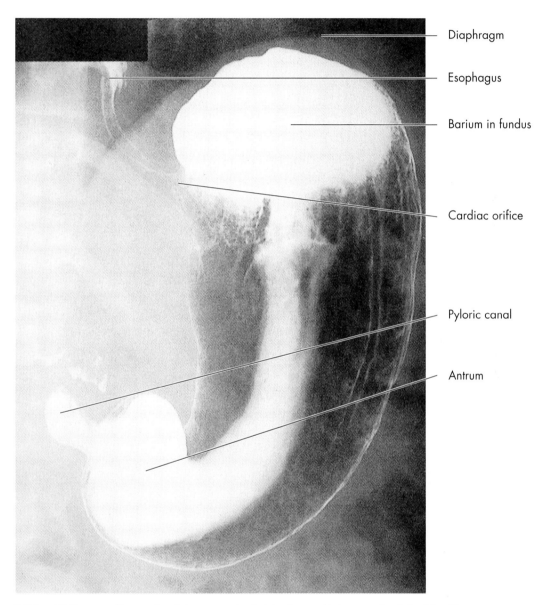

Diaphragm

Esophagus

Barium in fundus

Cardiac orifice

Pyloric canal

Antrum

Figure 5-51   Oblique radiograph of the same individual, now lying on the left side. The barium has flowed into the fundus of the stomach.

378

See DISSECTIONS, Section 5, p. 11
See PRINCIPLES, Figs. 5-18, 5-19

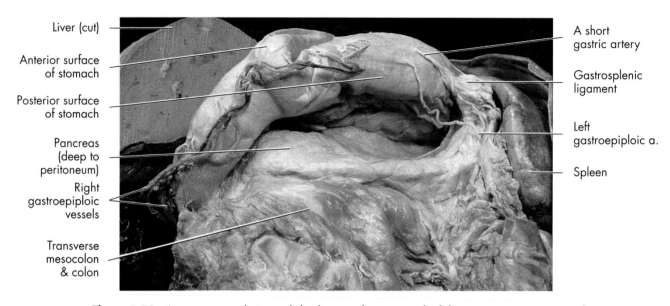

Liver (cut)

Anterior surface
of stomach

Posterior surface
of stomach

Pancreas
(deep to
peritoneum)

Right
gastroepiploic
vessels

Transverse
mesocolon
& colon

A short
gastric artery

Gastrosplenic
ligament

Left
gastroepiploic a.

Spleen

Figure 5-52 Lesser sac and stomach bed seen after removal of the greater omentum and lifting the greater curvature upward.

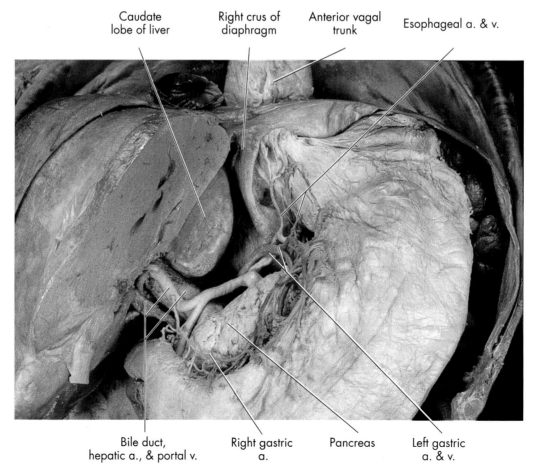

Caudate
lobe of liver

Right crus of
diaphragm

Anterior vagal
trunk

Esophageal a. & v.

Bile duct,
hepatic a., & portal v.

Right gastric
a.

Pancreas

Left gastric
a. & v.

Figure 5-53 Dissection of the lesser omentum showing structures along the lesser curvature of the stomach.

See **DISSECTIONS**, Section 5, p. 11

See **PRINCIPLES**, Figs. 5-27, 5-33

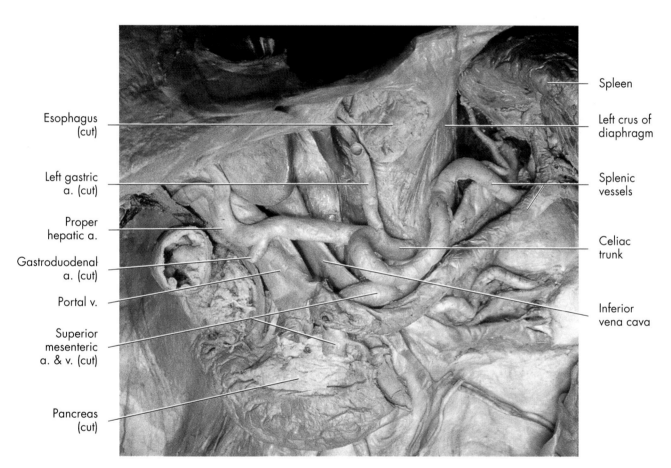

Esophagus (cut)

Left gastric a. (cut)

Proper hepatic a.

Gastroduodenal a. (cut)

Portal v.

Superior mesenteric a. & v. (cut)

Pancreas (cut)

Spleen

Left crus of diaphragm

Splenic vessels

Celiac trunk

Inferior vena cava

Figure 5-54 Stomach and most of the pancreas removed to reveal the celiac trunk and its branches.

SEE **DISSECTIONS**, SECTION 5, P. 13

SEE **PRINCIPLES**, FIG. 5-25

Gastric impression   Superior border   Notches

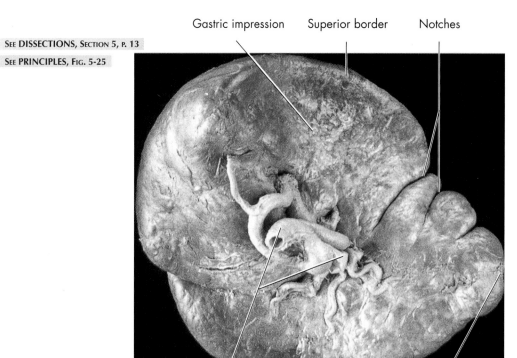

Splenic a. & v. (cut)   Inferior border   Anterior extremity

Figure 5-55   Visceral surface of the spleen. *Blunt trauma to the upper abdomen is most likely to injure solid organs such as the liver, spleen, or kidneys. The spleen, although protected by the lower ribcage, is subject to rupture because of its soft parenchyma and relatively delicate capsule. Rupture of the spleen results in intraperitoneal bleeding that can be life threatening if left unheeded. Surgical repair is sometimes successful, but often the spleen must be removed (splenectomy).*

Superior border

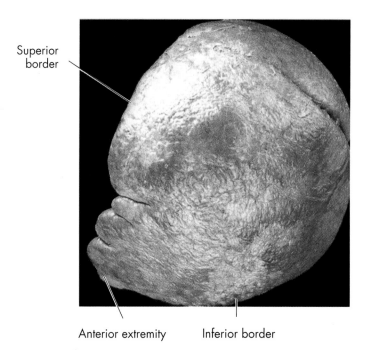

Anterior extremity   Inferior border

Figure 5-56   Diaphragmatic surface of the spleen. This specimen has several well-defined notches on its superior border and, in addition, a single notch on the inferior border.

SEE DISSECTIONS, SECTION 5, P. 13
SEE PRINCIPLES, FIG. 5-25

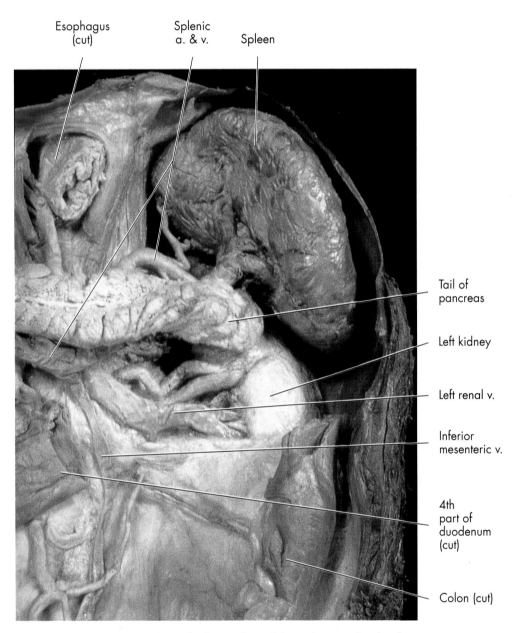

Esophagus (cut)

Splenic a. & v.

Spleen

Tail of pancreas

Left kidney

Left renal v.

Inferior mesenteric v.

4th part of duodenum (cut)

Colon (cut)

Figure 5-57 Spleen and its vessels and relationship of the spleen to the diaphragm, pancreas, and left kidney. The stomach, part of the colon, and all of the peritoneum have been removed.

382   **Clinical Anatomy Atlas**

SEE DISSECTIONS, SECTION 5, P. 13

SEE PRINCIPLES, FIGS. 5-27, 5-39

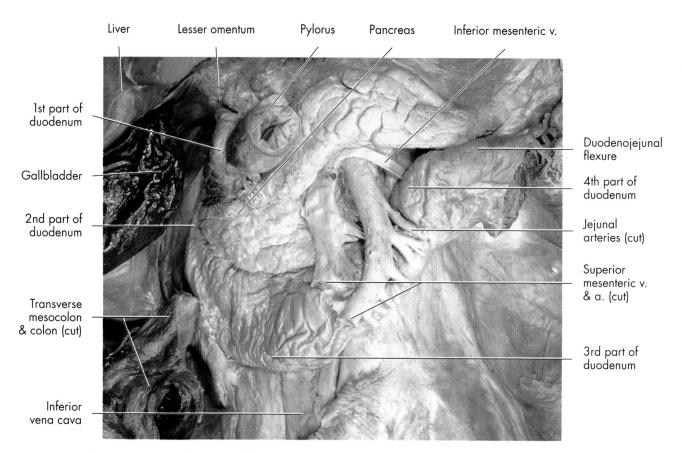

Figure 5-58   Duodenum and some related structures. The liver and gallbladder have been slightly displaced.

See DISSECTIONS, Section 5, p. 14

See PRINCIPLES, Fig. 5-17

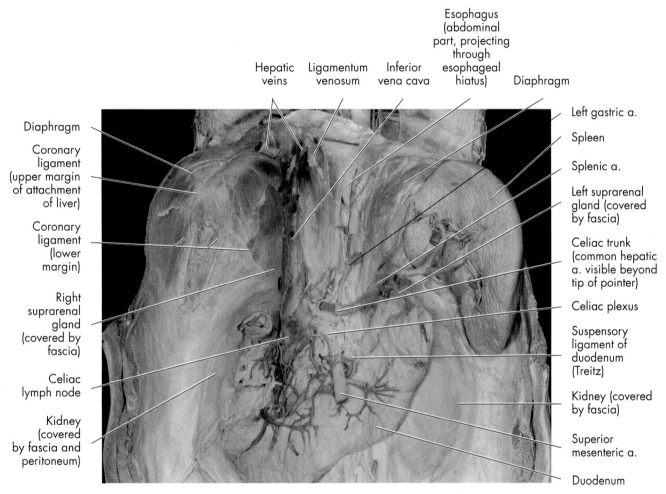

Hepatic veins

Ligamentum venosum

Inferior vena cava

Esophagus (abdominal part, projecting through esophageal hiatus)

Diaphragm

Diaphragm

Coronary ligament (upper margin of attachment of liver)

Coronary ligament (lower margin)

Right suprarenal gland (covered by fascia)

Celiac lymph node

Kidney (covered by fascia and peritoneum)

Left gastric a.

Spleen

Splenic a.

Left suprarenal gland (covered by fascia)

Celiac trunk (common hepatic a. visible beyond tip of pointer)

Celiac plexus

Suspensory ligament of duodenum (Treitz)

Kidney (covered by fascia)

Superior mesenteric a.

Duodenum

Figure 5-59 Coronary ligaments divided and the liver removed from the specimen. The course of the splenic artery and proximal part of the superior mesenteric artery are displayed. Note elongated downward extensions of the peritoneal reflection of the coronary ligament onto the liver. These reflections form the boundary of several peritoneal recesses between the diaphragm and the liver.

See **DISSECTIONS**, Section 5, p. 14

See **PRINCIPLES**, Fig. 5-24

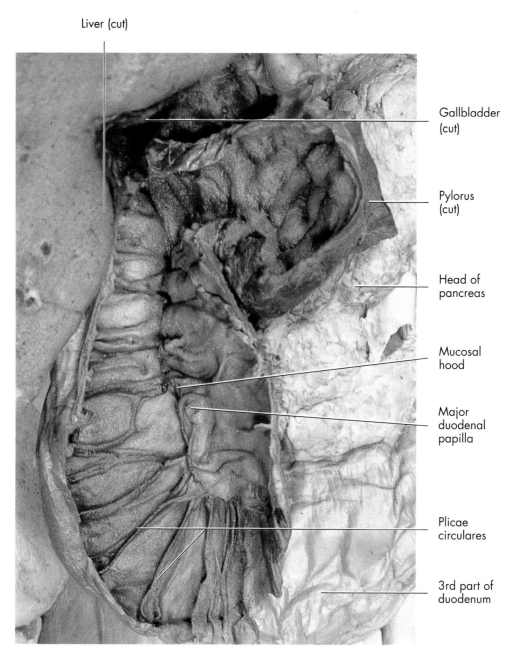

Liver (cut)

Gallbladder (cut)

Pylorus (cut)

Head of pancreas

Mucosal hood

Major duodenal papilla

Plicae circulares

3rd part of duodenum

Figure 5-60   First and second parts of the duodenum opened to show the plicae circulares and the major duodenal papilla.

SEE DISSECTIONS, SECTION 5, P. 14

SEE PRINCIPLES, FIG. 5-24

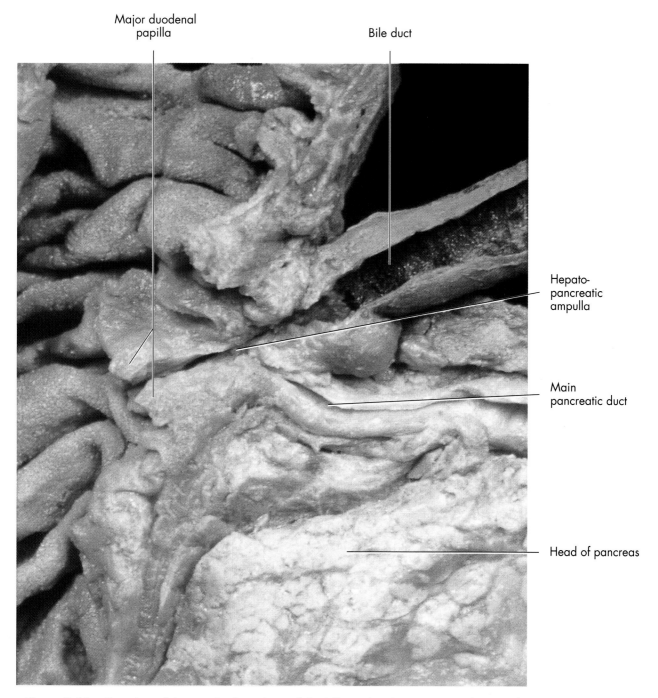

Figure 5-61 Opening of the terminal portions of the bile and main pancreatic ducts and the hepatopancreatic ampulla.

SEE DISSECTIONS, SECTION 5, P. 14

SEE PRINCIPLES, FIG. 5-27

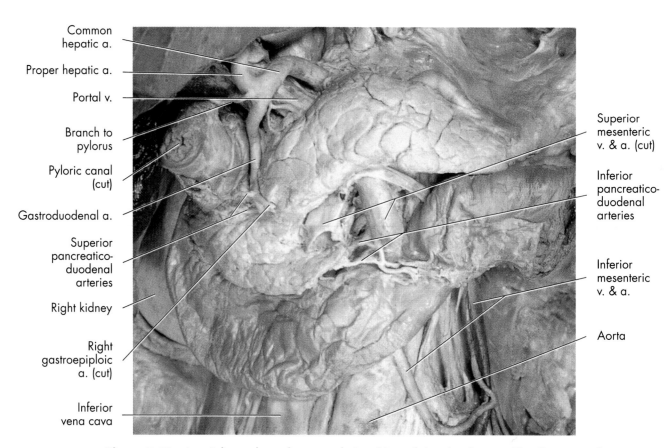

Common
hepatic a.

Proper hepatic a.

Portal v.

Branch to
pylorus

Pyloric canal
(cut)

Gastroduodenal a.

Superior
pancreatico-
duodenal
arteries

Right kidney

Right
gastroepiploic
a. (cut)

Inferior
vena cava

Superior
mesenteric
v. & a. (cut)

Inferior
pancreatico-
duodenal
arteries

Inferior
mesenteric
v. & a.

Aorta

Figure 5-62 Arterial supply and some relationships of the duodenum. The first part of
the duodenum has been displaced laterally to reveal the gastroduodenal artery, bile duct,
and portal vein.

See DISSECTIONS, Section 5, p. 14
See PRINCIPLES, Fig. 5-27

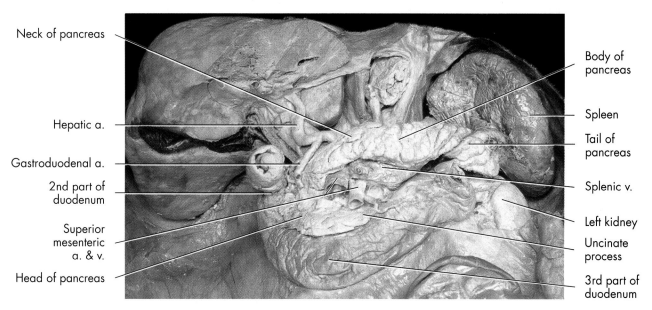

Neck of pancreas

Hepatic a.

Gastroduodenal a.

2nd part of
duodenum

Superior
mesenteric
a. & v.

Head of pancreas

Body of
pancreas

Spleen

Tail of
pancreas

Splenic v.

Left kidney

Uncinate
process

3rd part of
duodenum

Figure 5-63   Principal relationships and parts of the pancreas.

SEE DISSECTIONS, SECTION 5, P. 14
SEE PRINCIPLES, FIG. 5-28

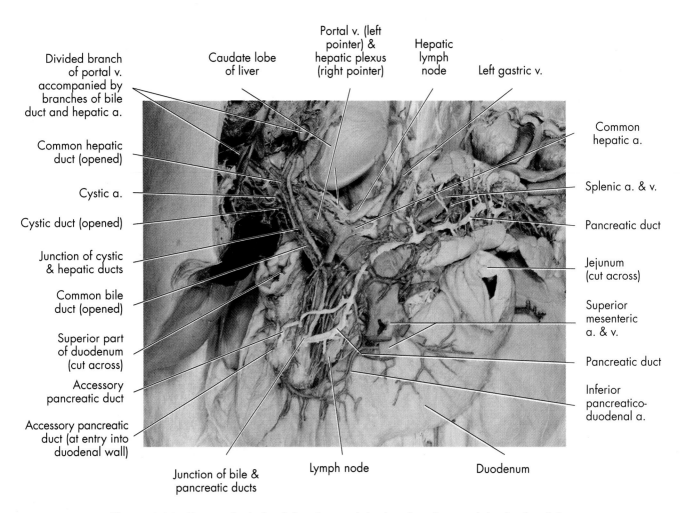

Figure 5-64   Removal of glandular tissue of the head and part of the body of the pancreas. Openings have been cut in the bile ducts, gallbladder, and main pancreatic duct. Blood vessels to the anterior and posterior aspects of the duodenum have been preserved.

S<small>EE</small> **DISSECTIONS**, S<small>ECTION</small> 5, <small>P.</small> 14
S<small>EE</small> **PRINCIPLES**, F<small>IG.</small> 5-28

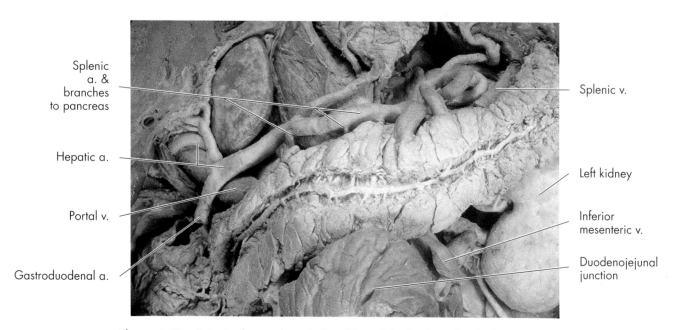

Splenic
a. &
branches
to pancreas

Hepatic a.

Portal v.

Gastroduodenal a.

Splenic v.

Left kidney

Inferior
mesenteric v.

Duodenojejunal
junction

Figure 5-65   Principal vascular relationships of the body and tail of the pancreas.

See **DISSECTIONS**, Section 5, p. 14

See **PRINCIPLES**, Fig. 5-24

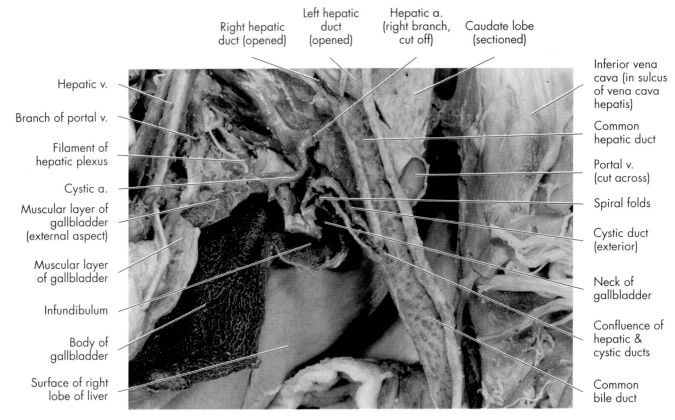

Right hepatic duct (opened)

Left hepatic duct (opened)

Hepatic a. (right branch, cut off)

Caudate lobe (sectioned)

Hepatic v.

Branch of portal v.

Filament of hepatic plexus

Cystic a.

Muscular layer of gallbladder (external aspect)

Muscular layer of gallbladder

Infundibulum

Body of gallbladder

Surface of right lobe of liver

Inferior vena cava (in sulcus of vena cava hepatis)

Common hepatic duct

Portal v. (cut across)

Spiral folds

Cystic duct (exterior)

Neck of gallbladder

Confluence of hepatic & cystic ducts

Common bile duct

Figure 5-66   Close-up view of the interior of the biliary tract and gallbladder. Note plicae tunicae mucosae in the body of the gallbladder. *Gallstones sometimes form within the gallbladder (cholecystolithiasis), a site where bile is stored and concentrated. Such stones may incite inflammation of the gallbladder (cholecystitis) or pass down the cystic duct to the common bile duct (choledocholithiasis). If such stones fail to pass into the duodenum, they may block the flow of bile in the common bile duct and cause jaundice.*

SEE DISSECTIONS, SECTION 5, P. 14

SEE PRINCIPLES, FIG. 5-24

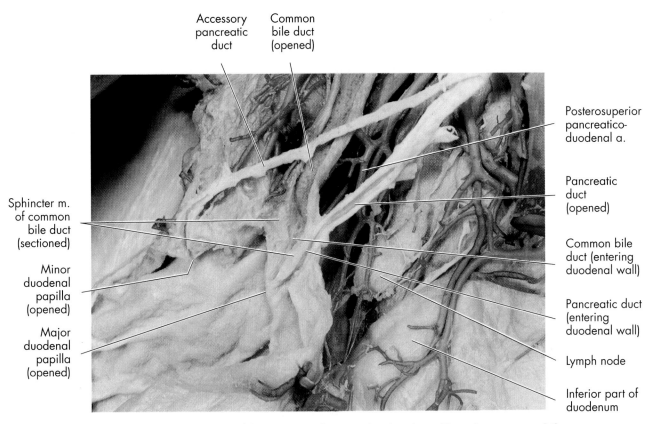

Accessory
pancreatic
duct

Common
bile duct
(opened)

Posterosuperior
pancreatico-
duodenal a.

Pancreatic
duct
(opened)

Common bile
duct (entering
duodenal wall)

Pancreatic duct
(entering
duodenal wall)

Lymph node

Inferior part of
duodenum

Sphincter m.
of common
bile duct
(sectioned)

Minor
duodenal
papilla
(opened)

Major
duodenal
papilla
(opened)

Figure 5-67   Close-up view of the major and minor duodenal papillae, the common bile duct, and the main and accessory pancreatic ducts.

See DISSECTIONS, Section 5, p. 12
See PRINCIPLES, Fig. 5-21

Falciform ligament   Left lobe of liver

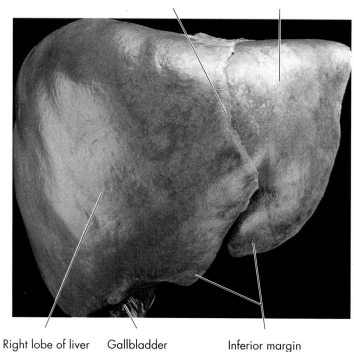

Right lobe of liver   Gallbladder   Inferior margin

Figure 5-68   Anterior view of the liver.

Right lobe   Diaphragm   Falciform ligament & edge cut   Left lobe
of liver   (cut)   from anterior abdominal wall   of liver

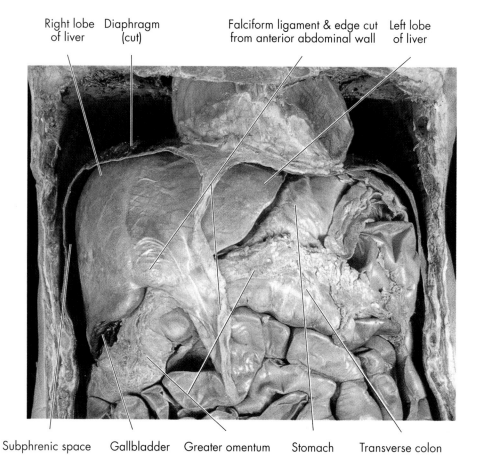

Subphrenic space   Gallbladder   Greater omentum   Stomach   Transverse colon

Figure 5-69   Liver and some of its relationships. In this specimen the greater omentum is adherent to the liver and stomach.

SEE **DISSECTIONS**, SECTION 5, P. 12

SEE **PRINCIPLES**, FIG. 5-23

Left triangular ligament — Openings of hepatic veins — Inferior vena cava (partially removed) — Bare area

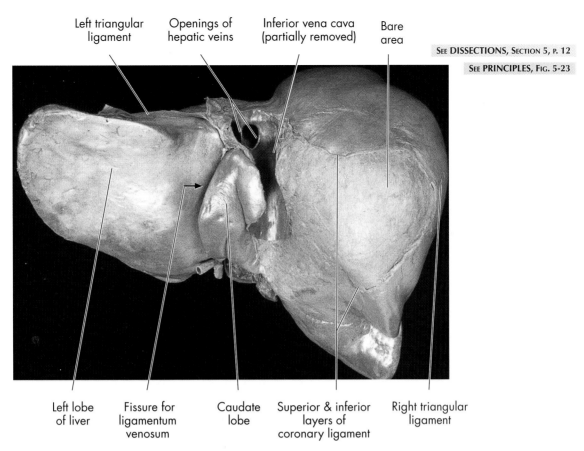

Left lobe of liver — Fissure for ligamentum venosum — Caudate lobe — Superior & inferior layers of coronary ligament — Right triangular ligament

Figure 5-70   Posterior view of the liver.

Portal v. — Caudate lobe — Bare area — Hepatic ducts — Indentation for right kidney

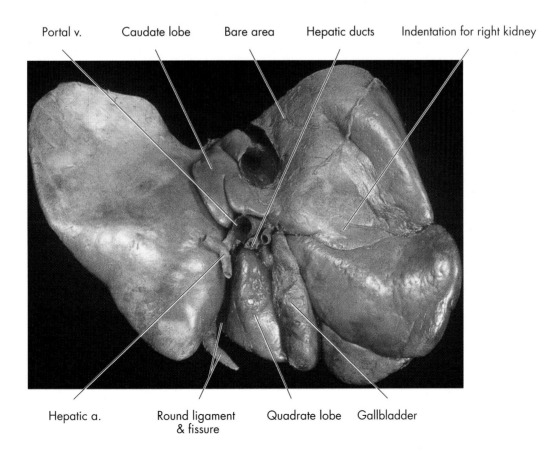

Hepatic a. — Round ligament & fissure — Quadrate lobe — Gallbladder

Figure 5-71   Inferior view of the liver and gallbladder showing the porta hepatis and visceral surface.

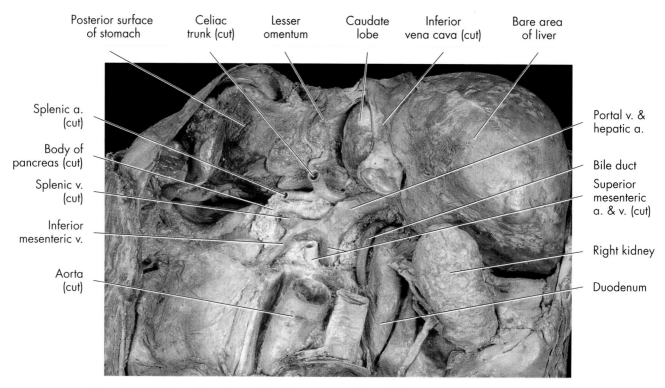

Posterior surface of stomach

Celiac trunk (cut)

Lesser omentum

Caudate lobe

Inferior vena cava (cut)

Bare area of liver

Splenic a. (cut)

Body of pancreas (cut)

Splenic v. (cut)

Inferior mesenteric v.

Aorta (cut)

Portal v. & hepatic a.

Bile duct

Superior mesenteric a. & v. (cut)

Right kidney

Duodenum

Figure 5-72   Posterior view of the liver, stomach, and lesser omentum. The spleen, left kidney, parts of the pancreas, aorta, and inferior vena cava have been removed.

See DISSECTIONS, Section 5, p. 11

See PRINCIPLES, Fig. 5-23

Liver (cut)   Common hepatic duct   Right & left hepatic ducts   Left branch of portal v.   Caudate lobe   Celiac trunk

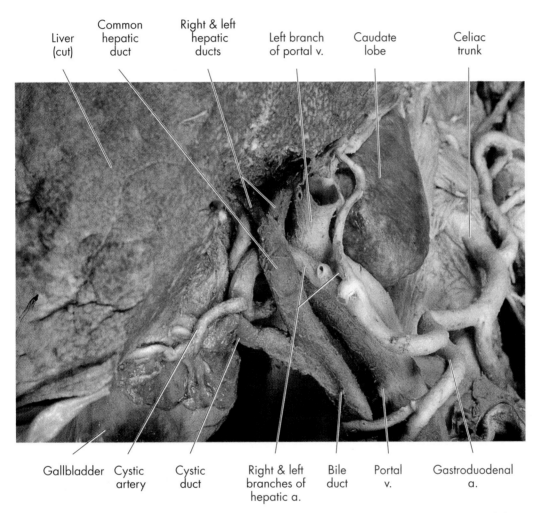

Gallbladder   Cystic artery   Cystic duct   Right & left branches of hepatic a.   Bile duct   Portal v.   Gastroduodenal a.

Figure 5-73   Porta hepatis including the right, left, and common hepatic ducts and the cystic branch of the hepatic artery.

See DISSECTIONS, SECTION 5, P. 11

See PRINCIPLES, FIG. 5-33

Bile duct

Right & left branches of hepatic a.

Caudate lobe of liver

Portal v.

Left gastric a. & v.

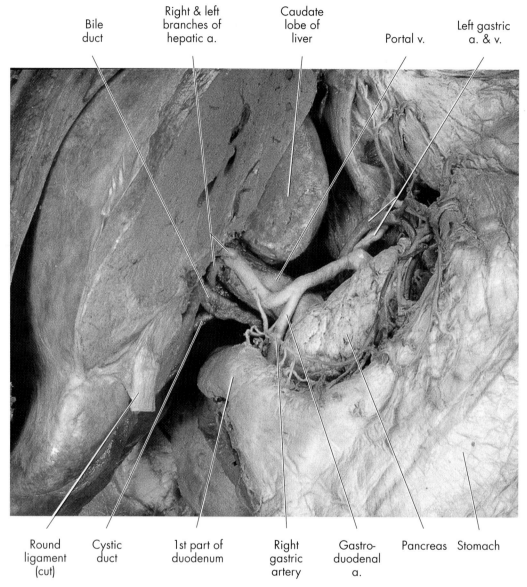

Round ligament (cut)

Cystic duct

1st part of duodenum

Right gastric artery

Gastro-duodenal a.

Pancreas   Stomach

Figure 5-74 Course and branches of the hepatic artery. The lesser omentum has been removed. *Portal hypertension occurs when there is partial or complete obstruction of blood flow from the hepatic portal vein through the liver to the inferior vena cava. The obstruction causes pressure in the portal venous system to rise. Portal blood returns to the systemic (vena caval) system through a number of collateral anastomotic channels. In the most important of these, blood from the gastric portal branches passes into the esophageal veins, which drain to the azygos system and thence to the superior vena cava. Large esophageal varicose veins are the result, which can easily rupture and cause massive hemorrhage.*

See **DISSECTIONS**, **Section 5**, p. 9
See **PRINCIPLES**, Fig. 5-38

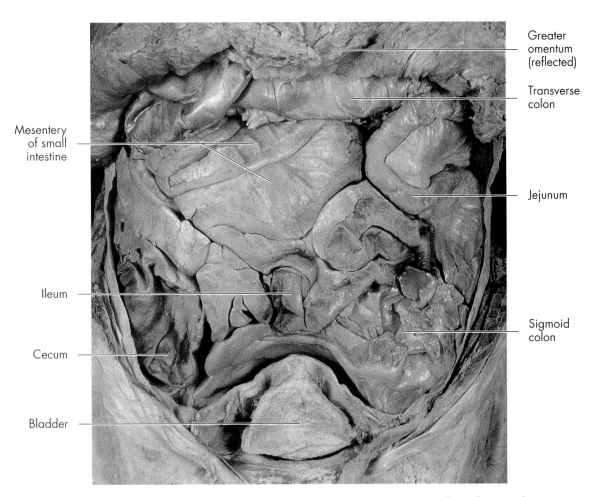

Figure 5-75   Jejunum and ileum. The greater omentum has been reflected upwards.

See DISSECTIONS, Section 5, p. 14

See PRINCIPLES, Table 5-9

Peritoneum
of mesentery
(cut)

Jejunal
arteries
& veins

Plicae
circulares

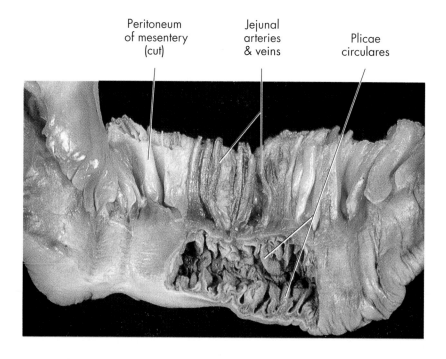

Ileal arteries
& veins

Mucosal
folds

Peritoneum
of mesentery (cut)

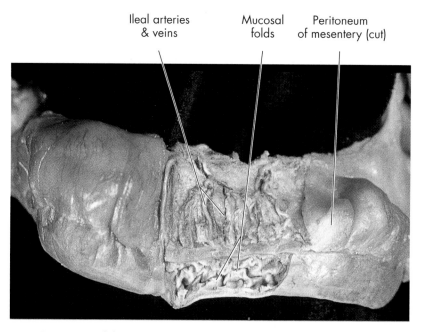

Figure 5-76 Segments of the jejunum (upper figure) and the ileum (lower figure) opened to show their mucosae. Their mesenteries have been dissected to reveal the blood vessels. *A surgeon exploring the abdomen through a limited incision must be able to differentiate a loop of jejunum from a loop of ileum. The jejunal wall is thick and velvety on palpation, and it has fewer arterial arcades and longer vasa recta in its mesentery than does the ileum.*

See DISSECTIONS, Section 5, p. 14
See PRINCIPLES, Fig. 5-18

Ileal
vessels
(cut)

Mesentery
of small
intestine

Transverse
colon

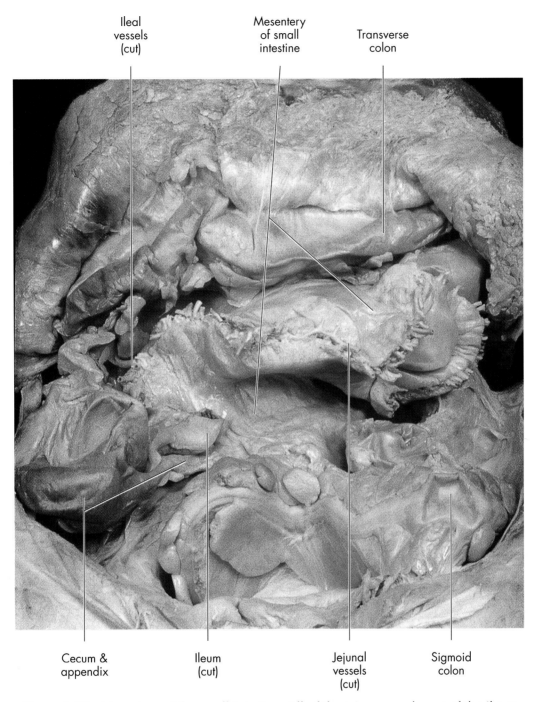

Cecum &
appendix

Ileum
(cut)

Jejunal
vessels
(cut)

Sigmoid
colon

Figure 5-77 Mesentery of the small intestine. All of the jejunum and most of the ileum have been excised and the cut edge of the mesentery trimmed to reveal the jejunal and ileal vessels.

See **DISSECTIONS**, Section 5, p. 14
See **PRINCIPLES**, p. 510, Table 5-9

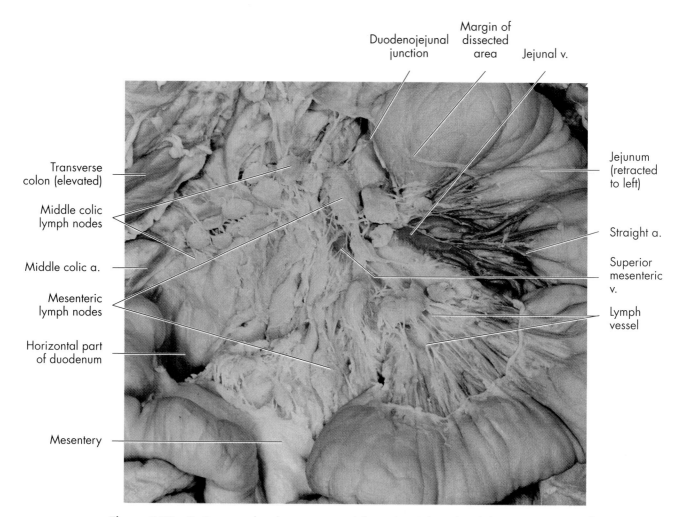

Duodenojejunal junction

Margin of dissected area

Jejunal v.

Transverse colon (elevated)

Middle colic lymph nodes

Middle colic a.

Mesenteric lymph nodes

Horizontal part of duodenum

Mesentery

Jejunum (retracted to left)

Straight a.

Superior mesenteric v.

Lymph vessel

Figure 5-78   Peritoneum has been removed from the right side of the mesentery in this loop of jejunum and from the lower surface of the transverse mesocolon to show blood vessels and lymphatics.

SEE DISSECTIONS, SECTION 5, P. 14
SEE PRINCIPLES, P. 509, TABLE 5-9

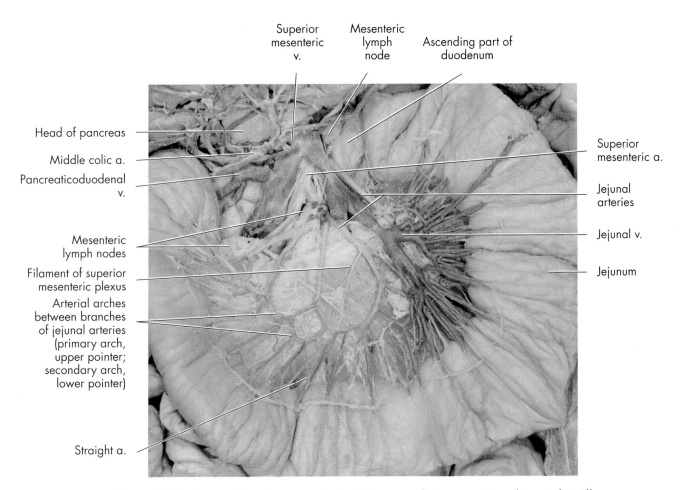

Figure 5-79 Loop of the first part of the jejunum with its mesentery dissected to illustrate the manner in which vessels and nerves approach the intestinal wall. Note that the superior mesenteric artery is accompanied by filaments of the superior mesenteric plexus.

See **DISSECTIONS**, Section 5, p. 14
See **PRINCIPLES**, Table 5-9

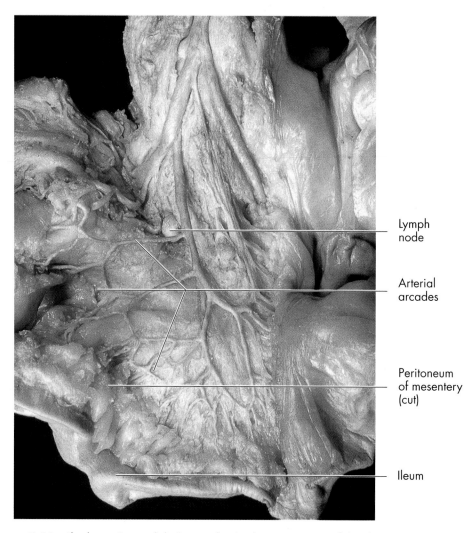

Lymph
node

Arterial
arcades

Peritoneum
of mesentery
(cut)

Ileum

Figure 5-80   Ileal arteries and their arcades in the mesentery of the ileum.

See **DISSECTIONS, Section 5, p. 14**

See **PRINCIPLES, Fig. 5-18**

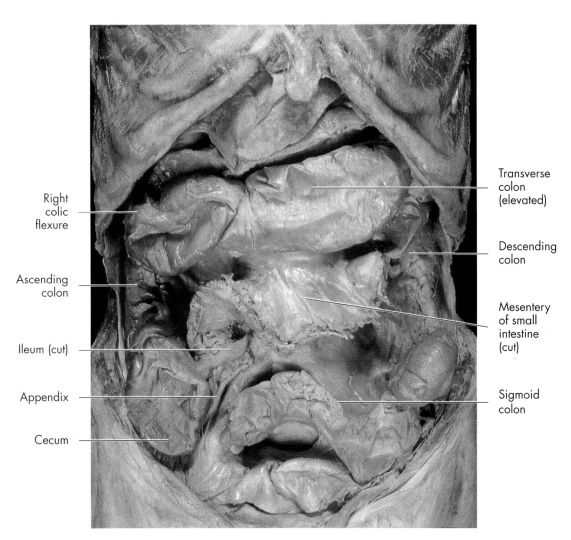

Right colic flexure

Ascending colon

Ileum (cut)

Appendix

Cecum

Transverse colon (elevated)

Descending colon

Mesentery of small intestine (cut)

Sigmoid colon

Figure 5-81 Cecum, appendix, and colon after removal of the greater omentum and most of the small intestine. The transverse colon has been raised.

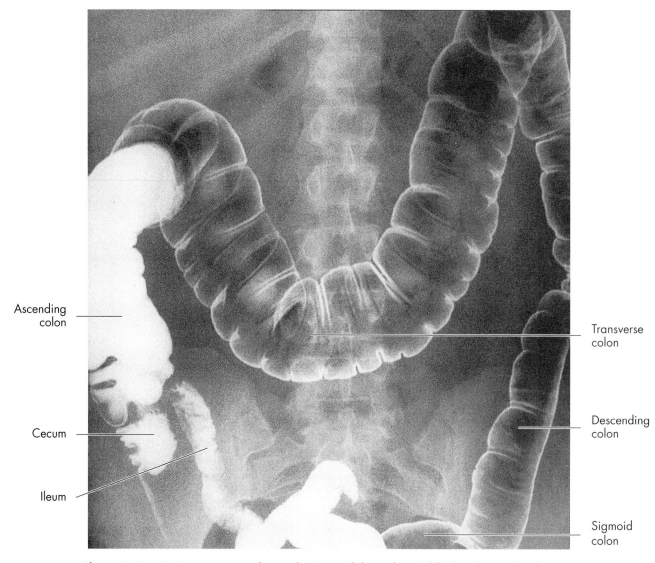

Figure 5-82　Barium enema radiograph. Most of the colon is filled with gas, but barium coats its mucosa and has passed proximally into the ileum.

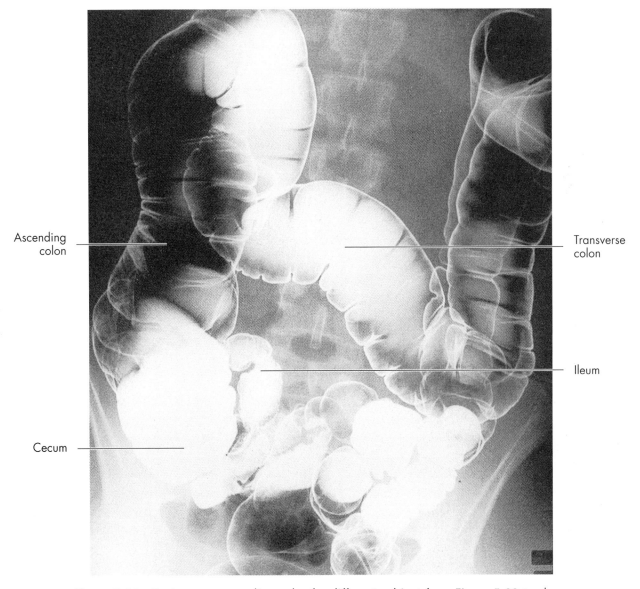

Ascending colon

Transverse colon

Ileum

Cecum

Figure 5-83 Barium enema radiograph of a different subject from Figure 5-82 to show variation in bowel anatomy. The transverse colon is more dependent, and coils of the sigmoid colon overlap each other.

See DISSECTIONS, Section 5, p. 14

See PRINCIPLES, Fig. 5-42

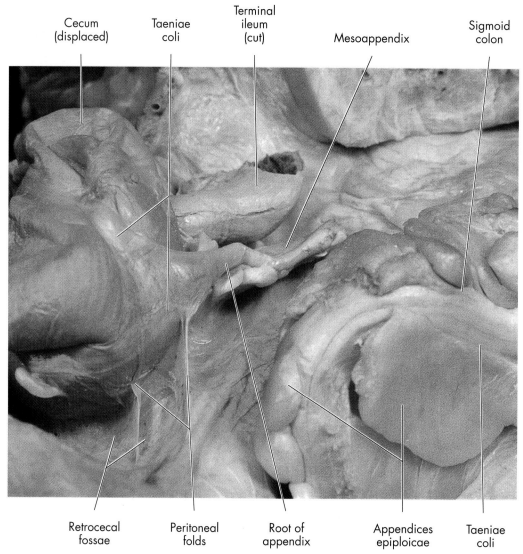

Cecum (displaced) · Taeniae coli · Terminal ileum (cut) · Mesoappendix · Sigmoid colon

Retrocecal fossae · Peritoneal folds · Root of appendix · Appendices epiploicae · Taeniae coli

Figure 5-84 Base of the appendix and retrocecal folds and fossae after pulling the cecum forward. *The appendix is the vestigal remnant of the long cecum found in herbivorous animals. It is a frequent site of infection (appendicitis), particularly if its lumen is obstructed by stone-like hardened feces (fecolith). The surgeon may find the base of the appendix by following one of the cecal taeniae coli to the point where it meets the other two taeniae at the dependent portion of the cecum. The appendix may extend from its base over the brim of the pelvis (pelvic appendix; see Figure 5-86), upward behind the cecum (retrocecal appendix; see Figure 5-87), or it may lie free in the peritoneal cavity.*

See DISSECTIONS, SECTION 5, P. 14
See PRINCIPLES, FIG. 5-42

Ascending colon   Cecal a.   Ileocolic a.   Mesoappendix

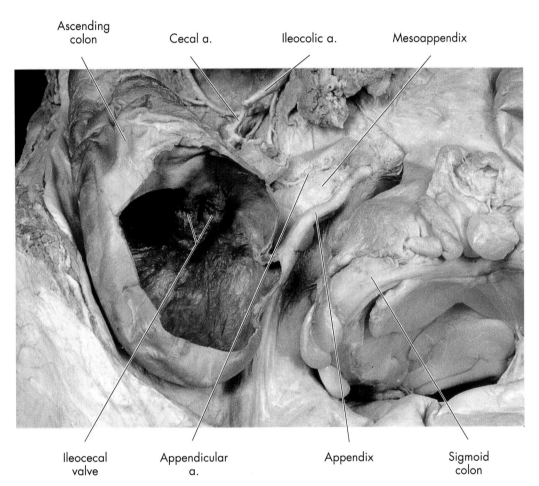

Ileocecal valve   Appendicular a.   Appendix   Sigmoid colon

Figure 5-85   Ileocecal valve revealed by removal of the anterior wall of the cecum. The mesoappendix has been dissected to show the appendicular artery.

SEE DISSECTIONS, SECTION 5, P. 14
SEE PRINCIPLES, FIG. 5-42

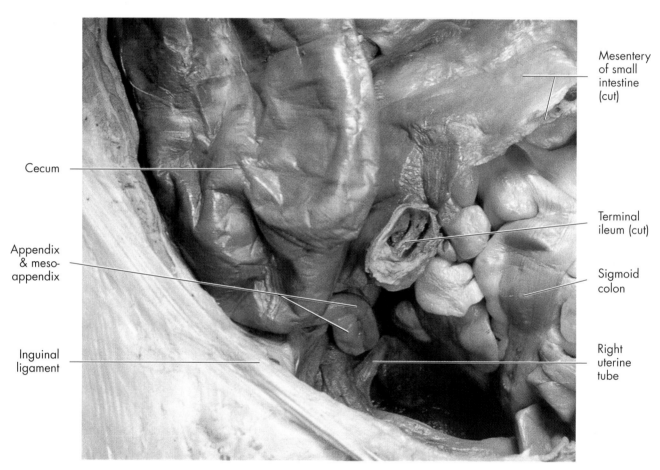

Mesentery
of small
intestine
(cut)

Cecum

Terminal
ileum (cut)

Appendix
& meso-
appendix

Sigmoid
colon

Inguinal
ligament

Right
uterine
tube

Figure 5-86 After removal of most of the small intestine, this appendix can be seen descending over the pelvic brim.

See **DISSECTIONS**, **Section** 5, p. 14

See **PRINCIPLES**, **Fig.** 5-42

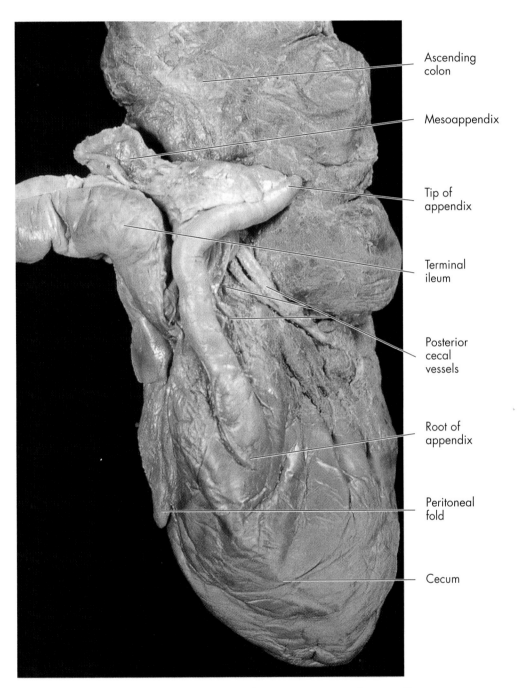

Ascending colon

Mesoappendix

Tip of appendix

Terminal ileum

Posterior cecal vessels

Root of appendix

Peritoneal fold

Cecum

Figure 5-87 Posterior aspect of the cecum showing a retrocecal appendix.

See **DISSECTIONS**, Section 5, p. 14
See **PRINCIPLES**, Fig. 5-43

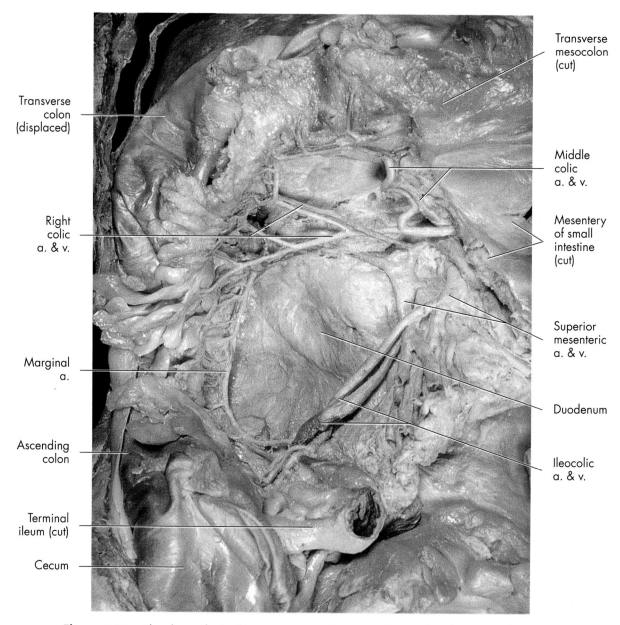

Transverse mesocolon (cut)

Transverse colon (displaced)

Middle colic a. & v.

Right colic a. & v.

Mesentery of small intestine (cut)

Superior mesenteric a. & v.

Marginal a.

Duodenum

Ascending colon

Ileocolic a. & v.

Terminal ileum (cut)

Cecum

Figure 5-88 Blood supply to the cecum and the ascending and transverse colon. The transverse mesocolon and the mesentery of the small intestine have been dissected to reveal the ileocolic, right colic, and middle colic vessels.

Sᴇᴇ **DISSECTIONS, Sᴇᴄᴛɪᴏɴ 5, ᴘ. 14**

Sᴇᴇ **PRINCIPLES, Fɪɢ. 5-47**

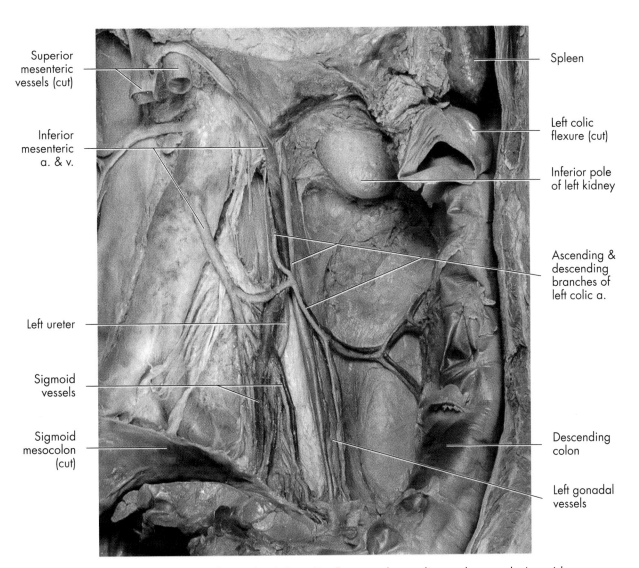

Superior
mesenteric
vessels (cut)

Inferior
mesenteric
a. & v.

Left ureter

Sigmoid
vessels

Sigmoid
mesocolon
(cut)

Spleen

Left colic
flexure (cut)

Inferior pole
of left kidney

Ascending &
descending
branches of
left colic a.

Descending
colon

Left gonadal
vessels

Figure 5-89   Blood supply to the left colic flexure, descending colon, and sigmoid colon. Removal of peritoneum from the posterior abdominal wall to the left of the aorta displays the inferior mesenteric vessels.

SEE DISSECTIONS, SECTION 5, PP. 11 AND 14

SEE PRINCIPLES, FIG. 5-19

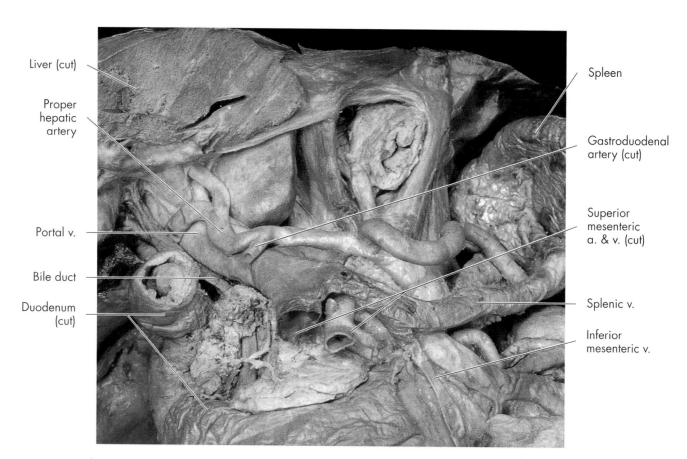

Liver (cut)

Proper
hepatic
artery

Portal v.

Bile duct

Duodenum
(cut)

Spleen

Gastroduodenal
artery (cut)

Superior
mesenteric
a. & v. (cut)

Splenic v.

Inferior
mesenteric v.

Figure 5-90   Portal and splenic veins. Most of the pancreas has been removed and the first part of the duodenum turned aside.

See DISSECTIONS, Section 5, pp. 11 and 14

See PRINCIPLES, Fig. 5-19

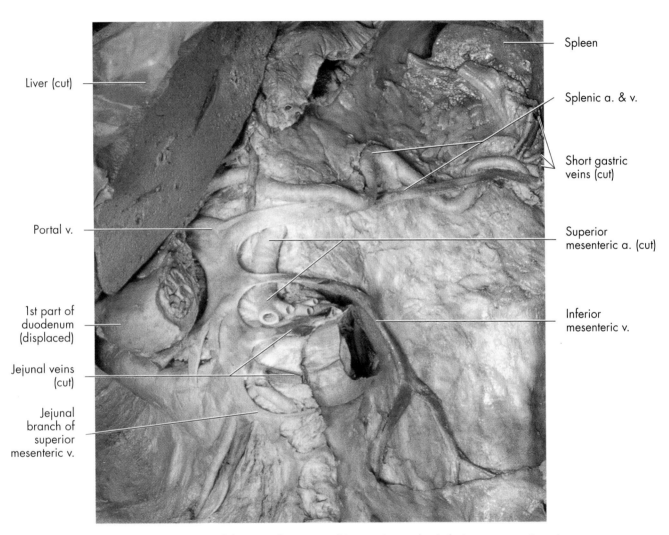

Spleen

Liver (cut)

Splenic a. & v.

Short gastric
veins (cut)

Portal v.

Superior
mesenteric a. (cut)

1st part of
duodenum
(displaced)

Inferior
mesenteric v.

Jejunal veins
(cut)

Jejunal
branch of
superior
mesenteric v.

Figure 5-91   Tributaries of the portal vein. In this specimen the inferior mesenteric vein joins the superior mesenteric vein.

414   Clinical Anatomy Atlas

See DISSECTIONS, Section 5, p. 15

See PRINCIPLES, Figs. 5-54, 5-60

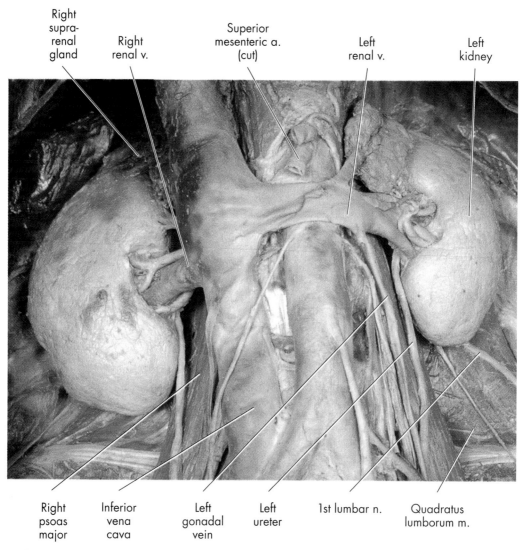

Right supra-renal gland   Right renal v.   Superior mesenteric a. (cut)   Left renal v.   Left kidney

Right psoas major   Inferior vena cava   Left gonadal vein   Left ureter   1st lumbar n.   Quadratus lumborum m.

Figure 5-92   Kidneys, suprarenal glands, and some of the vessels associated with them.

See DISSECTIONS, Section 5, p. 15

See PRINCIPLES, Fig. 5-53

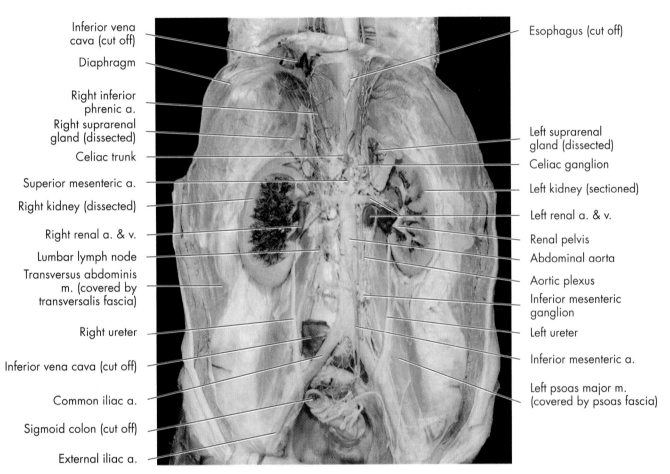

Inferior vena cava (cut off)

Diaphragm

Right inferior phrenic a.

Right suprarenal gland (dissected)

Celiac trunk

Superior mesenteric a.

Right kidney (dissected)

Right renal a. & v.

Lumbar lymph node

Transversus abdominis m. (covered by transversalis fascia)

Right ureter

Inferior vena cava (cut off)

Common iliac a.

Sigmoid colon (cut off)

External iliac a.

Esophagus (cut off)

Left suprarenal gland (dissected)

Celiac ganglion

Left kidney (sectioned)

Left renal a. & v.

Renal pelvis

Abdominal aorta

Aortic plexus

Inferior mesenteric ganglion

Left ureter

Inferior mesenteric a.

Left psoas major m. (covered by psoas fascia)

Figure 5-93 Right kidney dissected from its anterior surface to demonstrate distribution of the renal blood vessels. The left kidney has been sectioned longitudinally to display the vessels and the renal pelvis with its major and minor calyces. The central area of each suprarenal gland has been resected to expose the tributaries of the suprarenal veins.

See DISSECTIONS, SECTION 5, P. 15

See PRINCIPLES, FIG. 5-52

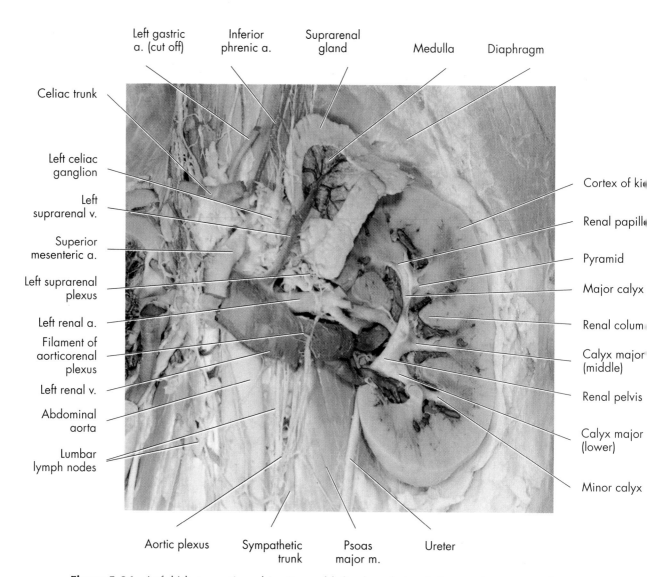

Left gastric a. (cut off)

Inferior phrenic a.

Suprarenal gland

Medulla

Diaphragm

Celiac trunk

Left celiac ganglion

Left suprarenal v.

Superior mesenteric a.

Left suprarenal plexus

Left renal a.

Filament of aorticorenal plexus

Left renal v.

Abdominal aorta

Lumbar lymph nodes

Cortex of ki[...]

Renal papill[...]

Pyramid

Major calyx

Renal colum[...]

Calyx major (middle)

Renal pelvis

Calyx major (lower)

Minor calyx

Aortic plexus

Sympathetic trunk

Psoas major m.

Ureter

Figure 5-94   Left kidney sectioned in situ and left adrenal gland dissected to expose the medulla. Anterior branches of the left renal artery are cut off near the sectioned kidney.

SEE PRINCIPLES, FIG. 5-53

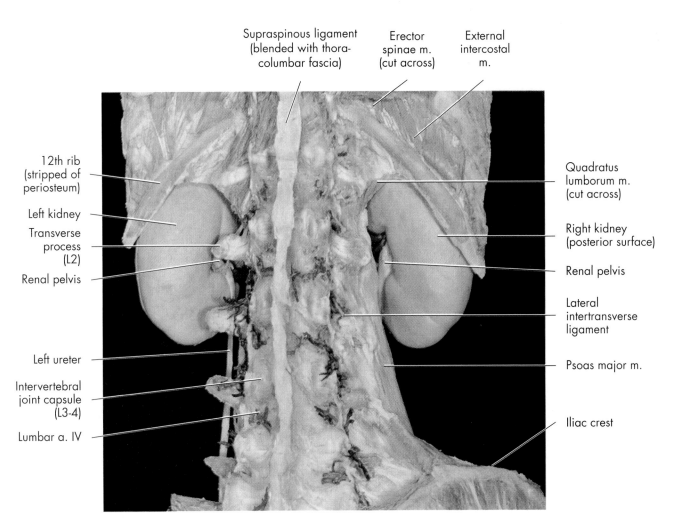

Figure 5-95 Kidneys exposed from behind by removal of spinal musculature and muscles of the abdominal wall. Fascia and fat related to the kidney have also been excised. *The kidneys are moderately well protected from blunt trauma injury because they lie in front of the twelfth rib, the upper two lumbar vertebral transverse processes, and the large psoas major and quadratus lumborum muscles with the surrounding lumbar fascia. Because of the kidney's retroperitoneal position, trauma to the kidney rarely causes bleeding into the peritoneal cavity (unlike trauma to the spleen).*

SEE PRINCIPLES, FIG. 5-51

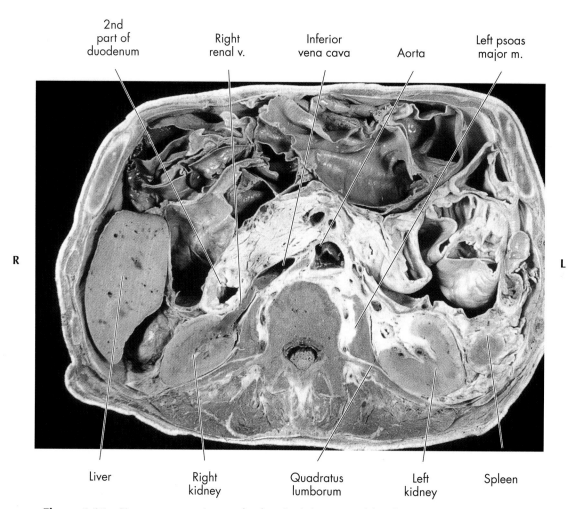

| 2nd part of duodenum | Right renal v. | Inferior vena cava | Aorta | Left psoas major m. |

R   L

| Liver | Right kidney | Quadratus lumborum | Left kidney | Spleen |

Figure 5-96   Transverse section at the level of the second lumbar vertebra viewed from below showing the relationships of the kidneys to the lumbar vertebrae and some of the digestive organs.

See DISSECTIONS, Section 5, p. 15

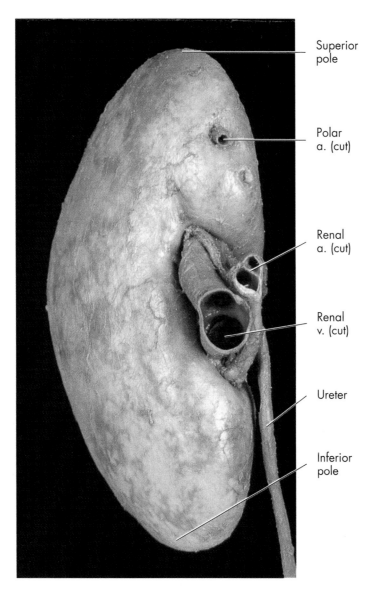

Superior
pole

Polar
a. (cut)

Renal
a. (cut)

Renal
v. (cut)

Ureter

Inferior
pole

Figure 5-97   Medial aspect of the right kidney showing the renal vessels passing through the hilum. *Accessory polar renal arteries represent vessels that in fetal life supplied separate kidney lobules. The parenchymal blood supply has a tendency to remain lobular so that, if a polar artery is ligated or blocked, the portion of the kidney supplied by that vessel may die (kidney infarct).*

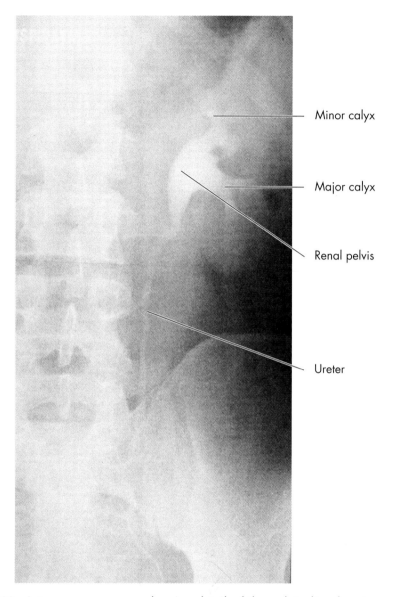

Minor calyx

Major calyx

Renal pelvis

Ureter

Figure 5-98   Intravenous urogram showing detail of the pelvicaliceal system. *Blockage of a ureter may be caused either by a stone (ureteral calculus) or external compression. When this occurs, the ureter proximal to the obstruction becomes enlarged (hydroureter) and may extend to include the renal pelvis (hydronephrosis). Such obstruction should be released to avoid loss of function or infection (pyelonephritis) of the affected kidney.*

See DISSECTIONS, Section 5, p. 15
See PRINCIPLES, Fig. 5-52

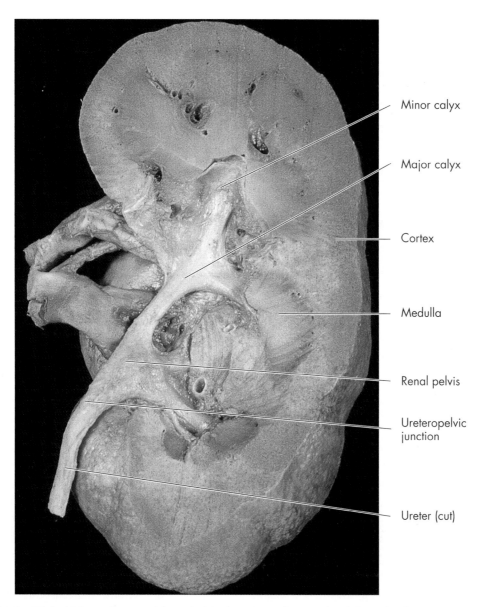

Minor calyx

Major calyx

Cortex

Medulla

Renal pelvis

Ureteropelvic
junction

Ureter (cut)

Figure 5-99   Right kidney dissected from behind to show the renal pelvis and calyces.

See **DISSECTIONS**, Section 5, p. 15

See **PRINCIPLES**, Fig. 5-51

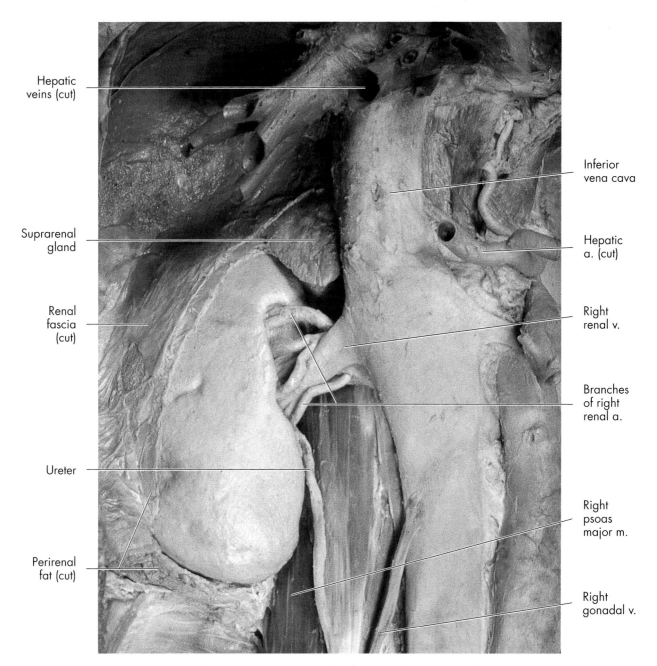

Hepatic veins (cut)

Suprarenal gland

Renal fascia (cut)

Ureter

Perirenal fat (cut)

Inferior vena cava

Hepatic a. (cut)

Right renal v.

Branches of right renal a.

Right psoas major m.

Right gonadal v.

Figure 5-100   Right kidney and suprarenal gland seen within the renal fascia and perirenal fat, part of which has been removed.

See **DISSECTIONS**, Section 5, p. 15

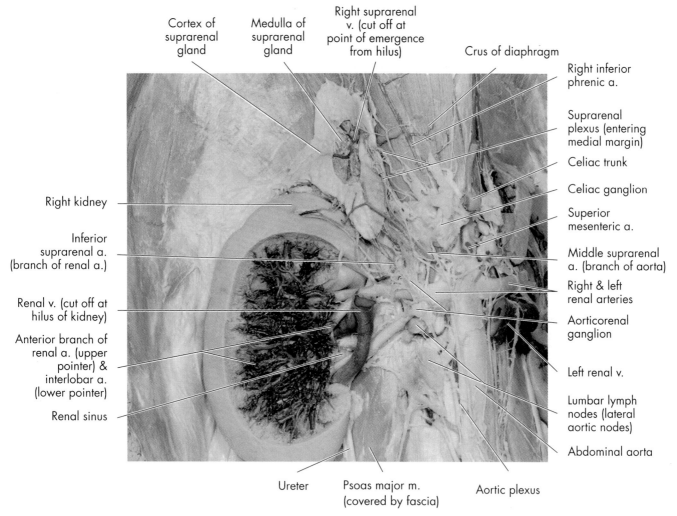

Figure 5-101 Dissection of the renal parenchyma of the right kidney exposing the latex-filled arteries and veins. The cortex has been removed near the center of the adrenal gland to expose the brownish medullary tissue.

See **DISSECTIONS**, Section 5, p. 15
See **PRINCIPLES**, Fig. 5-55

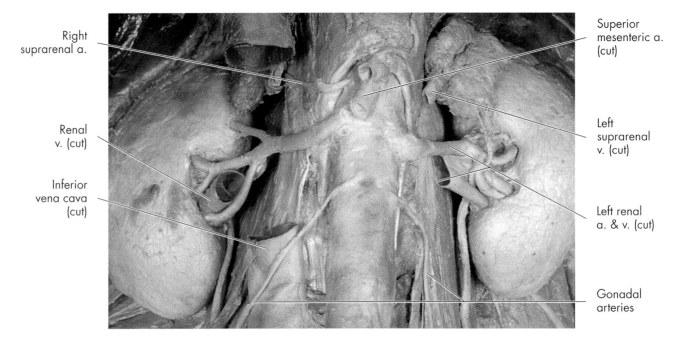

Right
suprarenal a.

Renal
v. (cut)

Inferior
vena cava
(cut)

Superior
mesenteric a.
(cut)

Left
suprarenal
v. (cut)

Left renal
a. & v. (cut)

Gonadal
arteries

Figure 5-102   Renal arteries exposed by removal of the renal veins and a portion of the inferior vena cava.

See DISSECTIONS, Section 5, p. 15

See PRINCIPLES, Fig. 5-54

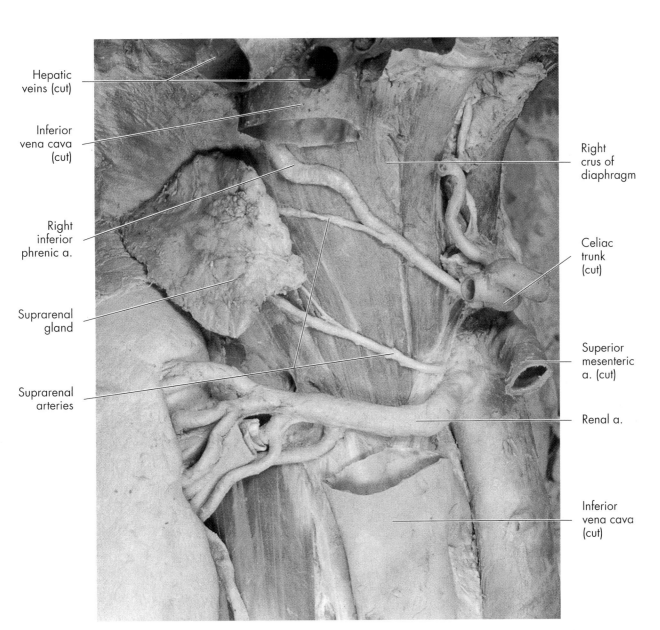

Hepatic
veins (cut)

Inferior
vena cava
(cut)

Right
inferior
phrenic a.

Suprarenal
gland

Suprarenal
arteries

Right
crus of
diaphragm

Celiac
trunk
(cut)

Superior
mesenteric
a. (cut)

Renal a.

Inferior
vena cava
(cut)

Figure 5-103   Right suprarenal gland and its arteries exposed by removal of the renal vein and a portion of the inferior vena cava.

See DISSECTIONS, SECTION 5, P. 15
See PRINCIPLES, FIG. 5-60

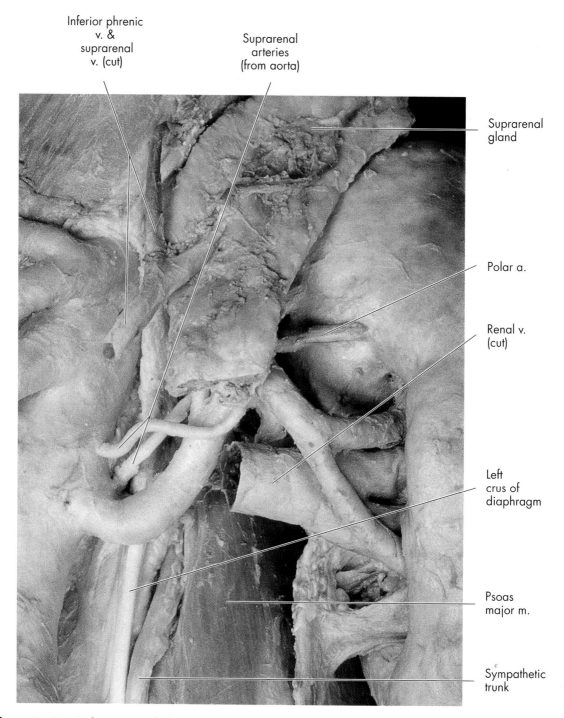

Inferior phrenic
v. &
suprarenal
v. (cut)

Suprarenal
arteries
(from aorta)

Suprarenal
gland

Polar a.

Renal v.
(cut)

Left
crus of
diaphragm

Psoas
major m.

Sympathetic
trunk

Figure 5-104   Left suprarenal gland and its vessels. The renal vein and inferior tip of the gland have been excised to reveal the suprarenal arteries.

See DISSECTIONS, Section 5, p. 17
See PRINCIPLES, Fig. 5-12

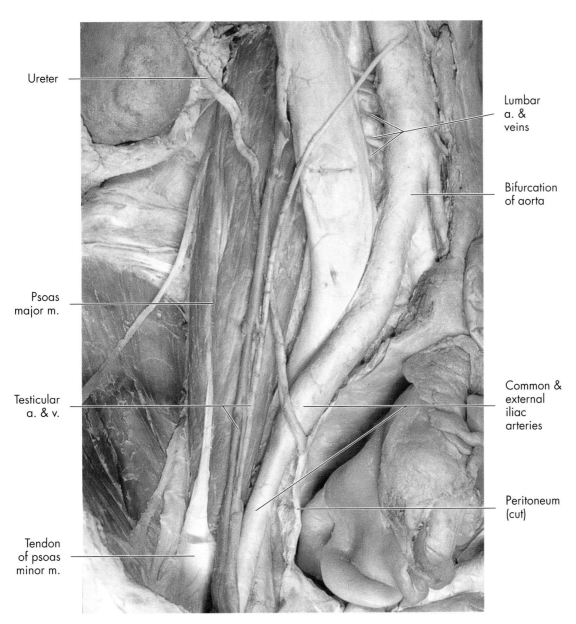

Ureter

Lumbar
a. &
veins

Bifurcation
of aorta

Psoas
major m.

Testicular
a. & v.

Common &
external
iliac
arteries

Peritoneum
(cut)

Tendon
of psoas
minor m.

Figure 5-105 Right testicular vessels within the abdomen. Several lumbar vessels are also seen.

See DISSECTIONS, Section 5, p. 17
See PRINCIPLES, Fig. 5-12

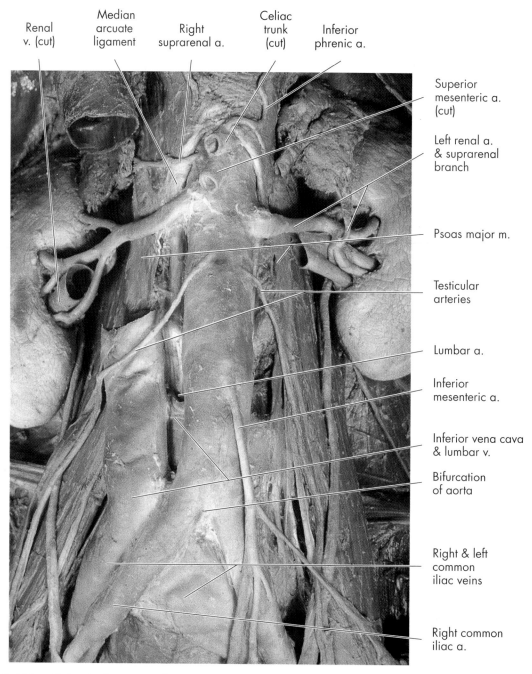

Figure 5-106　Abdominal aorta and its branches seen after removal of the renal veins and part of the inferior vena cava.

SEE DISSECTIONS, SECTION 5, P. 17
SEE PRINCIPLES, FIG. 5-12

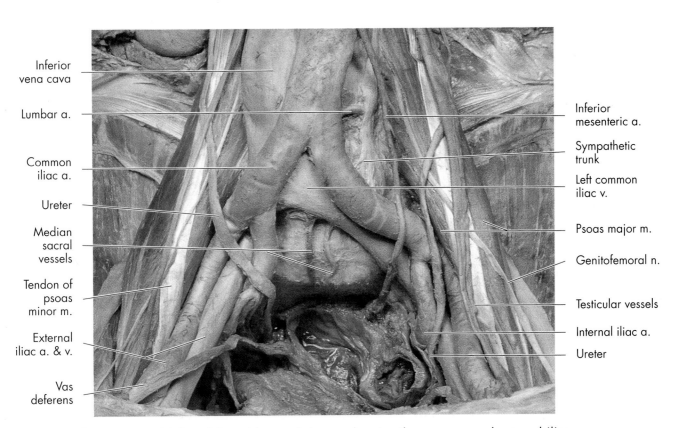

Inferior
vena cava

Lumbar a.

Common
iliac a.

Ureter

Median
sacral
vessels

Tendon of
psoas
minor m.

External
iliac a. & v.

Vas
deferens

Inferior
mesenteric a.

Sympathetic
trunk

Left common
iliac v.

Psoas major m.

Genitofemoral n.

Testicular vessels

Internal iliac a.

Ureter

Figure 5-107 Male pelvis and lower abdomen showing the common and external iliac vessels and some of their relationships.

See DISSECTIONS, Section 5, p. 17
See PRINCIPLES, Fig. 5-60

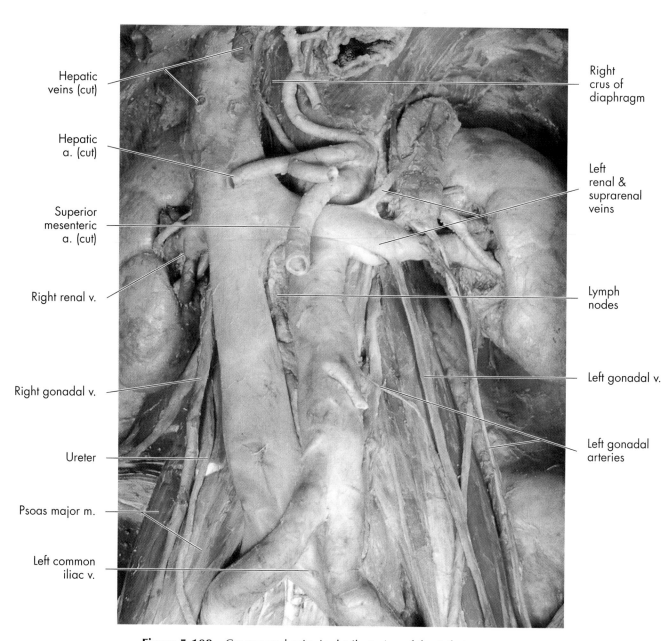

Hepatic veins (cut)

Hepatic a. (cut)

Superior mesenteric a. (cut)

Right renal v.

Right gonadal v.

Ureter

Psoas major m.

Left common iliac v.

Right crus of diaphragm

Left renal & suprarenal veins

Lymph nodes

Left gonadal v.

Left gonadal arteries

Figure 5-108   Course and principal tributaries of the inferior vena cava.

Sᴇᴇ **DISSECTIONS, Sᴇᴄᴛɪᴏɴ 5, ᴘ. 17**
Sᴇᴇ **PRINCIPLES, Fɪɢ. 5-60**

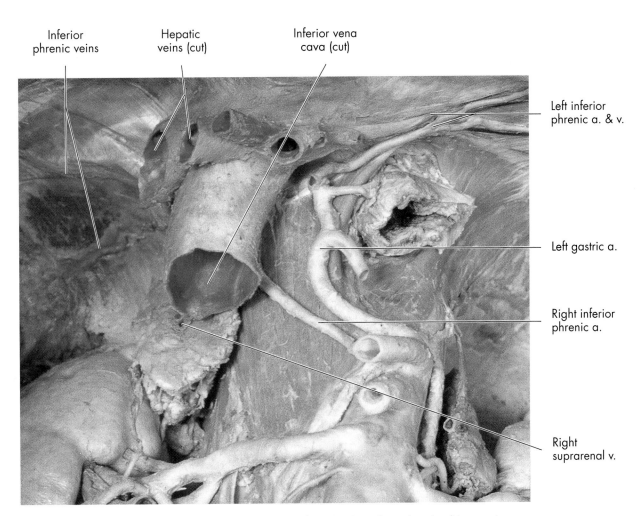

Inferior
phrenic veins

Hepatic
veins (cut)

Inferior vena
cava (cut)

Left inferior
phrenic a. & v.

Left gastric a.

Right inferior
phrenic a.

Right
suprarenal v.

Figure 5-109 Upper part of inferior vena cava showing its tributaries. In this specimen the left inferior phrenic artery arises from the left gastric artery.

SEE DISSECTIONS, SECTION 5, P. 17

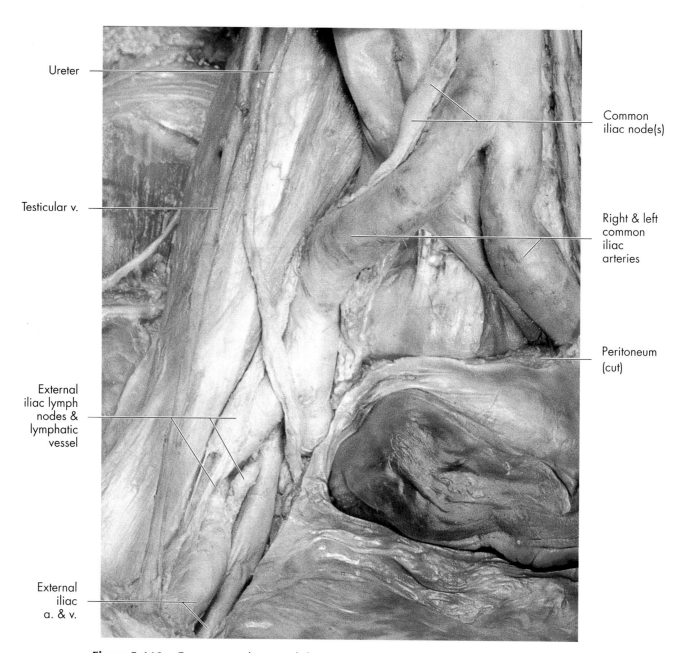

Ureter

Testicular v.

External
iliac lymph
nodes &
lymphatic
vessel

External
iliac
a. & v.

Common
iliac node(s)

Right & left
common
iliac
arteries

Peritoneum
(cut)

Figure 5-110   Common and external iliac arteries accompanied by a chain of lymphatic
vessels and nodes.

S<small>EE</small> **DISSECTIONS**, S<small>ECTION</small> 5, p. 17

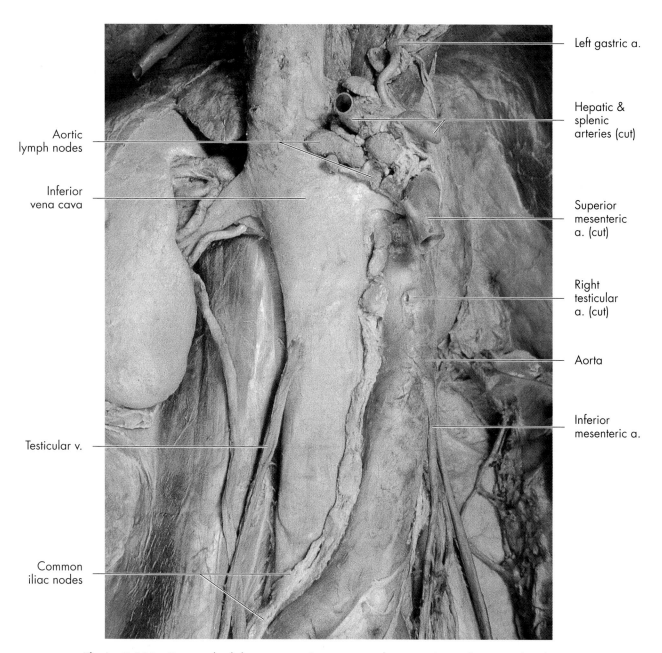

Left gastric a.

Hepatic &
splenic
arteries (cut)

Aortic
lymph nodes

Inferior
vena cava

Superior
mesenteric
a. (cut)

Right
testicular
a. (cut)

Aorta

Inferior
mesenteric a.

Testicular v.

Common
iliac nodes

Figure 5-111   Removal of the autonomic nerves and retroperitoneal connective tissues revealing the lymphatic vessels and nodes lying on the right side of the aorta.

See **DISSECTIONS**, Section 5, p. 17

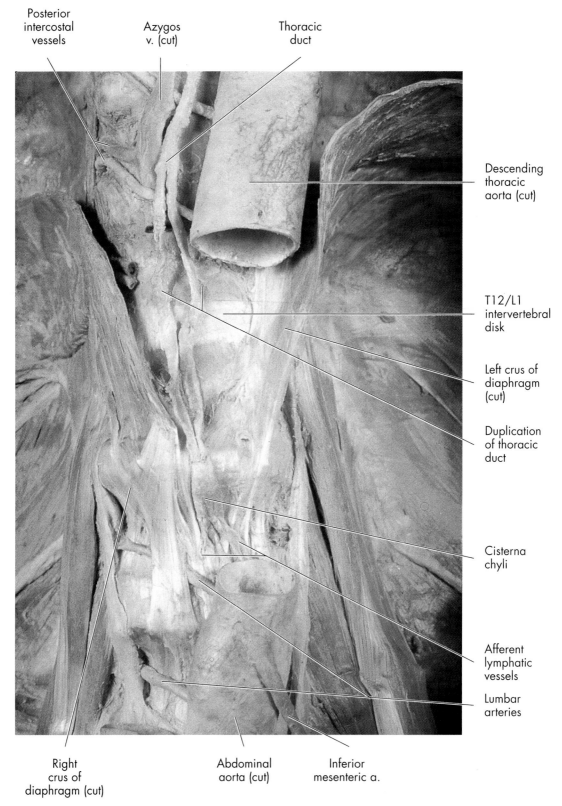

Posterior
intercostal
vessels

Azygos
v. (cut)

Thoracic
duct

Descending
thoracic
aorta (cut)

T12/L1
intervertebral
disk

Left crus of
diaphragm
(cut)

Duplication
of thoracic
duct

Cisterna
chyli

Afferent
lymphatic
vessels

Lumbar
arteries

Right
crus of
diaphragm (cut)

Abdominal
aorta (cut)

Inferior
mesenteric a.

Figure 5-112   Cisterna chyli revealed by removal of parts of the diaphragmatic crura and
a segment of the aorta.

SEE DISSECTIONS, SECTION 5, P. 14

SEE PRINCIPLES, FIG. 5-35

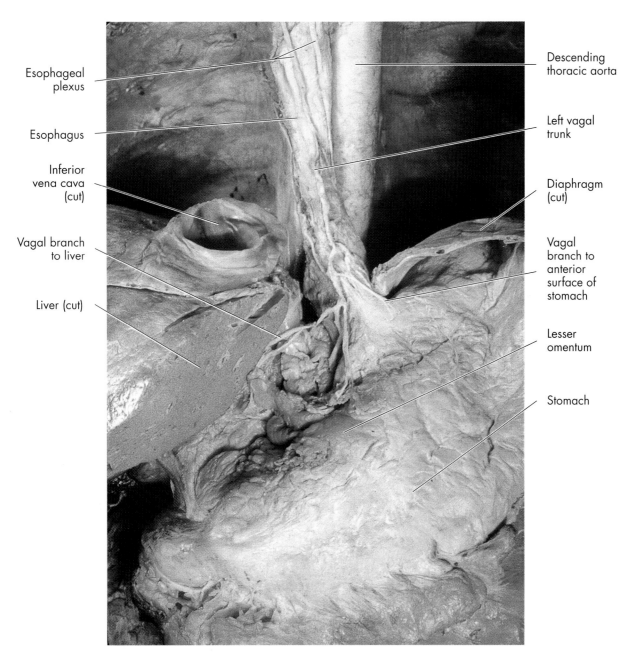

Esophageal plexus

Esophagus

Inferior vena cava (cut)

Vagal branch to liver

Liver (cut)

Descending thoracic aorta

Left vagal trunk

Diaphragm (cut)

Vagal branch to anterior surface of stomach

Lesser omentum

Stomach

Figure 5-113 Anterior vagal trunk revealed by removal of part of the diaphragm and exposure of the lower esophagus.

SEE DISSECTIONS, SECTION 5, P. 17

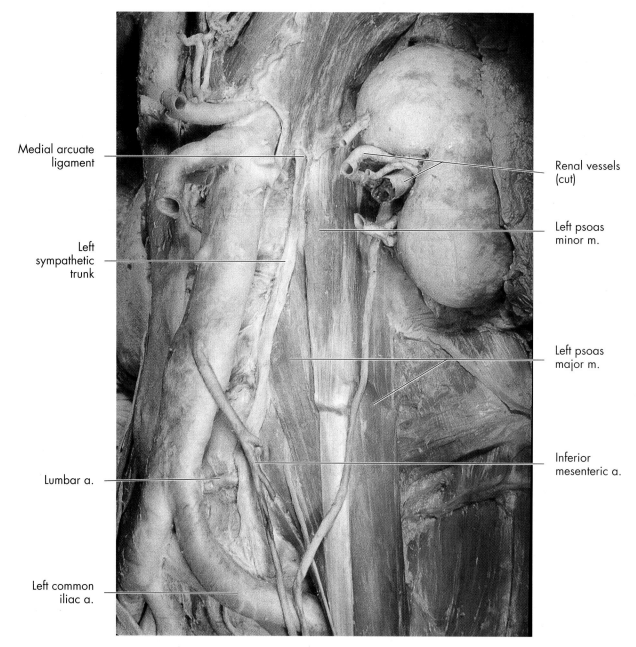

Medial arcuate ligament

Renal vessels (cut)

Left sympathetic trunk

Left psoas minor m.

Left psoas major m.

Lumbar a.

Inferior mesenteric a.

Left common iliac a.

Figure 5-114   Lumbar portion of the left sympathetic trunk after removal of the aortic nerve plexuses.

See **DISSECTIONS**, **Section 5, p. 17**

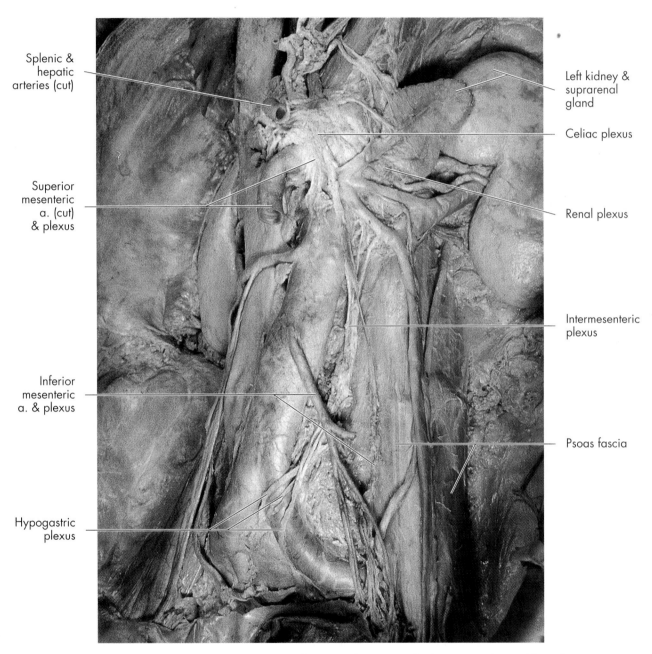

Splenic & hepatic arteries (cut)

Superior mesenteric a. (cut) & plexus

Inferior mesenteric a. & plexus

Hypogastric plexus

Left kidney & suprarenal gland

Celiac plexus

Renal plexus

Intermesenteric plexus

Psoas fascia

Figure 5-115   Aortic autonomic nerve plexuses after removal of aortic nodes and lymph vessels.

See DISSECTIONS, Section 5, p. 17

See PRINCIPLES, Fig. 5-59

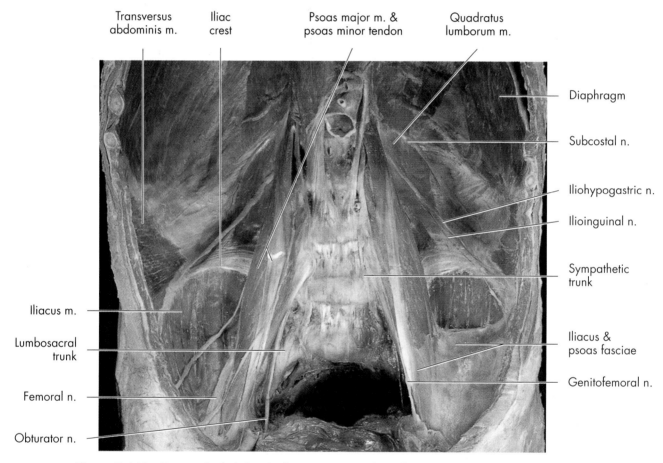

Transversus abdominis m.

Iliac crest

Psoas major m. & psoas minor tendon

Quadratus lumborum m.

Diaphragm

Subcostal n.

Iliohypogastric n.

Ilioinguinal n.

Sympathetic trunk

Iliacus m.

Lumbosacral trunk

Femoral n.

Obturator n.

Iliacus & psoas fasciae

Genitofemoral n.

Figure 5-116 Removal of abdominal contents revealing the muscles and nerves of the posterior abdominal wall. On one side some iliac and psoas fasciae have been preserved.

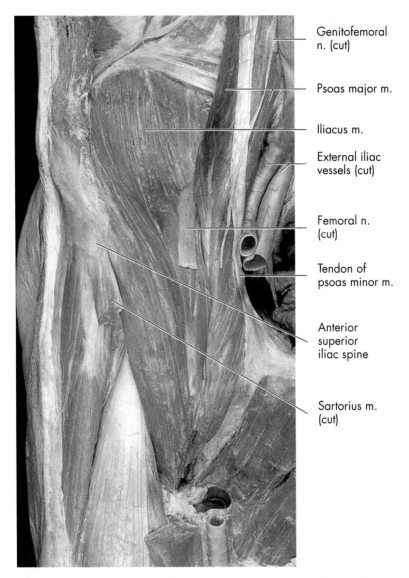

Genitofemoral
n. (cut)

Psoas major m.

Iliacus m.

External iliac
vessels (cut)

Femoral n.
(cut)

Tendon of
psoas minor m.

Anterior
superior
iliac spine

Sartorius m.
(cut)

Figure 5-117 Iliacus and psoas major, seen after removal of the inguinal ligament and part of sartorius muscle, attaching to the lesser trochanter of the femur. The psoas minor tendon descends to the iliopubic eminence of the hip bone.

SEE DISSECTIONS, SECTION 5, P. 17
SEE PRINCIPLES, FIG. 5-59

1st lumbar n.

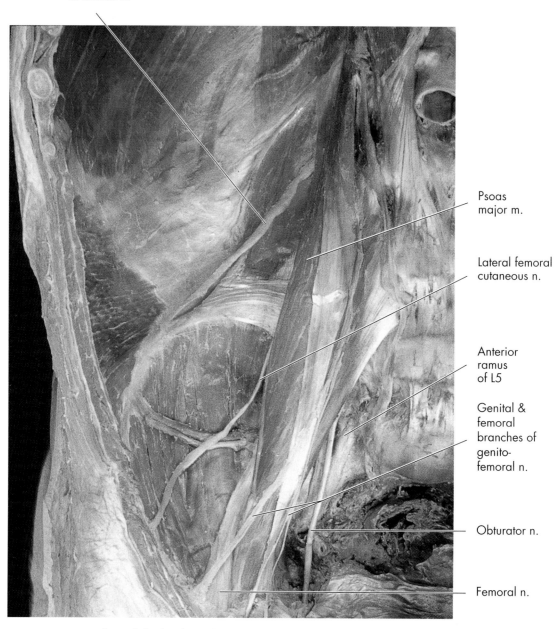

Psoas major m.

Lateral femoral cutaneous n.

Anterior ramus of L5

Genital & femoral branches of genito-femoral n.

Obturator n.

Femoral n.

Figure 5-118. Branches of the lumbar plexus emerging from the substance of the psoas major.

See PRINCIPLES, Fig. 5-59

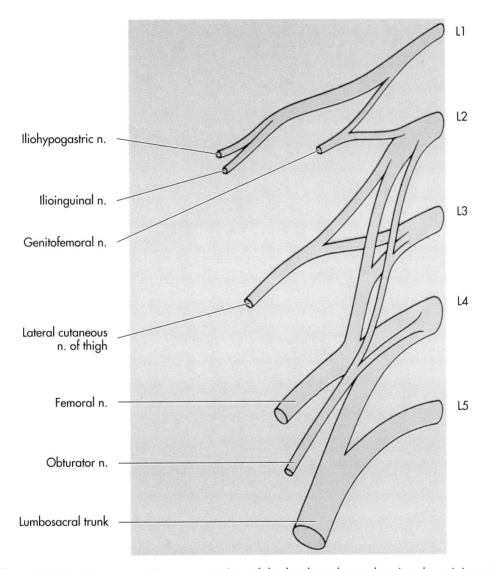

Figure 5-119   Diagrammatic representation of the lumbar plexus showing the origins of each of its branches. *The genitofemoral nerve has sensory branches that supply the medial aspect of the thigh and motor branches to the cremaster muscle. Stroking the inner thigh, therefore, results in active elevation of the testicle (cremasteric reflex).*

See **DISSECTIONS**, Section 5, p. 17

See **PRINCIPLES**, Fig. 5-59

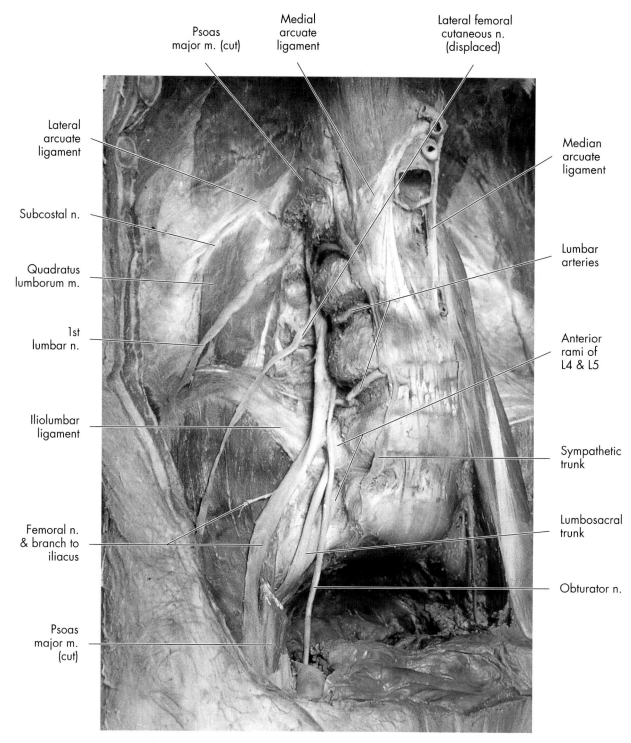

Figure 5-120   Removal of most of psoas major and the genitofemoral nerve exposing the lumbar plexus.

See Dissections, Section 5, p. 16
See Principles, Fig. 5-57

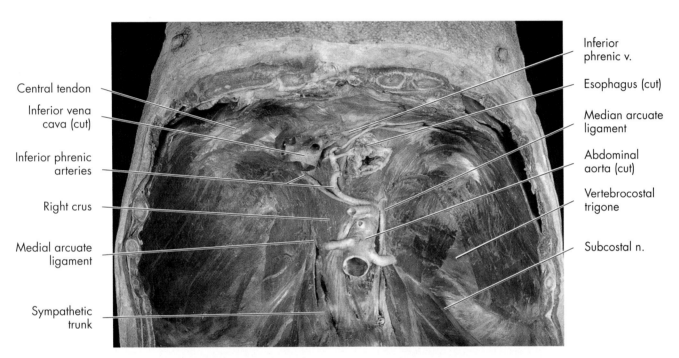

Central tendon

Inferior vena cava (cut)

Inferior phrenic arteries

Right crus

Medial arcuate ligament

Sympathetic trunk

Inferior phrenic v.

Esophagus (cut)

Median arcuate ligament

Abdominal aorta (cut)

Vertebrocostal trigone

Subcostal n.

Figure 5-121   Abdominal surface of the diaphragm after removal of the peritoneum. The xiphisternum and anterior costal margin have been excised, including part of the anterior periphery of the diaphragm.

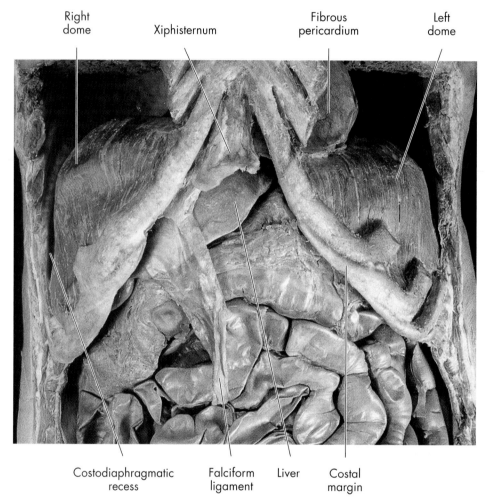

Figure 5-122 Anterior chest and abdominal walls removed (except for the costal margins) to reveal the diaphragm. The abdominal organs are undisturbed, but both lungs and diaphragmatic pleura have been removed.

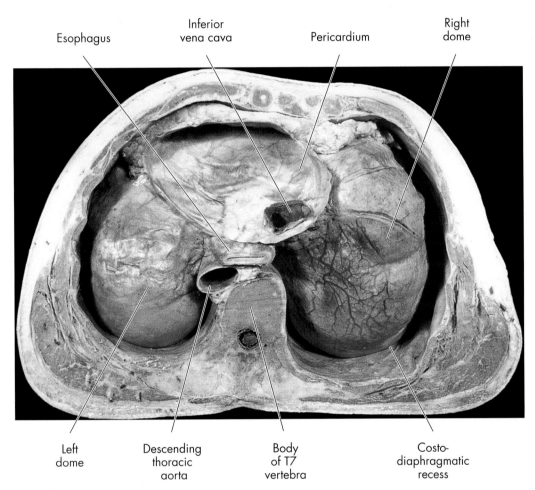

Esophagus

Inferior
vena cava

Pericardium

Right
dome

Left
dome

Descending
thoracic
aorta

Body
of T7
vertebra

Costo-
diaphragmatic
recess

Figure 5-123   Thoracic surface of the diaphragm. The parietal pleura remains in situ,
and the base of the fibrous pericardium has been retained.

See PRINCIPLES, Fig. 5-57

Pleura
(cut)

Posterior
intercostal
a. & v.

Azygos v.

Thoracic
duct

Descending
thoracic
aorta

Celiac trunk
(cut)

Cisterna
chyli

Superior
mesenteric
a. (cut)

Abdominal
aorta

Sympathetic
trunk

Psoas
major m.

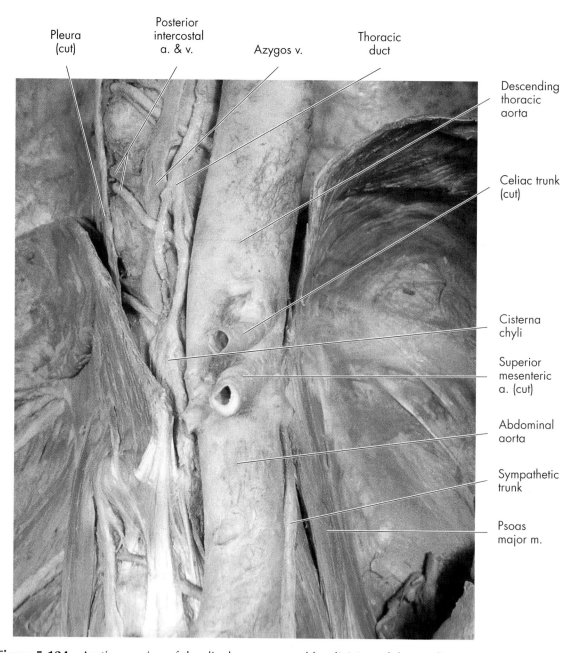

Figure 5-124   Aortic opening of the diaphragm opened by division of the median arcuate ligament and removal of parts of both crura. The aorta is accompanied by the azygos
vein and thoracic duct.

SECTION SIX

Pelvis and Perineum

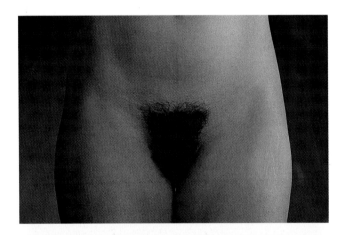
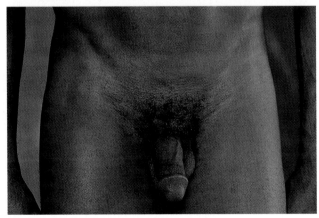
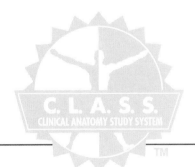

See PRINCIPLES, FIG. 6-14

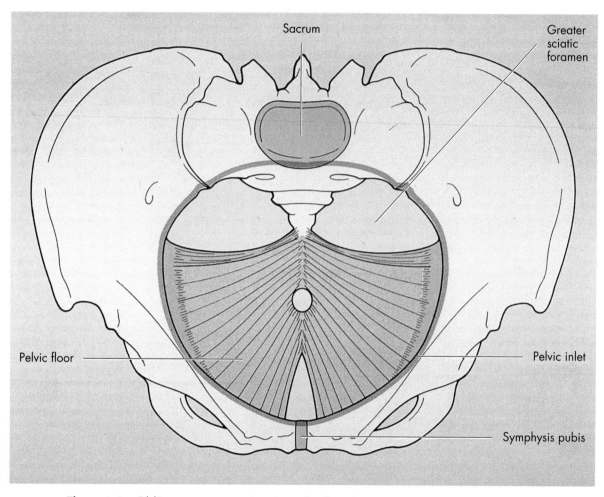

Figure 6-1   Oblique anterosuperior view of pelvis showing the inlet and pelvic floor.

SEE PRINCIPLES, FIG. 6-20, *B*

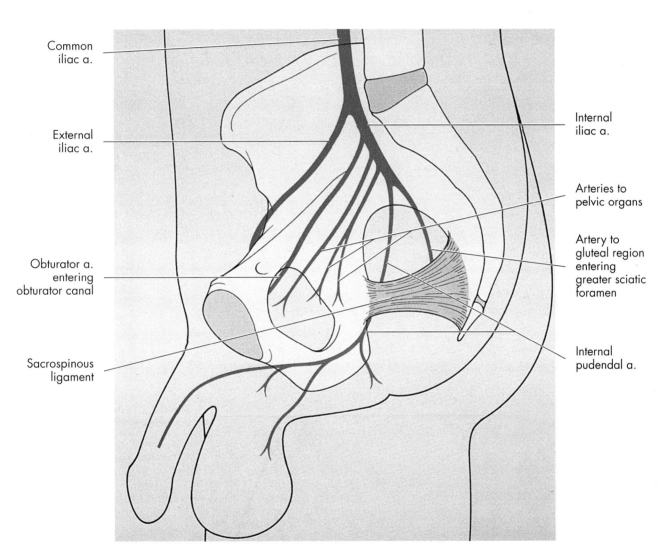

Common iliac a.

External iliac a.

Obturator a. entering obturator canal

Sacrospinous ligament

Internal iliac a.

Arteries to pelvic organs

Artery to gluteal region entering greater sciatic foramen

Internal pudendal a.

Figure 6-2   Internal iliac artery and some of its branches to the pelvis, perineum, and lower limb.

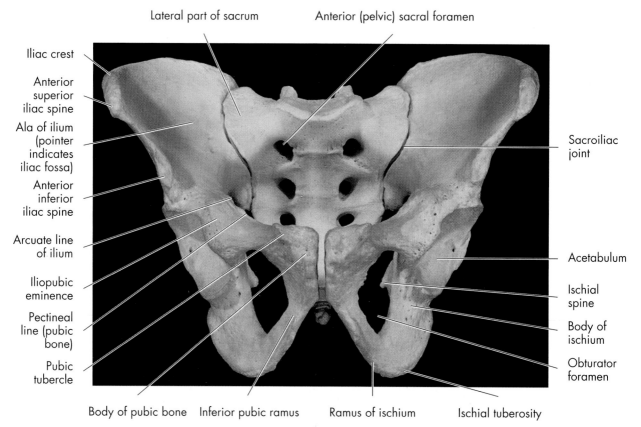

Lateral part of sacrum

Anterior (pelvic) sacral foramen

Iliac crest

Anterior superior iliac spine

Ala of ilium (pointer indicates iliac fossa)

Anterior inferior iliac spine

Arcuate line of ilium

Iliopubic eminence

Pectineal line (pubic bone)

Pubic tubercle

Sacroiliac joint

Acetabulum

Ischial spine

Body of ischium

Obturator foramen

Body of pubic bone   Inferior pubic ramus   Ramus of ischium   Ischial tuberosity

Figure 6-3   Articulated male pelvis. Specimen is viewed from in front and slightly below in order that details of the obturator foramen may be seen.

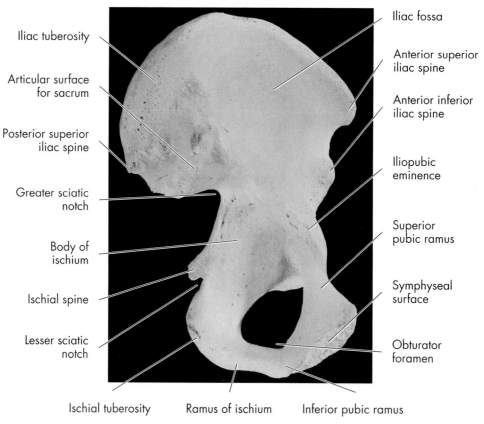

Iliac tuberosity

Articular surface for sacrum

Posterior superior iliac spine

Greater sciatic notch

Body of ischium

Ischial spine

Lesser sciatic notch

Iliac fossa

Anterior superior iliac spine

Anterior inferior iliac spine

Iliopubic eminence

Superior pubic ramus

Symphyseal surface

Obturator foramen

Ischial tuberosity   Ramus of ischium   Inferior pubic ramus

Figure 6-4   Left pelvic bones, medial aspect.

SEE PRINCIPLES, FIG. 6-22

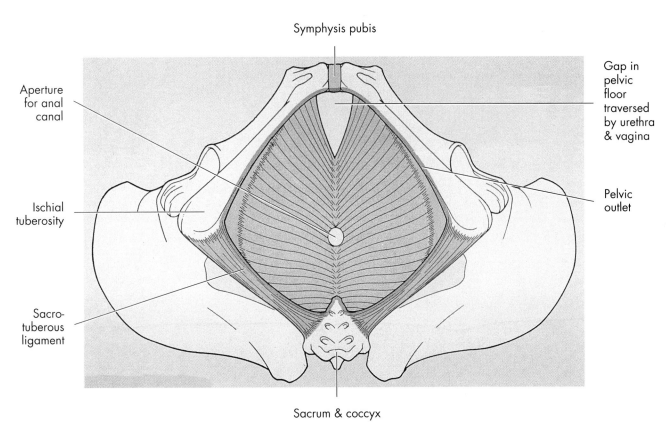

Symphysis pubis

Gap in
pelvic
floor
traversed
by urethra
& vagina

Aperture
for anal
canal

Pelvic
outlet

Ischial
tuberosity

Sacro-
tuberous
ligament

Sacrum & coccyx

Figure 6-5   Inferior aspect of the pelvic girdle showing the pelvic outlet and boundaries of the perineum.

See **DISSECTIONS**, Section 6, pp. 11 and 12

See **PRINCIPLES**, Fig. 6-19

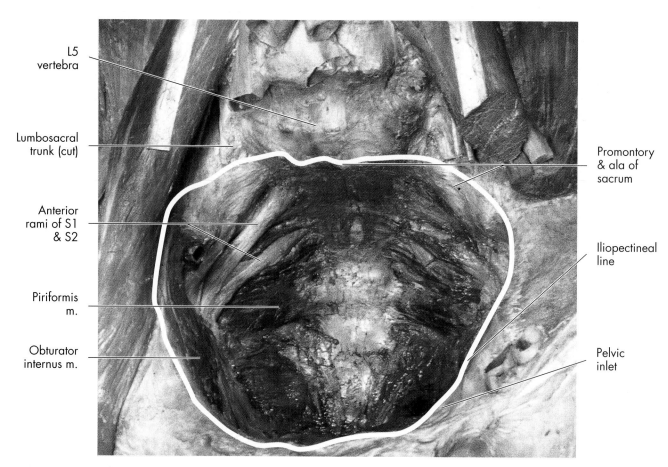

L5
vertebra

Lumbosacral
trunk (cut)

Anterior
rami of S1
& S2

Piriformis
m.

Obturator
internus m.

Promontory
& ala of
sacrum

Iliopectineal
line

Pelvic
inlet

Figure 6-6   Pelvis and lower abdomen after removal of all the organs and most of the vessels to demonstrate the pelvic inlet and cavity.

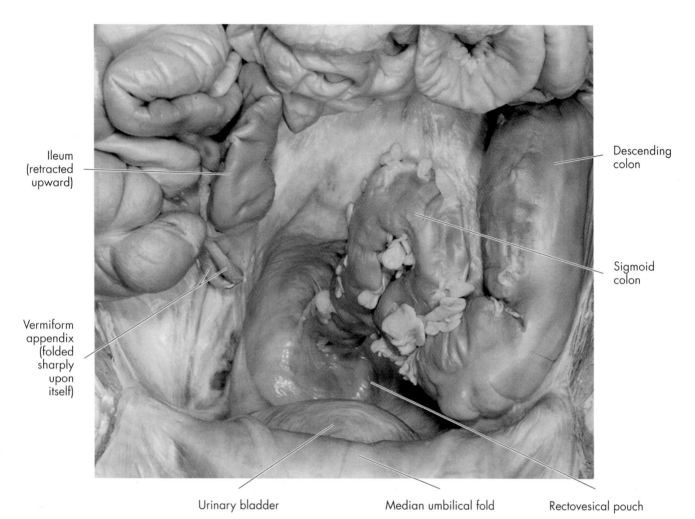

Figure 6-7 View of the pelvic part of the peritoneal cavity in a male showing the relations of organs within the pelvis. *Infection within the peritoneal cavity (peritonitis) may occur as a consequence of appendicitis, cholecystis (gallbladder infection), perforation of a viscus, salpingitis (infection progressing from vagina to uterine [fallopian] tube), pancreatitis, blood-borne infection, or a penetrating wound of the abdomen. Anatomically, such infections have a tendency to drain to and localize in certain areas. The most dependent (lowest) area in the peritoneal cavity is the rectouterine pouch (pouch of Douglas) in the female or its counterpart, the rectovesical pouch, in the male. Posterior perforated peptic ulcers, which may empty into the lesser sac, may drain out of the epiploic foramen (Winslow) tract along the gutter adjacent to the retroperitoneal ascending colon over the pelvic brim and collect in the pouch of Douglas or rectovesical pouch.*

See DISSECTIONS, Section 6, p. 9
See PRINCIPLES, Fig. 6-51

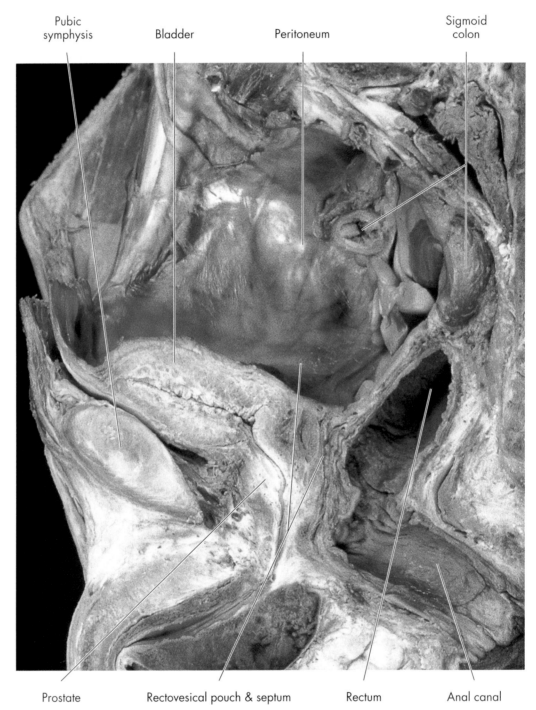

Pubic symphysis   Bladder   Peritoneum   Sigmoid colon

Prostate   Rectovesical pouch & septum   Rectum   Anal canal

Figure 6-8   Median sagittal section through the male pelvis showing the peritoneum and the principal pelvic viscera. *Digital examination of the rectum allows evaluation of the rectum itself and the prostate, seminal vesicles, bladder, and rectovesical pouch in the male.*

See **DISSECTIONS**, Section 6, p. 9
See **PRINCIPLES**, Fig. 6-26

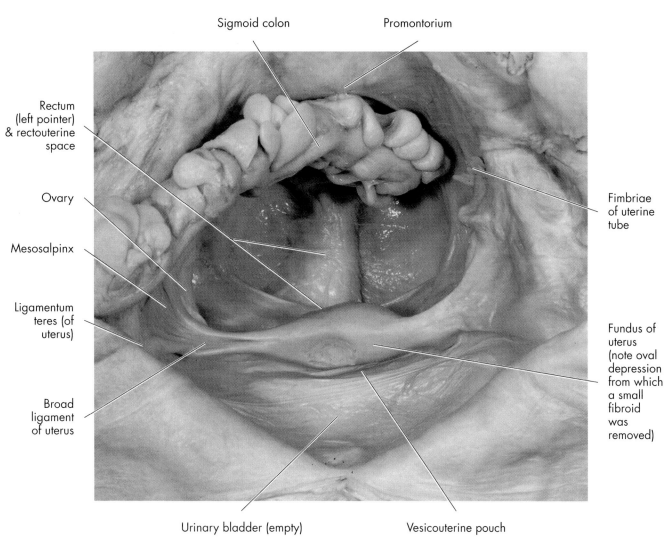

Sigmoid colon   Promontorium

Rectum
(left pointer)
& rectouterine
space

Ovary

Mesosalpinx

Ligamentum
teres (of
uterus)

Broad
ligament
of uterus

Fimbriae
of uterine
tube

Fundus of
uterus
(note oval
depression
from which
a small
fibroid
was
removed)

Urinary bladder (empty)   Vesicouterine pouch

Figure 6-9   Pelvic peritoneal cavity of a female. The bladder has been deflated to reveal the depth of the vesicouterine pouch.

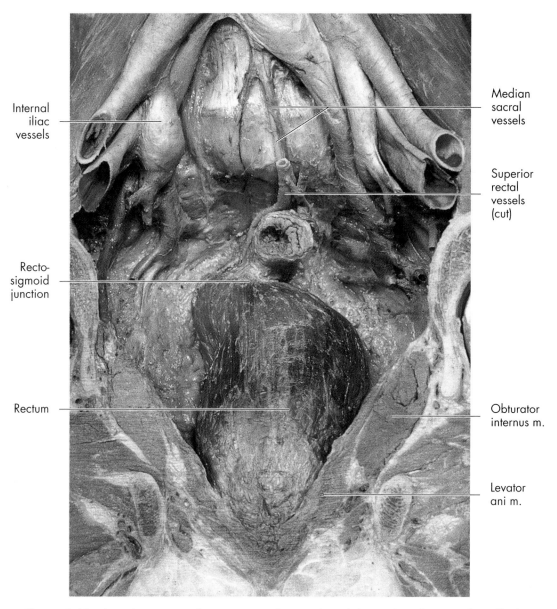

Internal
iliac
vessels

Median
sacral
vessels

Superior
rectal
vessels
(cut)

Recto-
sigmoid
junction

Rectum

Obturator
internus m.

Levator
ani m.

Figure 6-10   Anterior aspect of rectum seen in a male pelvis sectioned coronally. All of
the peritoneum has been removed.

See DISSECTIONS, Section 6, p. 9
See PRINCIPLES, Fig. 6-25

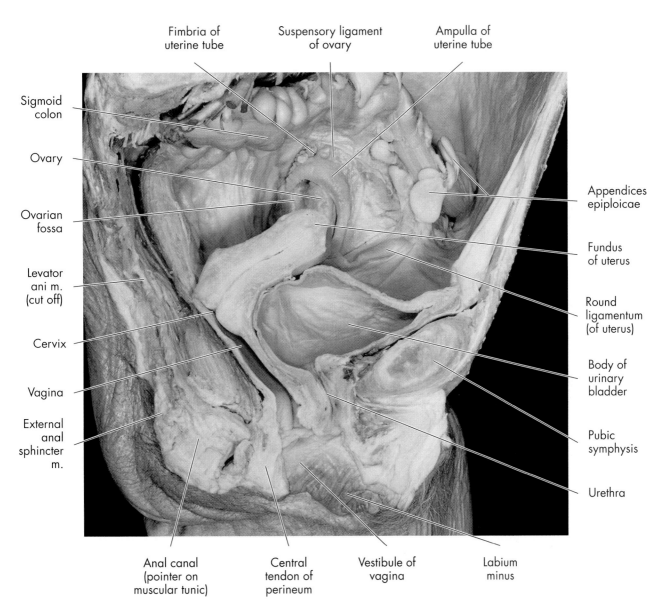

Fimbria of uterine tube · Suspensory ligament of ovary · Ampulla of uterine tube

Sigmoid colon · Ovary · Ovarian fossa · Levator ani m. (cut off) · Cervix · Vagina · External anal sphincter m.

Appendices epiploicae · Fundus of uterus · Round ligamentum (of uterus) · Body of urinary bladder · Pubic symphysis · Urethra

Anal canal (pointer on muscular tunic) · Central tendon of perineum · Vestibule of vagina · Labium minus

Figure 6-11 Median sagittal section of a female pelvis. The bladder, urethra, uterus, and vagina have been sectioned in the median plane. The rectum and anal canal have been exposed but not opened. Peritoneum remains intact in the left half of the pelvic cavity. *Digital examination of the rectum allows palpation of the vagina, cervix, uterus, ovaries, uterine tubes, and bladder (through the vaginal walls). In the female in labor, rectal examination allows evaluation of the extent of effacing and dilation of the cervix and thereby assessment of the progress of labor.*

See **DISSECTIONS,** Section 6, p. 9
See **PRINCIPLES,** Fig. 6-25

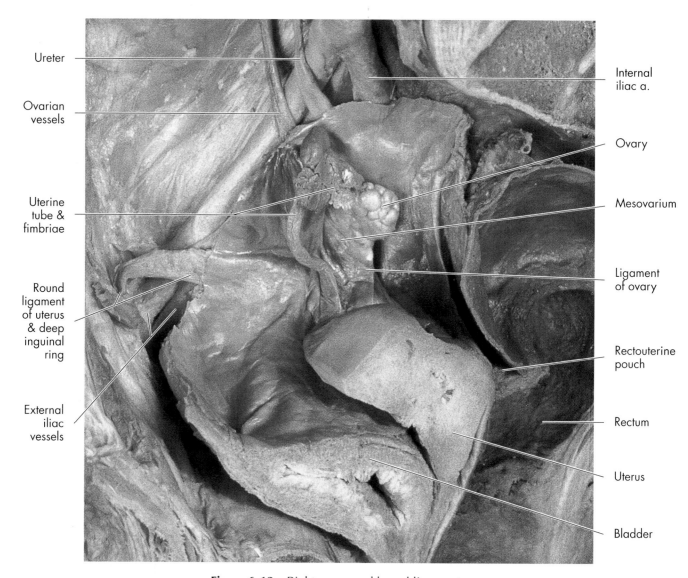

Ureter

Ovarian vessels

Uterine tube & fimbriae

Round ligament of uterus & deep inguinal ring

External iliac vessels

Internal iliac a.

Ovary

Mesovarium

Ligament of ovary

Rectouterine pouch

Rectum

Uterus

Bladder

Figure 6-12   Right ovary and broad ligament.

SEE DISSECTIONS, SECTION 6, PP. 9 AND 10

SEE PRINCIPLES, FIG. 6-57

Fundus

Uterine
cavity

Body

Cervical
canal

Cervix

Posterior
fornix

Vesicouterine
pouch

External os

Anterior
fornix

Bladder

Vagina

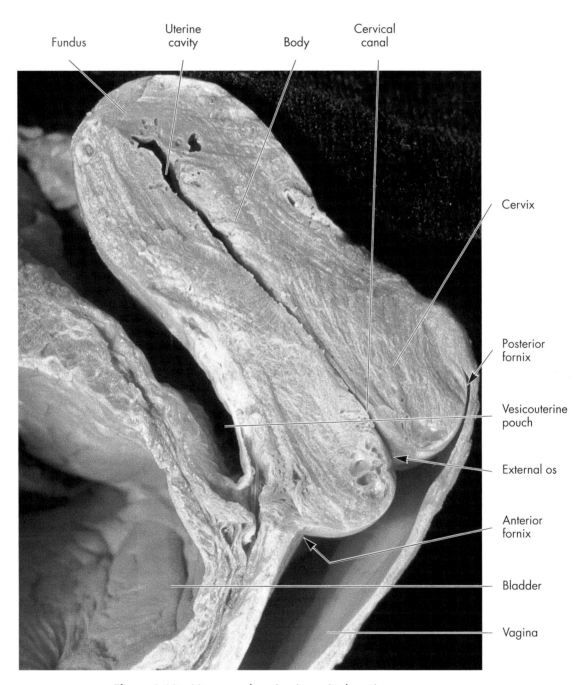

Figure 6-13   Uterus and vagina in sagittal section.

See DISSECTIONS, Section 6, p. 9
See PRINCIPLES, Fig. 6-57

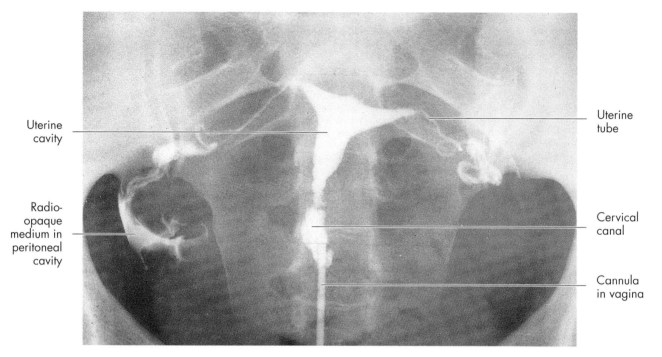

Uterine cavity

Radio-opaque medium in peritoneal cavity

Uterine tube

Cervical canal

Cannula in vagina

Figure 6-14 Hysterosalpingogram. Radio-opaque medium has been injected, via a cannula in the vagina, into the uterus and along the uterine tubes.

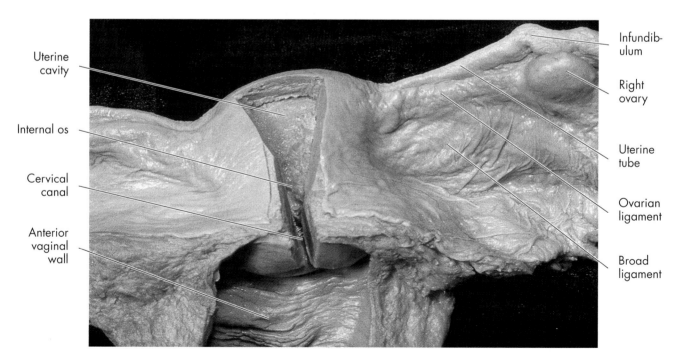

Uterine cavity

Internal os

Cervical canal

Anterior vaginal wall

Infundibulum

Right ovary

Uterine tube

Ovarian ligament

Broad ligament

Figure 6-15 Uterine cavity and cervical canal exposed by removal of parts of their posterior walls.

See DISSECTIONS, Section 6, pp. 9 and 10

See PRINCIPLES, Fig. 6-57

Postero-
superior
surface
of uterus

Lateral
fornix

External
os

Vaginal
wall (cut)

Anterior
fornix

Rugae

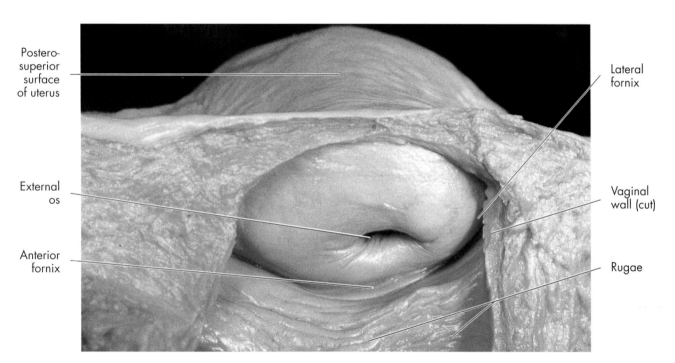

Figure 6-16   Intravaginal part of the cervix revealed by removal of the posterior wall of the vagina.

See DISSECTIONS, Section 6, pp. 10 and 11

See PRINCIPLES, Figs. 6-11, 6-20

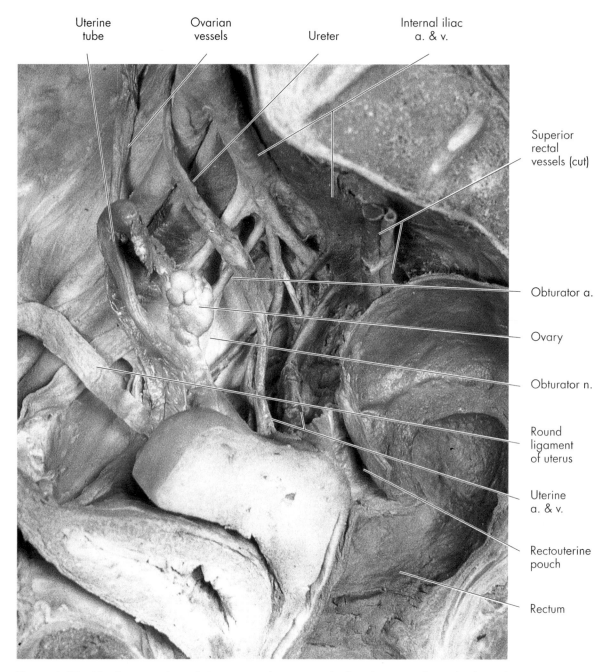

Uterine tube   Ovarian vessels   Ureter   Internal iliac a. & v.

Superior rectal vessels (cut)

Obturator a.

Ovary

Obturator n.

Round ligament of uterus

Uterine a. & v.

Rectouterine pouch

Rectum

Figure 6-17   Uterine vessels and the ureter after removal of peritoneum from the lateral pelvic wall.

See DISSECTIONS, Section 6, pp. 10 and 11

See PRINCIPLES, Fig. 6-20

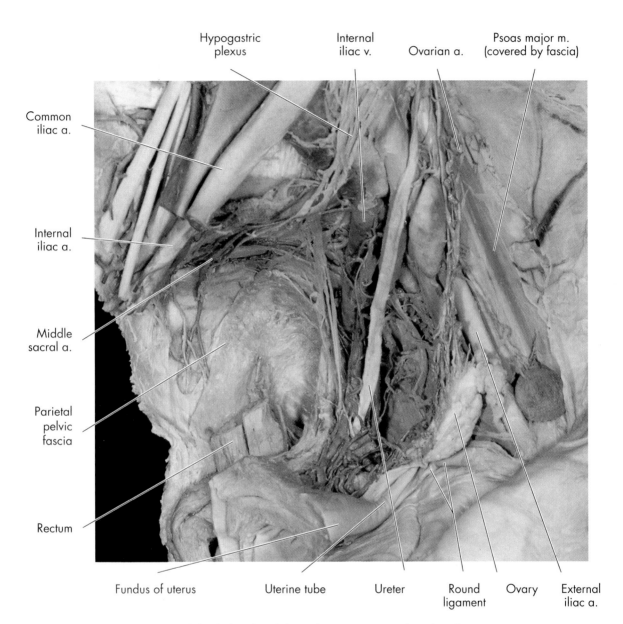

Figure 6-18   Interior of the left side of the pelvic cavity in a female. The ovary, ovarian vessels, and uterine tube have been displaced anteriorly.

SEE PRINCIPLES, FIG. 6-32

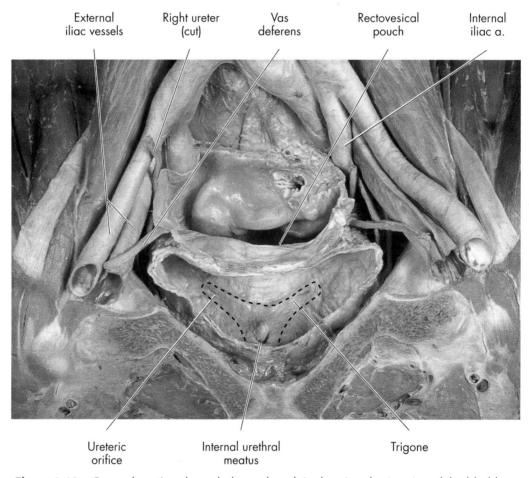

External   Right ureter   Vas   Rectovesical   Internal
iliac vessels   (cut)   deferens   pouch   iliac a.

Ureteric   Internal urethral   Trigone
orifice   meatus

Figure 6-19   Coronal section through the male pelvis showing the interior of the bladder and some of its relationships.

See DISSECTIONS, Section 6, pp. 9 and 10

See PRINCIPLES, Fig. 6-64

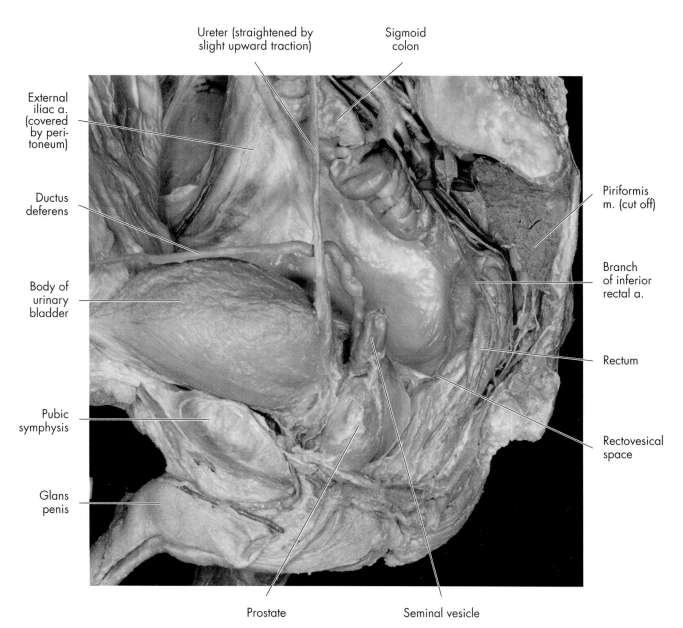

Ureter (straightened by slight upward traction)

Sigmoid colon

External iliac a. (covered by peritoneum)

Piriformis m. (cut off)

Ductus deferens

Branch of inferior rectal a.

Body of urinary bladder

Rectum

Pubic symphysis

Rectovesical space

Glans penis

Prostate

Seminal vesicle

Figure 6-20 Lateral view of the male pelvis showing the relationship of the bladder, prostate, seminal vesicles and rectovesical septum to the pelvic peritoneum. *Specimens of fluid from the prostate and seminal vesicles may be attained by digital massage of the seminal vessels and prostate through the rectal wall. After such massage, semen will appear at the urethral orifice of the penis, and it can then be analyzed.*

See PRINCIPLES, Fig. 6-25

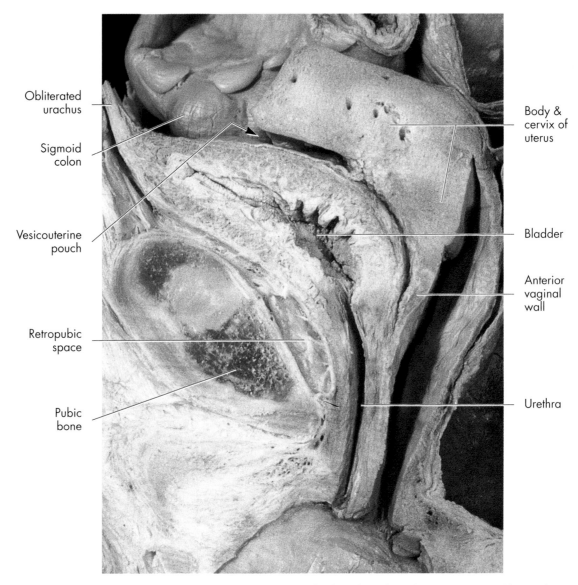

Obliterated
urachus

Sigmoid
colon

Vesicouterine
pouch

Retropubic
space

Pubic
bone

Body &
cervix of
uterus

Bladder

Anterior
vaginal
wall

Urethra

Figure 6-21   Median sagittal section through the female pelvis showing the bladder and
some of its relationships. *Once the urethral orifice is located in the anterior vaginal wall
at the introitus, the short, straight course of the urethra makes the passage of a catheter or
instrument quite simple in females.*

SEE DISSECTIONS, SECTION 6, PP. 10 AND 11
SEE PRINCIPLES, FIG. 6-20

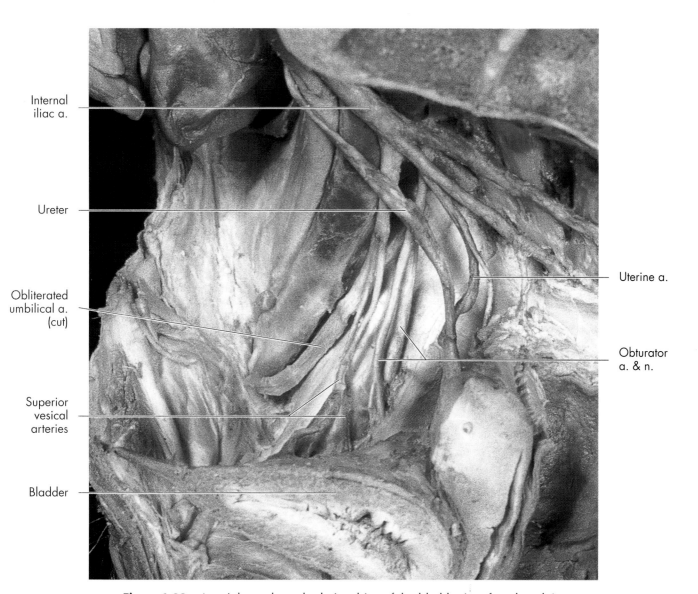

Figure 6-22 Arterial supply and relationships of the bladder in a female pelvis.

Internal iliac a.

Ureter

Obliterated umbilical a. (cut)

Superior vesical arteries

Bladder

Uterine a.

Obturator a. & n.

See PRINCIPLES, Fig. 6-55

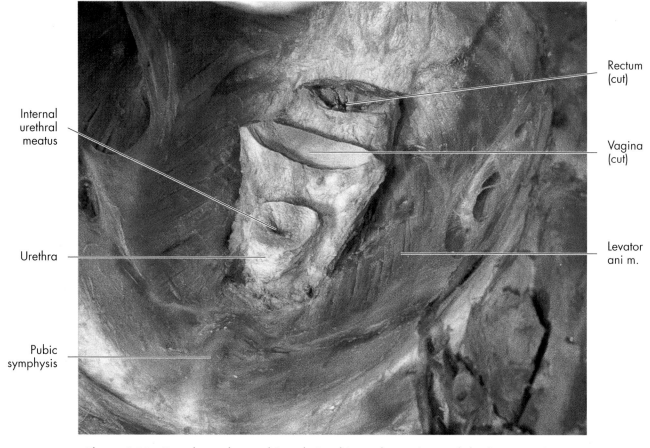

Figure 6-23   Female urethra and its relationship to the vagina and the levator ani muscles.

See DISSECTIONS, Section 6, p. 7
See PRINCIPLES, Fig. 6-31

Navicular fossa   Glans penis   Spongy urethra   Corpus spongiosum   Intrabulbar fossa   Puboprostatic ligaments   Bladder

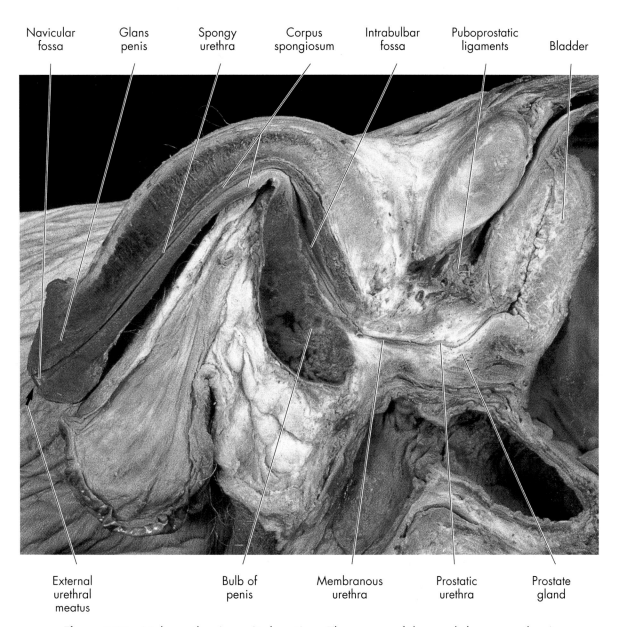

External urethral meatus   Bulb of penis   Membranous urethra   Prostatic urethra   Prostate gland

Figure 6-24   Male urethra in sagittal section. *The course of the much longer urethra in the male makes catherization of the bladder more complex. After passage through the penile urethra, there is an abrupt turn into the membranous urethra. To lessen the risk of urethral perforation in the male, sounds (probes) and catheter guides are curved to allow passage into the membranous urethra.*

See DISSECTIONS, Section 6, p. 12
See PRINCIPLES, Fig. 6-64

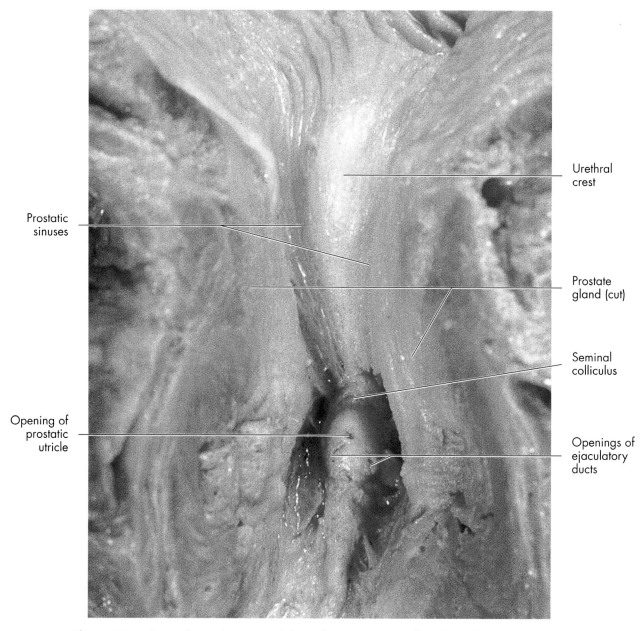

Urethral
crest

Prostatic
sinuses

Prostate
gland (cut)

Seminal
colliculus

Opening of
prostatic
utricle

Openings of
ejaculatory
ducts

Figure 6-25 Prostatic urethra opened through its anterior wall to show the urethral crest and seminal colliculus.

SEE PRINCIPLES, FIG. 6-64

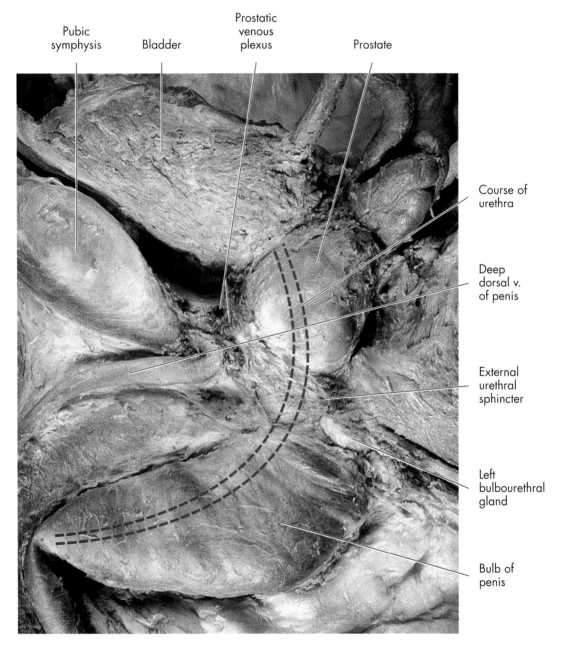

Figure 6-26 Left pelvic wall and levator ani muscles removed to show the prostate gland, external urethral sphincter, left bulbourethral gland, and the bulb of the penis. The course of the urethra through the prostate, the urogenital diaphragm, and the bulb of the penis is outlined by the dashed line.

SEE **DISSECTIONS**, SECTION 6, P. 12

SEE **PRINCIPLES**, FIGS. 6-46, 6-64

Ureters

Vasa deferentia

Bladder

Left seminal vesicle

Prostate

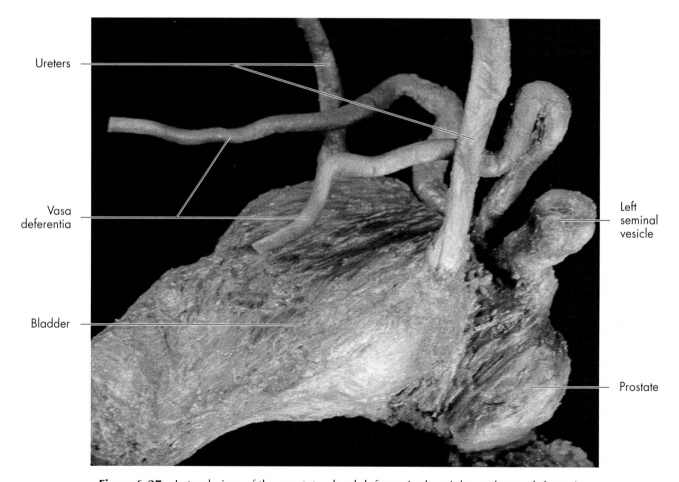

Figure 6-27   Lateral view of the prostate gland, left seminal vesicle, and vasa deferentia.

See **DISSECTIONS**, Section 6, p. 12
See **PRINCIPLES**, Figs. 6-46, 6-64

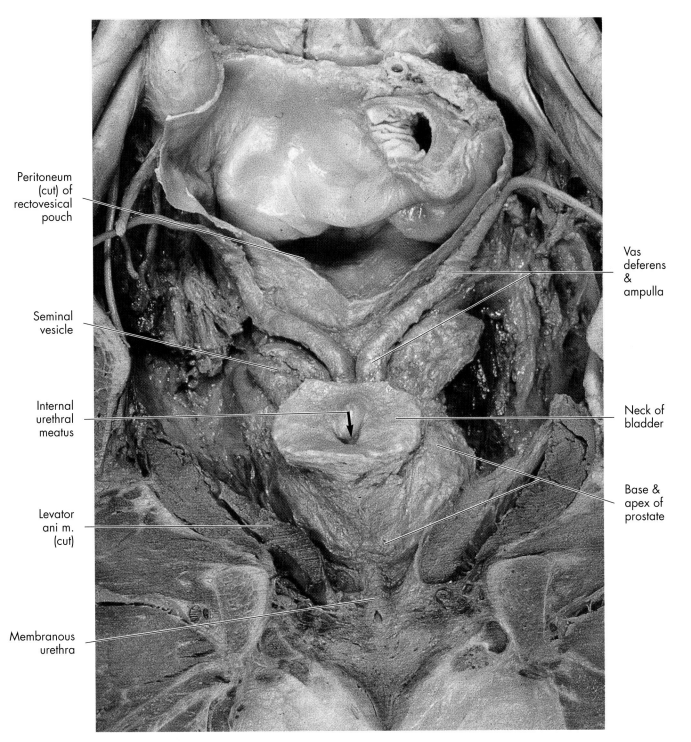

Peritoneum (cut) of rectovesical pouch

Seminal vesicle

Internal urethral meatus

Levator ani m. (cut)

Membranous urethra

Vas deferens & ampulla

Neck of bladder

Base & apex of prostate

Figure 6-28   Coronal section of the pelvic walls and floor. Most of the bladder has been removed to reveal the prostate, seminal vesicles, and vas deferens. The internal urethral meatus is visible at the labeled arrow.

SEE DISSECTIONS, SECTION 6, P. 12

SEE PRINCIPLES, FIG. 6-64

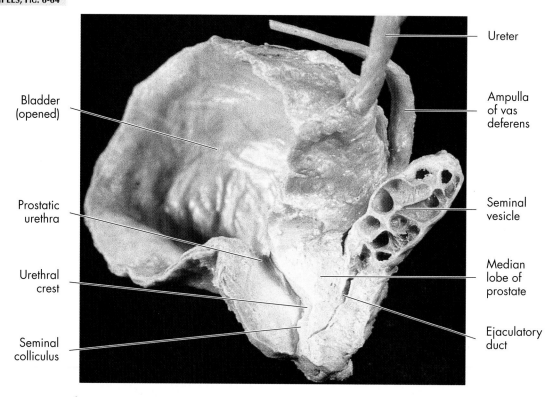

Ureter

Bladder
(opened)

Ampulla
of vas
deferens

Prostatic
urethra

Seminal
vesicle

Urethral
crest

Median
lobe of
prostate

Seminal
colliculus

Ejaculatory
duct

Figure 6-29 Dissection of the prostate gland and the left seminal vesicle.

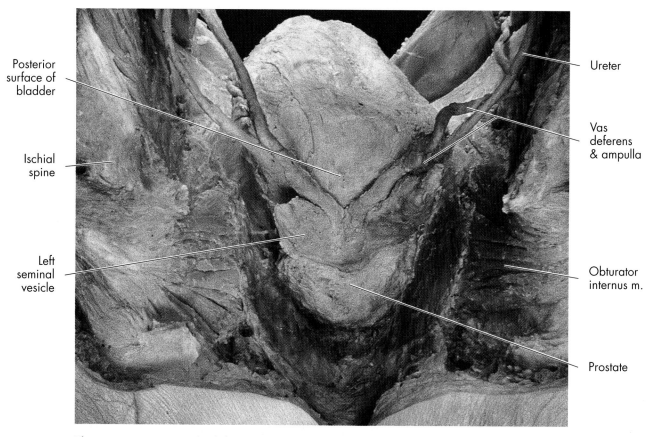

Posterior
surface of
bladder

Ureter

Vas
deferens
& ampulla

Ischial
spine

Left
seminal
vesicle

Obturator
internus m.

Prostate

Figure 6-30 Removal of the rectum and the posterior wall of the pelvis exposing the bladder, prostate, seminal vesicles, and vas deferens from behind.

See DISSECTIONS, Section 6, p. 12

See PRINCIPLES, Fig. 6-15

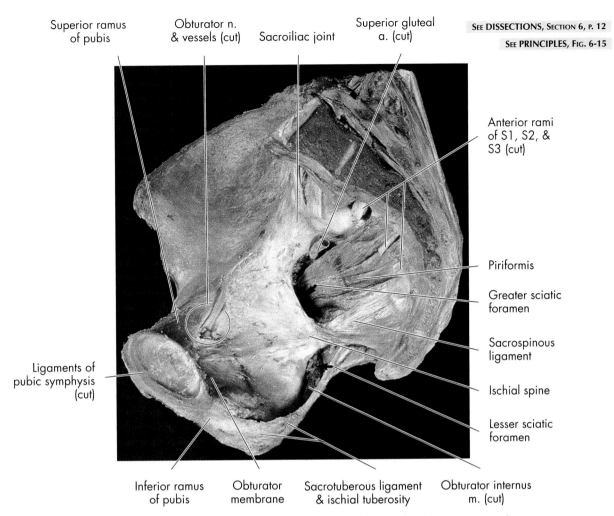

Superior ramus of pubis

Obturator n. & vessels (cut)

Sacroiliac joint

Superior gluteal a. (cut)

Anterior rami of S1, S2, & S3 (cut)

Piriformis

Greater sciatic foramen

Sacrospinous ligament

Ischial spine

Lesser sciatic foramen

Ligaments of pubic symphysis (cut)

Inferior ramus of pubis

Obturator membrane

Sacrotuberous ligament & ischial tuberosity

Obturator internus m. (cut)

Figure 6-31   Right hemipelvis showing the pubic symphysis, the obturator membrane, the ligaments, and the foramina.

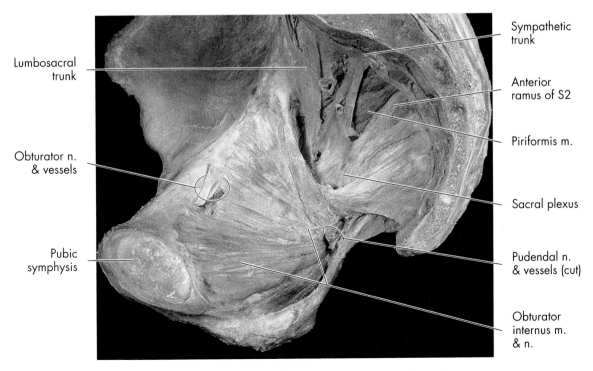

Lumbosacral trunk

Obturator n. & vessels

Pubic symphysis

Sympathetic trunk

Anterior ramus of S2

Piriformis m.

Sacral plexus

Pudendal n. & vessels (cut)

Obturator internus m. & n.

Figure 6-32   Right hemipelvis showing the pelvic attachment of the obturator internus.

SEE **DISSECTIONS**, SECTION 6, P. 11

SEE **PRINCIPLES**, FIG. 6-15

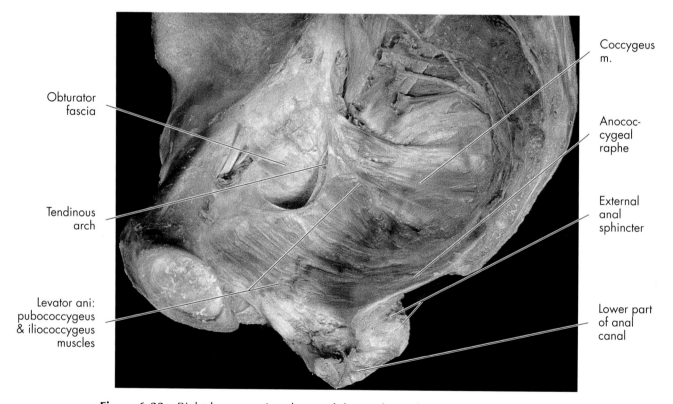

Obturator
fascia

Tendinous
arch

Levator ani:
pubococcygeus
& iliococcygeus
muscles

Coccygeus
m.

Anococ-
cygeal
raphe

External
anal
sphincter

Lower part
of anal
canal

Figure 6-33   Right levator ani and part of the anal canal seen in a median sagittal section of the pelvis.

See DISSECTIONS, Section 6, pp. 10 and 12

See PRINCIPLES, Fig. 6-36

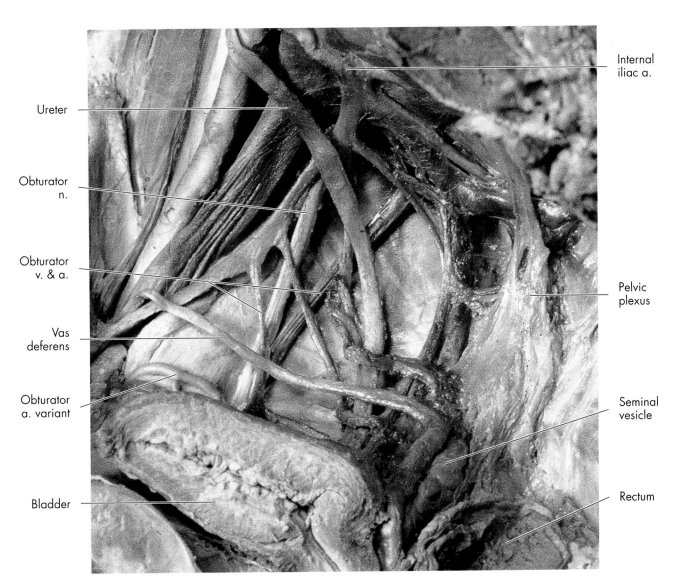

Ureter

Obturator
n.

Obturator
v. & a.

Vas
deferens

Obturator
a. variant

Bladder

Internal
iliac a.

Pelvic
plexus

Seminal
vesicle

Rectum

Figure 6-34   Right pelvic plexus of autonomic nerves. This specimen has an obturator artery variant.

See DISSECTIONS, Section 6, pp. 10 and 12

See PRINCIPLES, Figs. 6-20, 6-39, 6-42

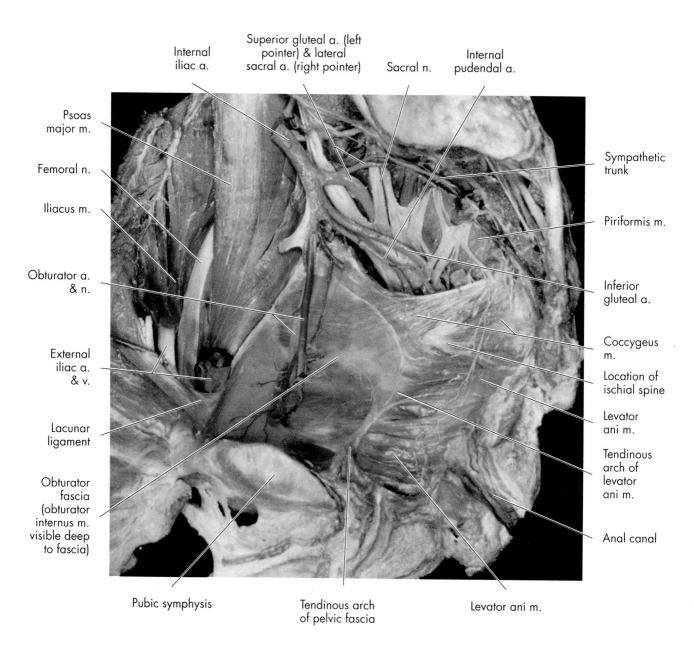

Figure 6-35 Lateral view of the male pelvis with the prostate removed. The superior fascia of the pelvic diaphragm has been dissected to expose branches from sacral nerves III and IV.

SEE DISSECTIONS, SECTION 6, P. 12
SEE PRINCIPLES, FIG. 6-40

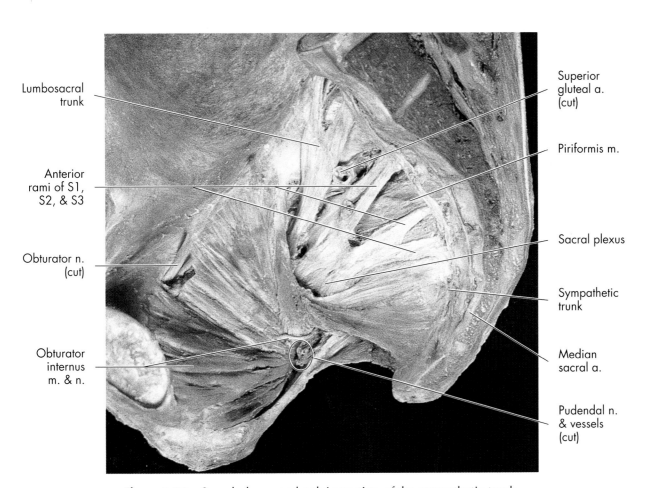

Lumbosacral
trunk

Anterior
rami of S1,
S2, & S3

Obturator n.
(cut)

Obturator
internus
m. & n.

Superior
gluteal a.
(cut)

Piriformis m.

Sacral plexus

Sympathetic
trunk

Median
sacral a.

Pudendal n.
& vessels
(cut)

Figure 6-36   Sacral plexus and pelvic portion of the sympathetic trunk.

See **DISSECTIONS**, Section 6, p. 12
See **PRINCIPLES**, Fig. 6-39

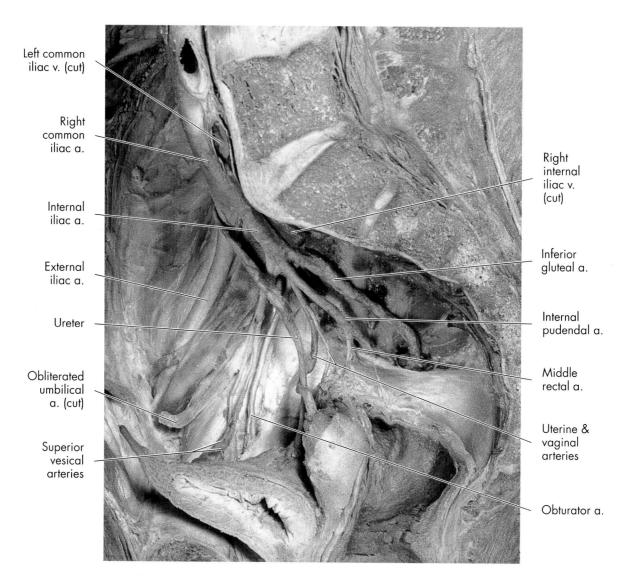

Left common
iliac v. (cut)

Right
common
iliac a.

Internal
iliac a.

External
iliac a.

Ureter

Obliterated
umbilical
a. (cut)

Superior
vesical
arteries

Right
internal
iliac v.
(cut)

Inferior
gluteal a.

Internal
pudendal a.

Middle
rectal a.

Uterine &
vaginal
arteries

Obturator a.

Figure 6-37   Right internal iliac artery and some of its branches.

SEE **DISSECTIONS,** SECTION 6, P. 12
SEE **PRINCIPLES,** FIG. 6-20, *A*

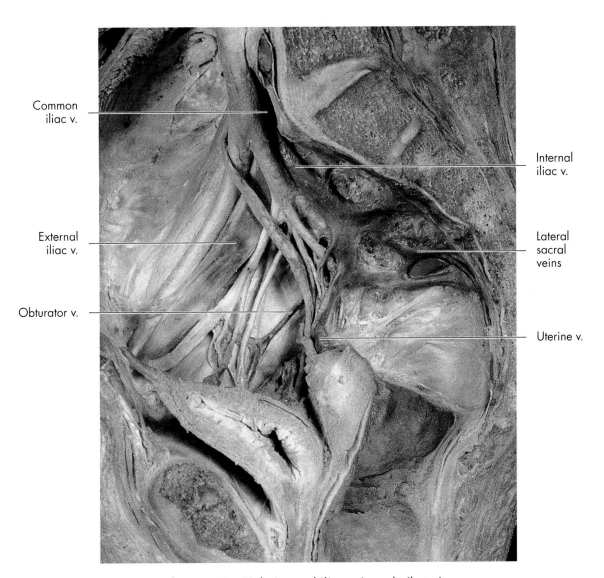

Common
iliac v.

External
iliac v.

Obturator v.

Internal
iliac v.

Lateral
sacral
veins

Uterine v.

Figure 6-38   Right internal iliac vein and tributaries.

SEE DISSECTIONS, SECTION 6, PP. 3 AND 4

SEE PRINCIPLES, FIG. 6-13

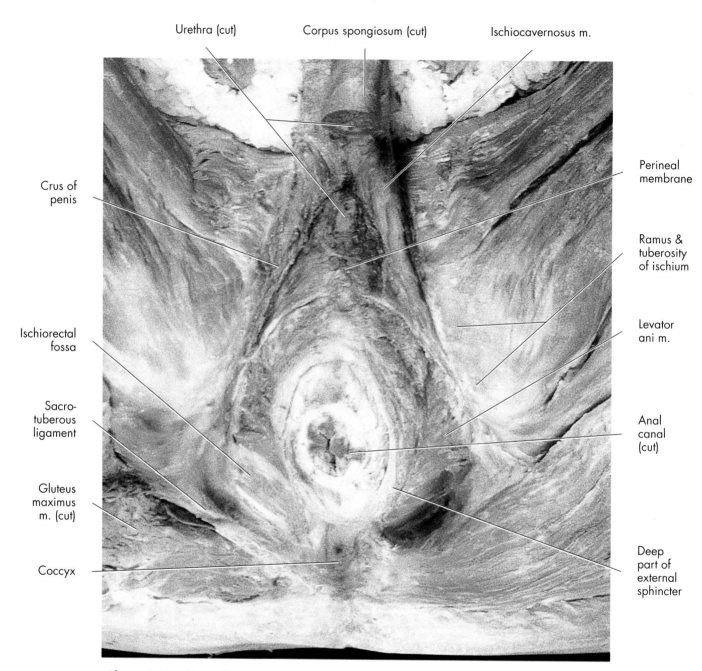

Urethra (cut)   Corpus spongiosum (cut)   Ischiocavernosus m.

Crus of penis

Perineal membrane

Ramus & tuberosity of ischium

Ischiorectal fossa

Levator ani m.

Sacro-tuberous ligament

Anal canal (cut)

Gluteus maximus m. (cut)

Coccyx

Deep part of external sphincter

Figure 6-39   Deep dissection of male perineum showing its boundaries. The bulb of the penis has been removed to expose the perineal membrane, and the gluteus maximus on one side has been resected to reveal the sacrotuberous ligament.

SEE PRINCIPLES, FIG. 6-19

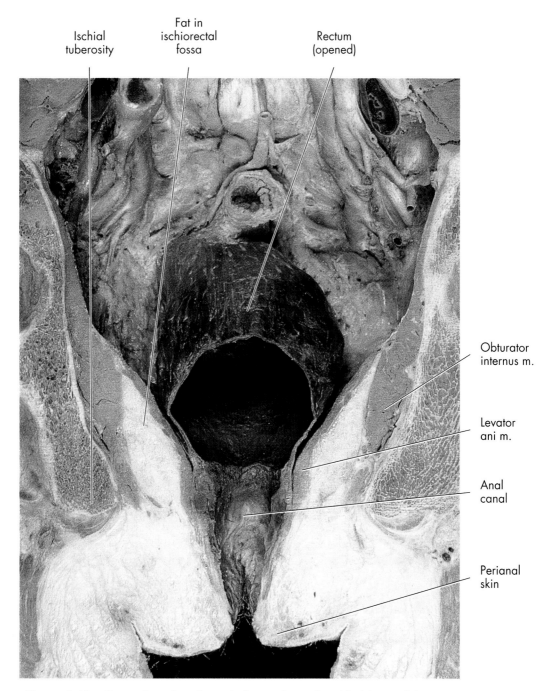

Ischial
tuberosity

Fat in
ischiorectal
fossa

Rectum
(opened)

Obturator
internus m.

Levator
ani m.

Anal
canal

Perianal
skin

Figure 6-40 Coronal section through the anal canal and ischiorectal fossae.

See **DISSECTIONS**, Section 6, pp. 3 and 4

See **PRINCIPLES**, Fig. 6-22

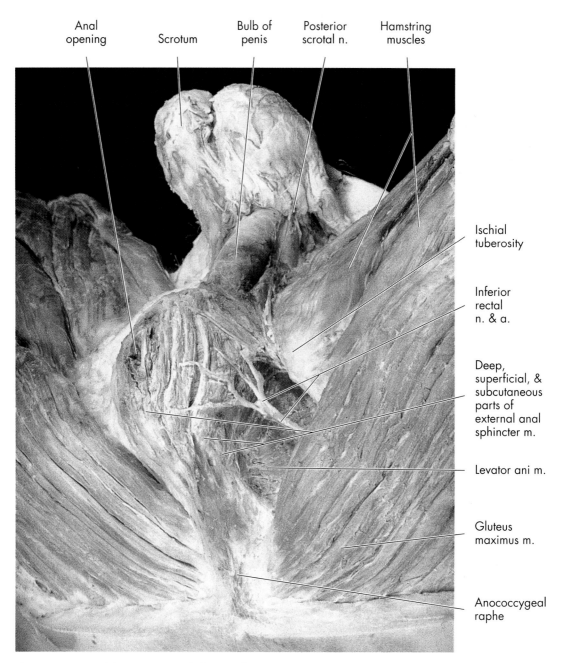

Anal
opening

Scrotum

Bulb of
penis

Posterior
scrotal n.

Hamstring
muscles

Ischial
tuberosity

Inferior
rectal
n. & a.

Deep,
superficial, &
subcutaneous
parts of
external anal
sphincter m.

Levator ani m.

Gluteus
maximus m.

Anococcygeal
raphe

Figure 6-41   Oblique view of the anal triangle showing parts of the external anal sphincter and the inferior rectal nerve and vessels.

See DISSECTIONS, Section 6, p. 7
See PRINCIPLES, Fig. 6-42

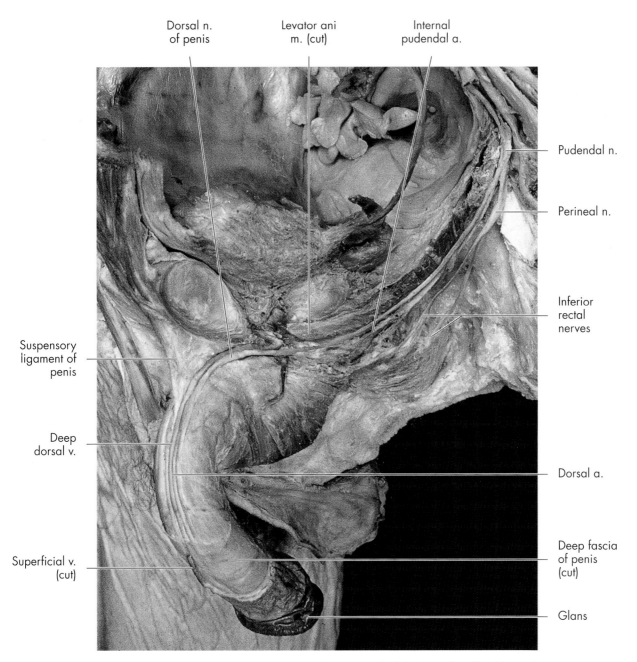

Dorsal n.
of penis

Levator ani
m. (cut)

Internal
pudendal a.

Pudendal n.

Perineal n.

Inferior
rectal
nerves

Suspensory
ligament of
penis

Deep
dorsal v.

Dorsal a.

Superficial v.
(cut)

Deep fascia
of penis
(cut)

Glans

Figure 6-42   Left pudendal nerve exposed by removal of the lateral wall of the pelvis.

SEE DISSECTIONS, SECTION 6, P. 7
SEE PRINCIPLES, FIG. 6-16

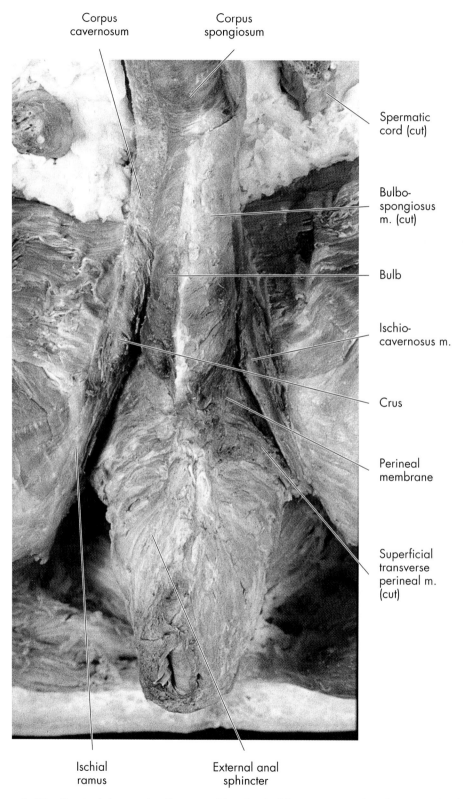

Corpus
cavernosum

Corpus
spongiosum

Spermatic
cord (cut)

Bulbo-
spongiosus
m. (cut)

Bulb

Ischio-
cavernosus m.

Crus

Perineal
membrane

Superficial
transverse
perineal m.
(cut)

Ischial
ramus

External anal
sphincter

Figure 6-43 Root of the penis. On one side, the ischiocavernosus has been excised to reveal the crus, and the bulbospongiosus has been removed to expose half of the bulb.

SEE DISSECTIONS, SECTION 6, P. 7

SEE PRINCIPLES, FIG. 6-27

Corpus spongiosum
of penis

Crus of penis
(cut across)

Bulbo-
spongio-
sus m.

Body of
pubic
bone

Duct of
bulbourethral
gland

Dorsal n.
of the
penis

Bulb of
penis (left
half dissected)

Dorsal a.
of penis

Ischiocaver-
nosus m.

Internal
pudendal
a.

Central
tendon of
perineum

Posterior
border of
urogenital
diaphragm

Inferior fascia of urogenital
diaphragm (tissue of bulb of
penis removed)

Artery of
bulb of penis

Deep transverse
perineal m.

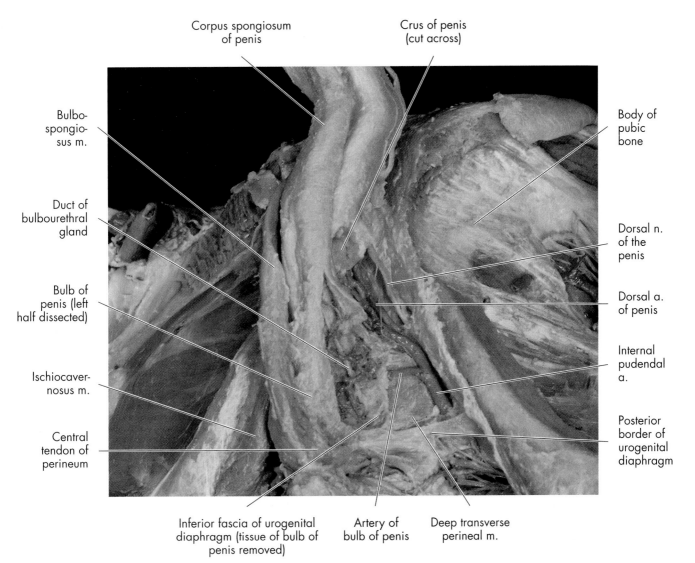

Figure 6-44   Male perineum dissected to show the bulb of the penis and the deep perineal space. The left half of the penile bulb has been opened and cleared of trabeculated
erectile tissue. The area of attachment of the bulb to the urogenital diaphragm has been
preserved with the artery of the bulb passing through it. The duct of the bulbourethral
gland has been dissected from the point at which it emerges from the urogenital
diaphragm to its site of penetration of the urethral wall.

See DISSECTIONS, Section 6, pp. 6 and 7
See PRINCIPLES, Fig. 6-29, *A* and *B*

Superficial v.   Skin

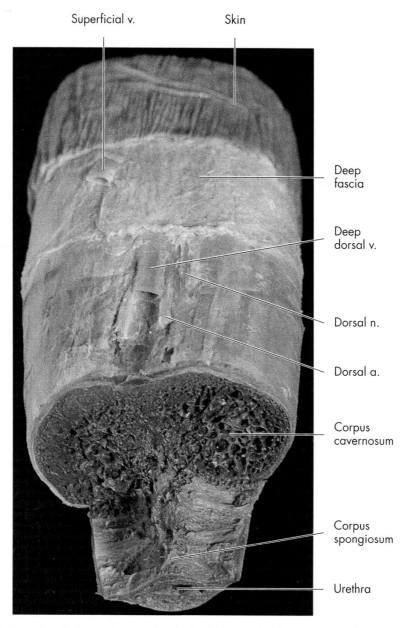

Deep
fascia

Deep
dorsal v.

Dorsal n.

Dorsal a.

Corpus
cavernosum

Corpus
spongiosum

Urethra

Figure 6-45   "Step" dissection of the shaft of the penis showing the three corpora and the dorsal vessels.

See **DISSECTIONS**, Section 6, p. 8
See **PRINCIPLES**, Fig. 6-27

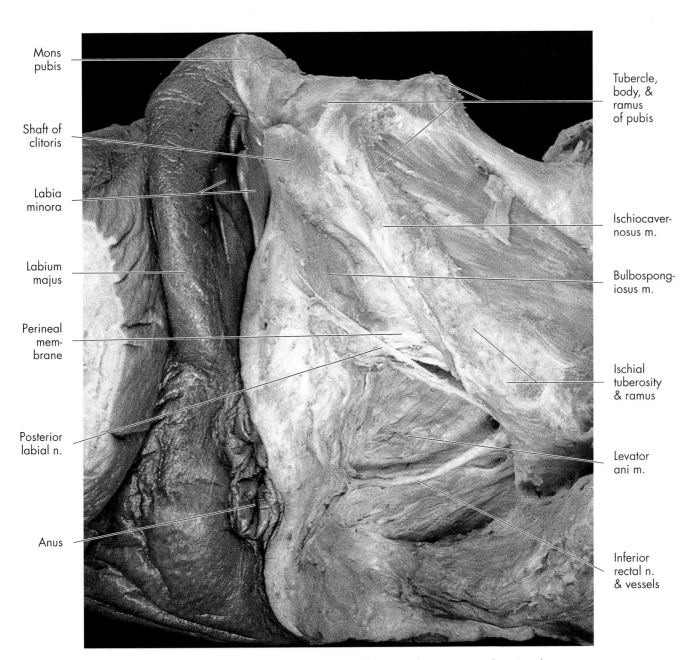

Figure 6-46 Superficial dissection of one side of the female perineum showing the muscles and cutaneous nerves.

See DISSECTIONS, Section 6, p. 8
See PRINCIPLES, Fig. 6-24

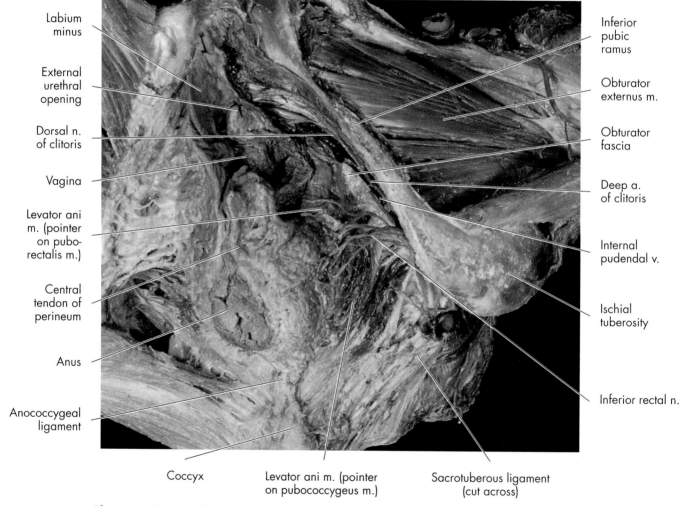

Labium minus

External urethral opening

Dorsal n. of clitoris

Vagina

Levator ani m. (pointer on pubo-rectalis m.)

Central tendon of perineum

Anus

Anococcygeal ligament

Inferior pubic ramus

Obturator externus m.

Obturator fascia

Deep a. of clitoris

Internal pudendal v.

Ischial tuberosity

Inferior rectal n.

Coccyx

Levator ani m. (pointer on pubococcygeus m.)

Sacrotuberous ligament (cut across)

Figure 6-47   Female perineum dissected to show the inferior aspect of the levator ani muscle. The left half of the urogenital diaphragm has been removed to show the anterior recess of the ischiorectal fossa. *Abscesses are prone to occur in the poorly vascularized fat that occupies the ischiorectal fossa. Infection often starts in the anal valves, progresses through the wall of the anal canal, and enters the ischiorectal space. Such abscesses may discharge through the skin in the anal area, thereby forming a tract from the anal to the perianal skin (anal fistula).*

SEE **DISSECTIONS**, SECTION 6, P. 8

SEE **PRINCIPLES**, FIG. 6-27

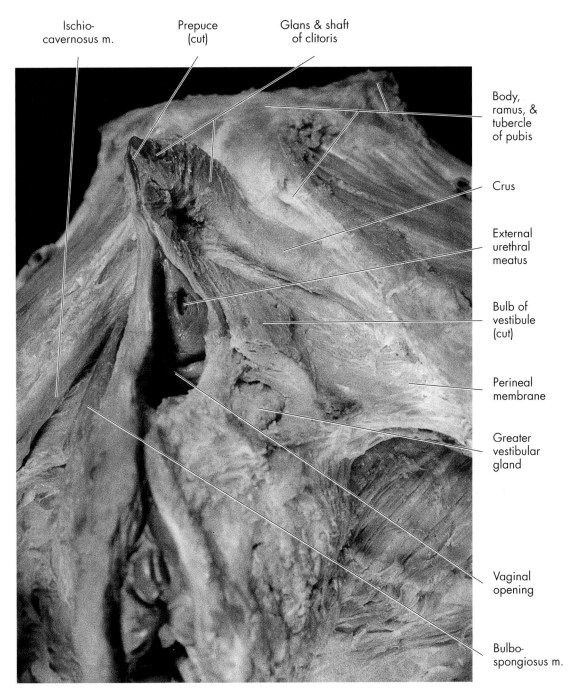

Ischio-
cavernosus m.

Prepuce
(cut)

Glans & shaft
of clitoris

Body,
ramus, &
tubercle
of pubis

Crus

External
urethral
meatus

Bulb of
vestibule
(cut)

Perineal
membrane

Greater
vestibular
gland

Vaginal
opening

Bulbo-
spongiosus m.

Figure 6-48   Deeper dissection of the female perineum. The glans, shaft, and left crus of
the clitoris have been exposed. The left bulb of the vestibule has been cut to reveal the
greater vestibular gland.

Lower Limb

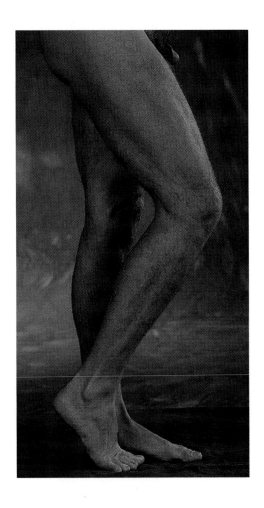

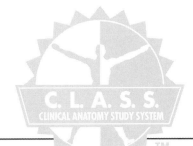

See PRINCIPLES, Fig. 7-2

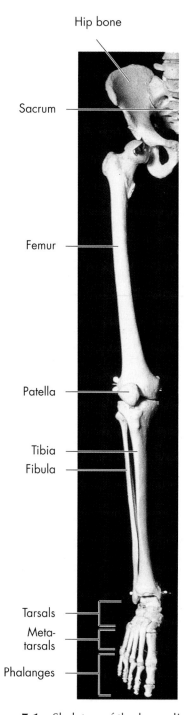

Hip bone

Sacrum

Femur

Patella

Tibia

Fibula

Tarsals

Meta-
tarsals

Phalanges

Figure 7-1   Skeleton of the lower limb.

See PRINCIPLES, Figs. 7-14, 7-15

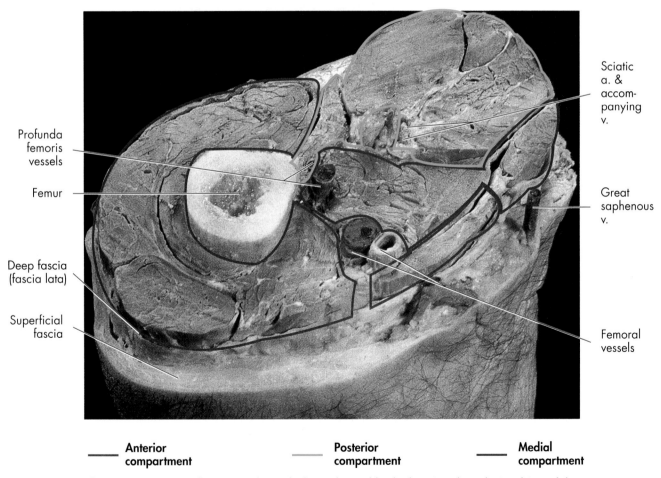

Profunda
femoris
vessels

Femur

Deep fascia
(fascia lata)

Superficial
fascia

Sciatic
a. &
accom-
panying
v.

Great
saphenous
v.

Femoral
vessels

_____ **Anterior**
compartment   _____ **Posterior**
compartment   _____ **Medial**
compartment

Figure 7-2 "Step" dissection through the right midthigh showing the relationships of the
compartments.

See PRINCIPLES, Figs. 7-53, 7-54

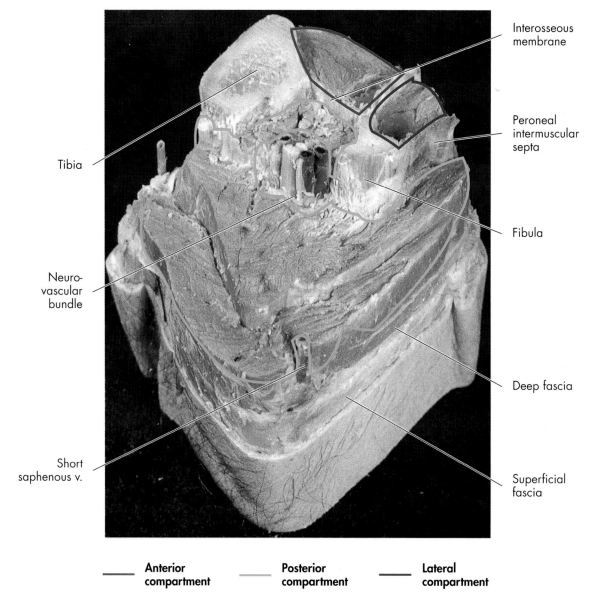

Interosseous
membrane

Peroneal
intermuscular
septa

Tibia

Fibula

Neuro-
vascular
bundle

Deep fascia

Short
saphenous v.

Superficial
fascia

_____ Anterior   _____ Posterior   _____ Lateral
        compartment   compartment   compartment

Figure 7-3   "Step" dissection through the right midcalf showing the relationships of the compartments. *The division of muscle groups into compartments by tough fascial partitions is the anatomic basis for "compartment syndrome." Increased, unrelieved pressure within a compartment may reach a level that causes interruption of arterial blood inflow. The result is compression of the muscles and nerves within a compartment. The initiating cause may be blunt trauma to the area, a fracture with bleeding confined to the space, or over-exercising a muscle or group of muscles within a compartment. For example, vigorous exercising without conditioning may result in swelling of muscles in the anterior compartment, an elevation of pressure, and consequent inadequate blood inflow. The patient will suffer temporary foot drop with paralysis of the extensor muscle group. Rest and elevation often reverse the problem, but some compartment syndromes require surgery to divide the deep fascia in order to relieve pressure on the enclosed structures (see also Figures 7-42 and 7-60).*

See **PRINCIPLES**, Fig. 7-8

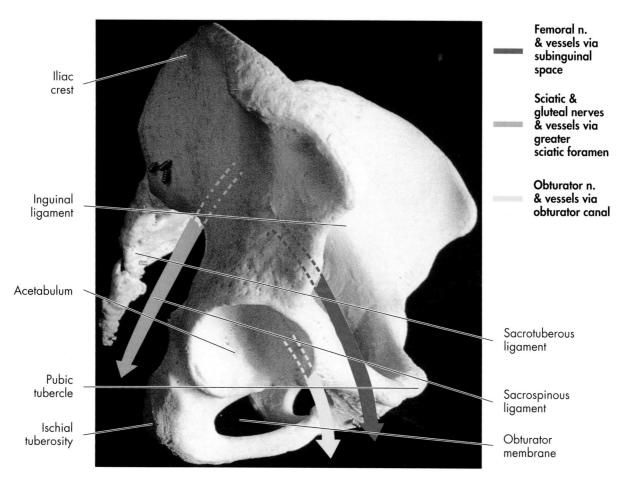

Femoral n. & vessels via subinguinal space

Sciatic & gluteal nerves & vessels via greater sciatic foramen

Obturator n. & vessels via obturator canal

Iliac crest

Inguinal ligament

Acetabulum

Pubic tubercle

Ischial tuberosity

Sacrotuberous ligament

Sacrospinous ligament

Obturator membrane

Figure 7-4 Sites of access of the principal nerves and vessels from the abdomen and pelvis into the root of the lower limb.

Sᴇᴇ **PRINCIPLES**, Fɪɢ. 7-78

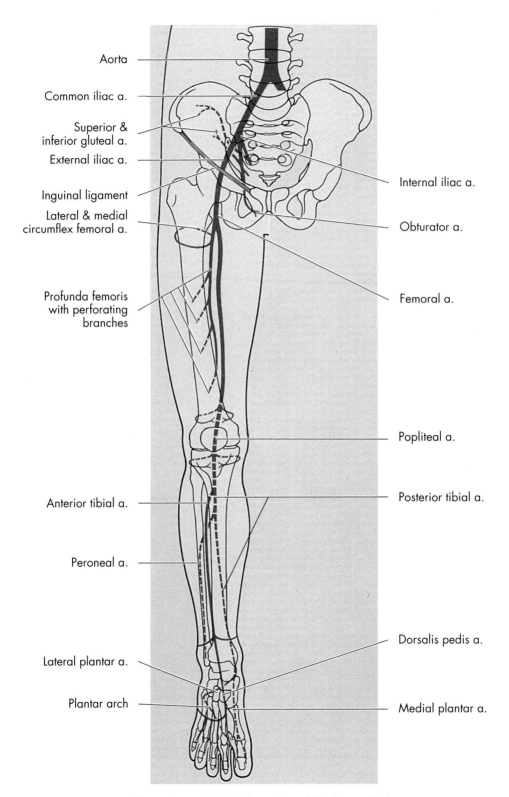

Aorta

Common iliac a.

Superior &
inferior gluteal a.

External iliac a.

Inguinal ligament

Lateral & medial
circumflex femoral a.

Profunda femoris
with perforating
branches

Anterior tibial a.

Peroneal a.

Lateral plantar a.

Plantar arch

Internal iliac a.

Obturator a.

Femoral a.

Popliteal a.

Posterior tibial a.

Dorsalis pedis a.

Medial plantar a.

Figure 7-5   Principal arteries of the lower limb.

SEE **PRINCIPLES**, FIGS. 7-17, 7-18

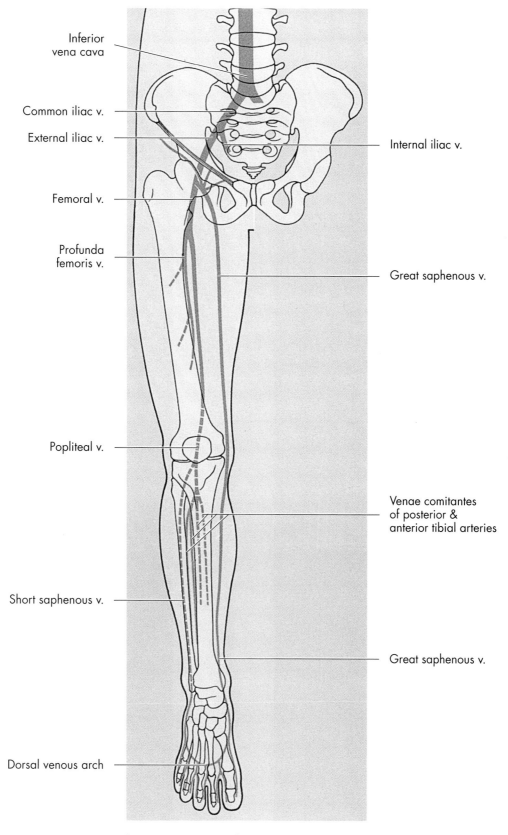

Inferior
vena cava

Common iliac v.

External iliac v.

Internal iliac v.

Femoral v.

Profunda
femoris v.

Great saphenous v.

Popliteal v.

Venae comitantes
of posterior &
anterior tibial arteries

Short saphenous v.

Great saphenous v.

Dorsal venous arch

Figure 7-6   Principal veins of the lower limb.

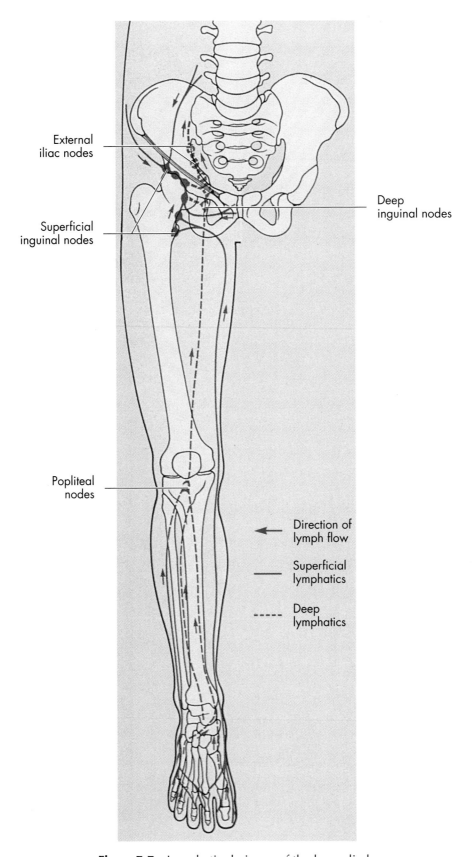

External
iliac nodes

Deep
inguinal nodes

Superficial
inguinal nodes

Popliteal
nodes

Direction of
lymph flow

Superficial
lymphatics

Deep
lymphatics

Figure 7-7 Lymphatic drainage of the lower limb.

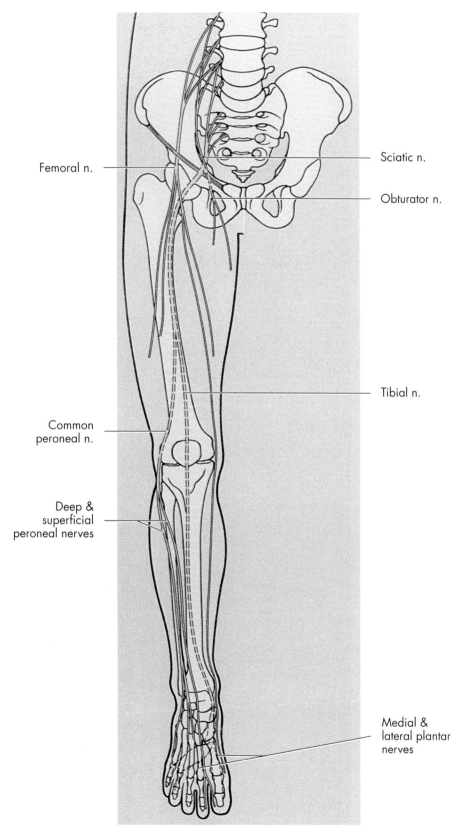

Femoral n.

Sciatic n.

Obturator n.

Tibial n.

Common peroneal n.

Deep & superficial peroneal nerves

Medial & lateral plantar nerves

Figure 7-8 Principal nerves of the lower limb.

See PRINCIPLES, Fig. 7-1

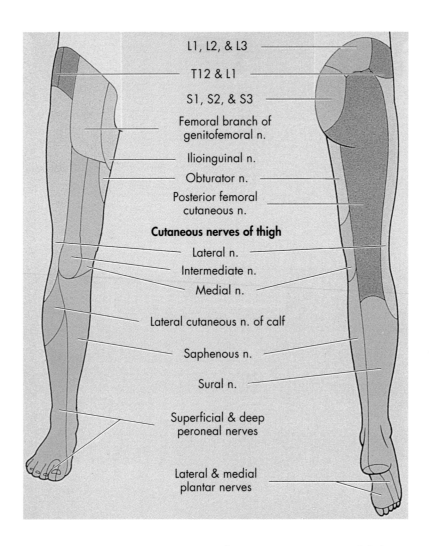

L1, L2, & L3

T12 & L1

S1, S2, & S3

Femoral branch of
genitofemoral n.

Ilioinguinal n.

Obturator n.

Posterior femoral
cutaneous n.

Cutaneous nerves of thigh

Lateral n.

Intermediate n.

Medial n.

Lateral cutaneous n. of calf

Saphenous n.

Sural n.

Superficial & deep
peroneal nerves

Lateral & medial
plantar nerves

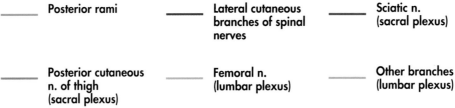

Posterior rami	Lateral cutaneous branches of spinal nerves	Sciatic n. (sacral plexus)
Posterior cutaneous n. of thigh (sacral plexus)	Femoral n. (lumbar plexus)	Other branches (lumbar plexus)

Figure 7-9   Areas of distribution of cutaneous nerves in the lower limb.

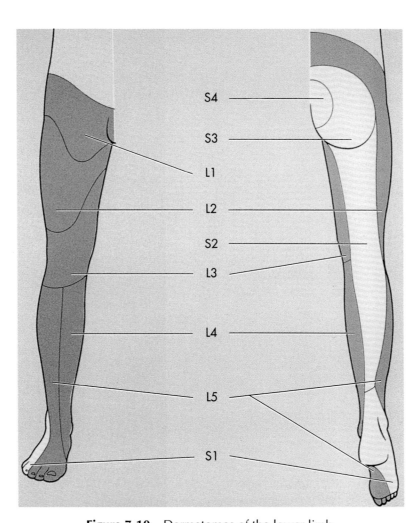

Figure 7-10 Dermatomes of the lower limb.

SEE DISSECTIONS, SECTION 6, PP. 5 AND 6; SECTION 7, P. 2

SEE PRINCIPLES, FIGS. 7-16, 7-17

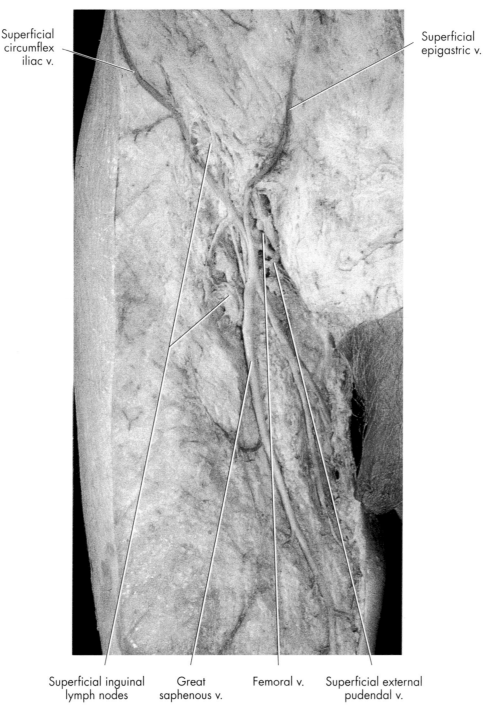

Superficial circumflex iliac v.

Superficial epigastric v.

Superficial inguinal lymph nodes

Great saphenous v.

Femoral v.

Superficial external pudendal v.

Figure 7-11 Great saphenous vein, its tributaries, and the superficial inguinal lymph nodes lying in the superficial fascia. *An upright posture results in high venous pressure in the lower limbs. Venous return depends on the competency of valves in both the deep and superficial veins of the lower limb. Incompetent valves in the saphenous system are the most common cause of enlargement with tortuosity (varicose veins) of the subcutaneous veins of the leg. Blood is pumped upward through the deep venous system by the muscles in the lower limb as long as valves in the system are competent. Blood remaining static in the venous system may clot (phlebothrombosis) and then break off to travel in the system (embolism) through the right side of the heart to the pulmonary arterial tree (pulmonary embolus) (see also Figures 7-43 and 7-62).*

See **DISSECTIONS**, Section 7, p. 2
See **PRINCIPLES**, Fig. 7-19

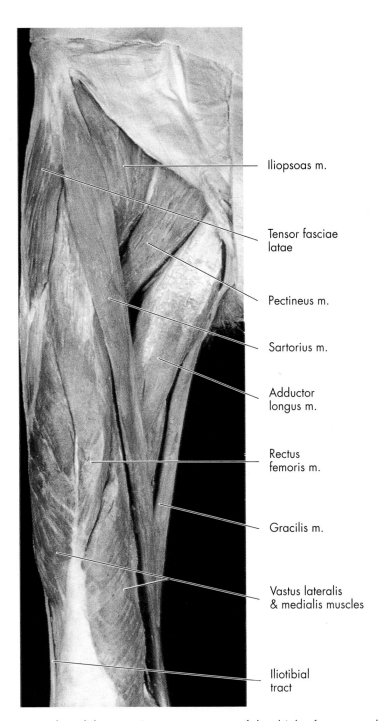

Iliopsoas m.

Tensor fasciae latae

Pectineus m.

Sartorius m.

Adductor longus m.

Rectus femoris m.

Gracilis m.

Vastus lateralis & medialis muscles

Iliotibial tract

Figure 7-12   Muscles of the anterior compartment of the thigh after removal of the skin and fascia lata.

SEE DISSECTIONS, SECTION 7, P. 4

SEE PRINCIPLES, FIG. 7-26, *A*

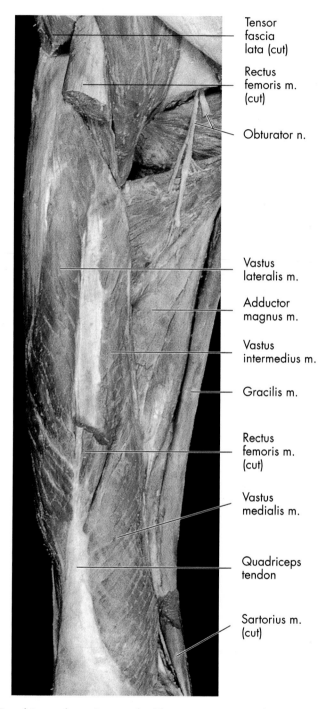

Tensor
fascia
lata (cut)

Rectus
femoris m.
(cut)

Obturator n.

Vastus
lateralis m.

Adductor
magnus m.

Vastus
intermedius m.

Gracilis m.

Rectus
femoris m.
(cut)

Vastus
medialis m.

Quadriceps
tendon

Sartorius m.
(cut)

Figure 7-13   Quadriceps femoris muscle. The vastus intermedius is partially revealed by removal of the rectus femoris.

SEE PRINCIPLES, FIG. 7-14

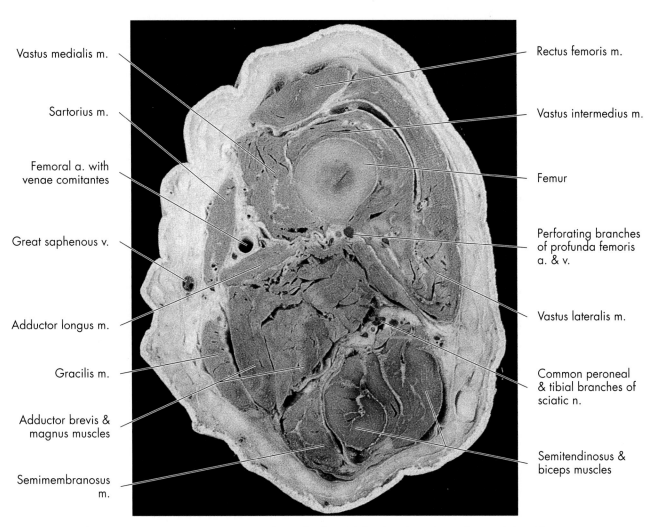

Figure 7-14 Transverse section through the thigh showing the subsartorial adductor canal and components of the quadriceps femoris muscle.

See PRINCIPLES, Figs. 7-2, 7-23

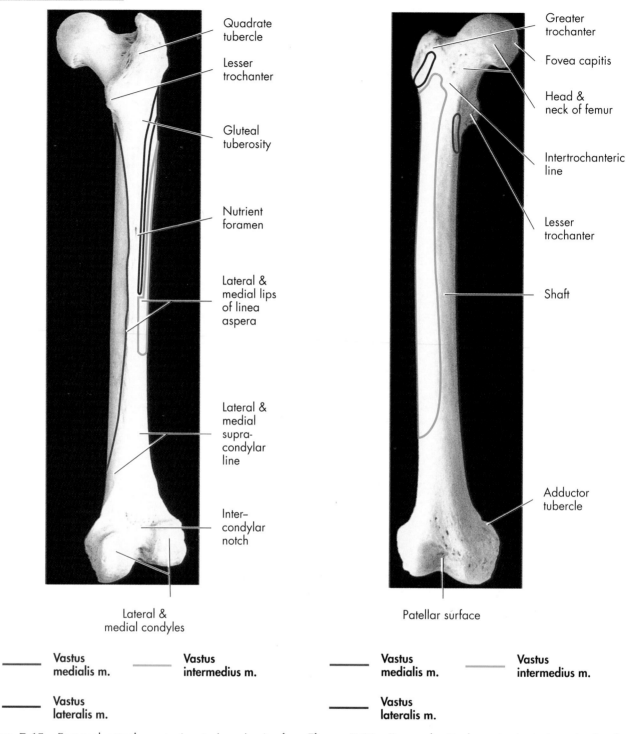

Quadrate
tubercle

Lesser
trochanter

Gluteal
tuberosity

Nutrient
foramen

Lateral &
medial lips
of linea
aspera

Lateral &
medial
supra-
condylar
line

Inter-
condylar
notch

Lateral &
medial condyles

_____ Vastus
medialis m.

_____ Vastus
intermedius m.

_____ Vastus
lateralis m.

Greater
trochanter

Fovea capitis

Head &
neck of femur

Intertrochanteric
line

Lesser
trochanter

Shaft

Adductor
tubercle

Patellar surface

_____ Vastus
medialis m.

_____ Vastus
intermedius m.

_____ Vastus
lateralis m.

Figure 7-15 Femoral attachments (posterior view) of the vasti muscles.

Figure 7-16 Femoral attachments (anterior view) of the vasti muscles. *The common term* hip fracture *actually refers to a fracture of the neck of the femur or a fracture through the intertrochanteric region. Hip fractures are treated surgically by securing a nail across the fracture site extended by a stabilizing plate along the femoral shaft. Alternatively, a partial or complete artificial hip joint (prosthesis) may be employed. This allows early mobilization, which helps avoid common complications of immobility in the elderly.*

SEE DISSECTIONS, SECTION 6,
PP. 5 AND 6; SECTION 7, P. 2

SEE PRINCIPLES, FIG. 7-19

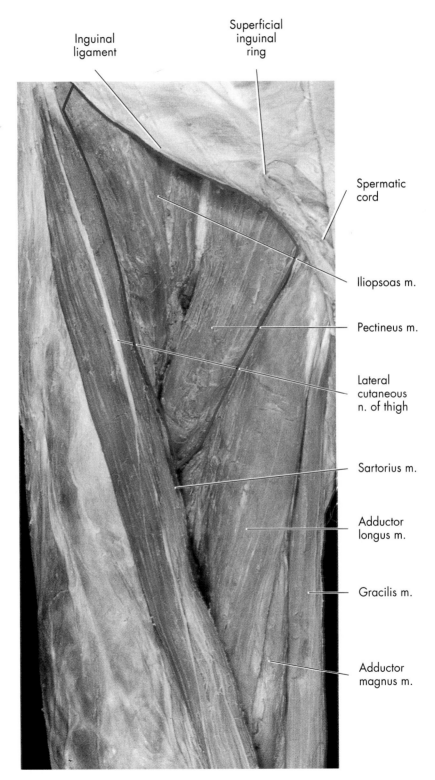

Figure 7-17   Boundaries and floor of the femoral triangle.

SEE DISSECTIONS, SECTION 7, P. 3

SEE PRINCIPLES, FIG. 7-11

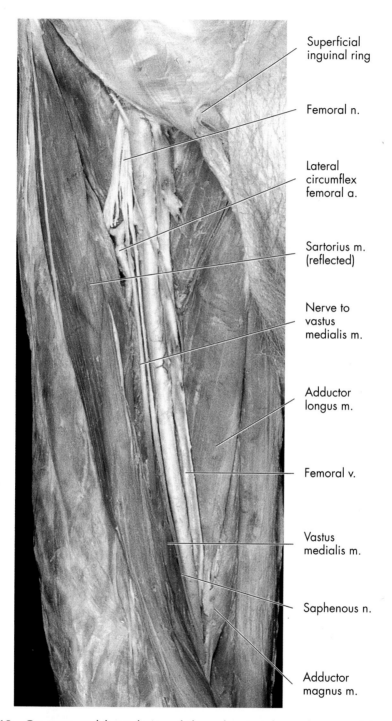

Superficial
inguinal ring

Femoral n.

Lateral
circumflex
femoral a.

Sartorius m.
(reflected)

Nerve to
vastus
medialis m.

Adductor
longus m.

Femoral v.

Vastus
medialis m.

Saphenous n.

Adductor
magnus m.

Figure 7-18 Contents and boundaries of the subsartorial canal exposed by displacement of the sartorius muscle laterally.

See **DISSECTIONS**, Section 7, p. 3
See **PRINCIPLES**, Fig. 7-11

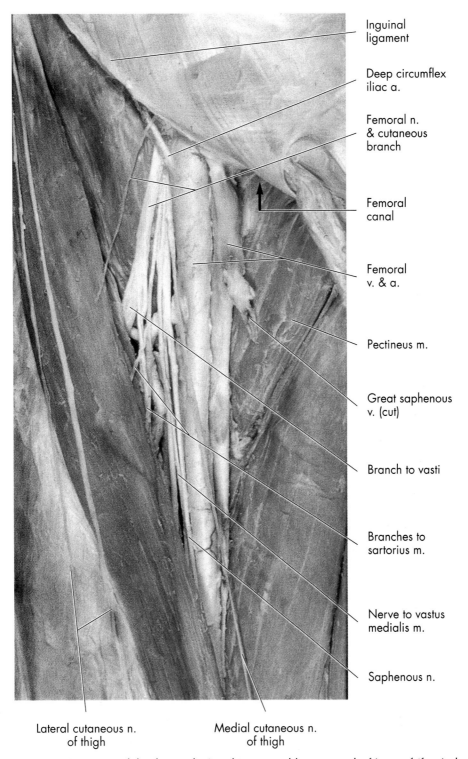

Inguinal
ligament

Deep circumflex
iliac a.

Femoral n.
& cutaneous
branch

Femoral
canal

Femoral
v. & a.

Pectineus m.

Great saphenous
v. (cut)

Branch to vasti

Branches to
sartorius m.

Nerve to vastus
medialis m.

Saphenous n.

Lateral cutaneous n.
of thigh

Medial cutaneous n.
of thigh

Figure 7-19   Contents of the femoral triangle exposed by removal of its roof (fascia lata).
The deep inguinal lymph nodes lie within the femoral canal.

SEE **DISSECTIONS**, SECTION 7, P. 3
SEE **PRINCIPLES**, FIGS. 7-24, 7-25

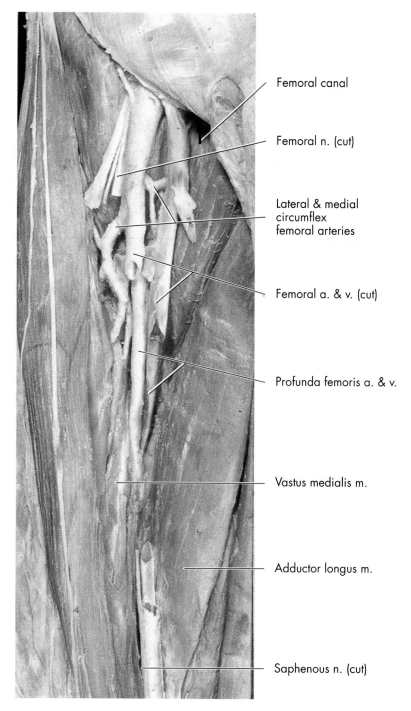

Femoral canal

Femoral n. (cut)

Lateral & medial circumflex femoral arteries

Femoral a. & v. (cut)

Profunda femoris a. & v.

Vastus medialis m.

Adductor longus m.

Saphenous n. (cut)

Figure 7-20   Profunda femoris vessels seen after removal of segments of the femoral artery and vein.

SEE **PRINCIPLES**, FIG. 7-19

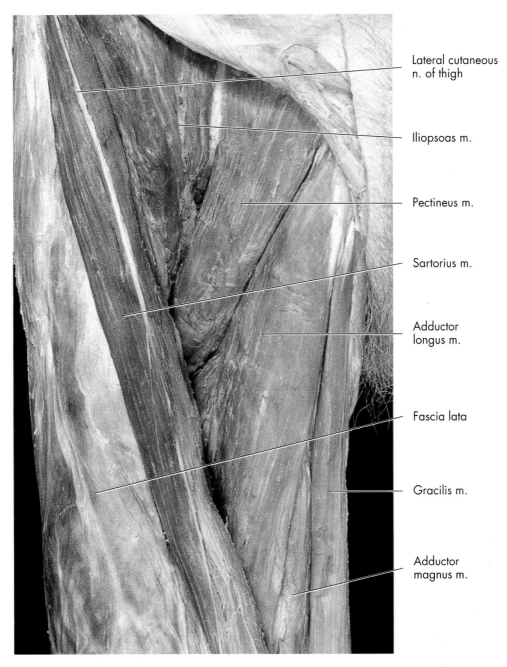

Lateral cutaneous
n. of thigh

Iliopsoas m.

Pectineus m.

Sartorius m.

Adductor
longus m.

Fascia lata

Gracilis m.

Adductor
magnus m.

Figure 7-21 Anterior layer of muscles of the medial compartment of the thigh.

SEE DISSECTIONS, SECTION 7, P. 4
SEE PRINCIPLES, FIG. 7-26, *B*

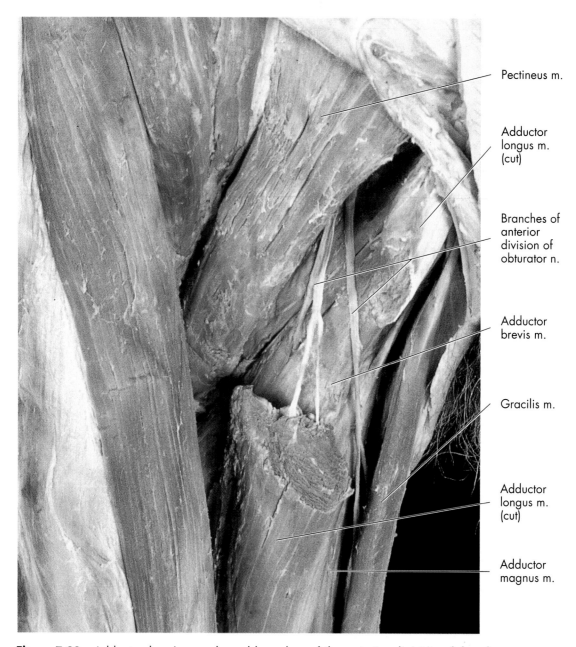

Pectineus m.

Adductor
longus m.
(cut)

Branches of
anterior
division of
obturator n.

Adductor
brevis m.

Gracilis m.

Adductor
longus m.
(cut)

Adductor
magnus m.

Figure 7-22 Adductor brevis muscle and branches of the anterior division of the obturator nerve revealed by removal of part of the adductor longus.

See DISSECTIONS, Section 7, p. 4

See PRINCIPLES, Fig. 7-26, *B*

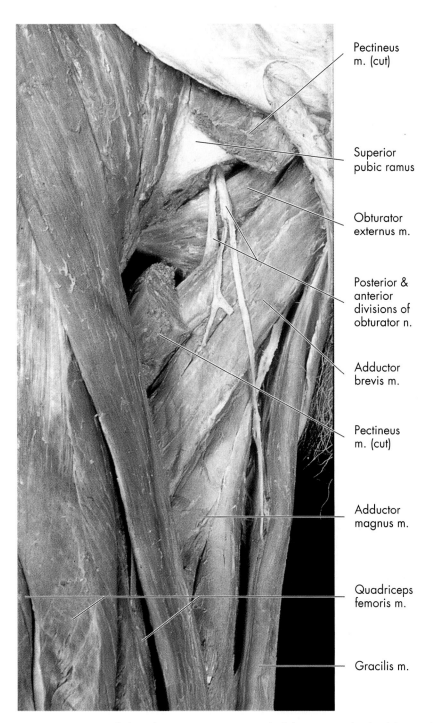

Pectineus
m. (cut)

Superior
pubic ramus

Obturator
externus m.

Posterior &
anterior
divisions of
obturator n.

Adductor
brevis m.

Pectineus
m. (cut)

Adductor
magnus m.

Quadriceps
femoris m.

Gracilis m.

Figure 7-23   Divisions of the obturator nerve revealed by removal of adductor longus muscle and part of the pectineus. In this specimen the posterior division lies in front of the obturator externus.

See DISSECTIONS, Section 7, p. 4
See PRINCIPLES, Fig. 7-26, *B*

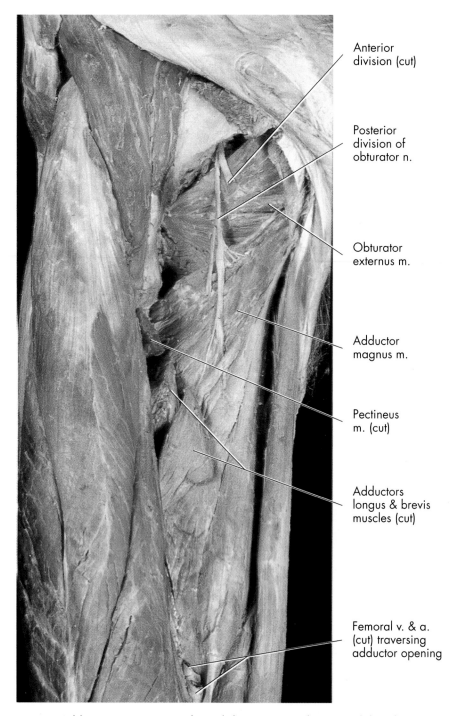

Anterior
division (cut)

Posterior
division of
obturator n.

Obturator
externus m.

Adductor
magnus m.

Pectineus
m. (cut)

Adductors
longus & brevis
muscles (cut)

Femoral v. & a.
(cut) traversing
adductor opening

Figure 7-24   Adductor magnus muscle and the posterior division of the obturator nerve.
The adductor brevis has been removed.

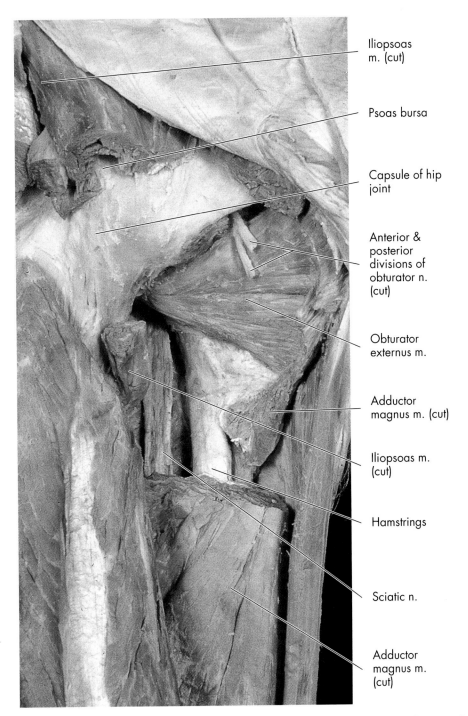

Iliopsoas
m. (cut)

Psoas bursa

Capsule of hip
joint

Anterior &
posterior
divisions of
obturator n.
(cut)

Obturator
externus m.

Adductor
magnus m. (cut)

Iliopsoas m.
(cut)

Hamstrings

Sciatic n.

Adductor
magnus m.
(cut)

Figure 7-25   Obturator externus muscle completely revealed by removal of parts of the iliopsoas and adductor magnus.

SEE PRINCIPLES, FIGS. 7-8, 7-23

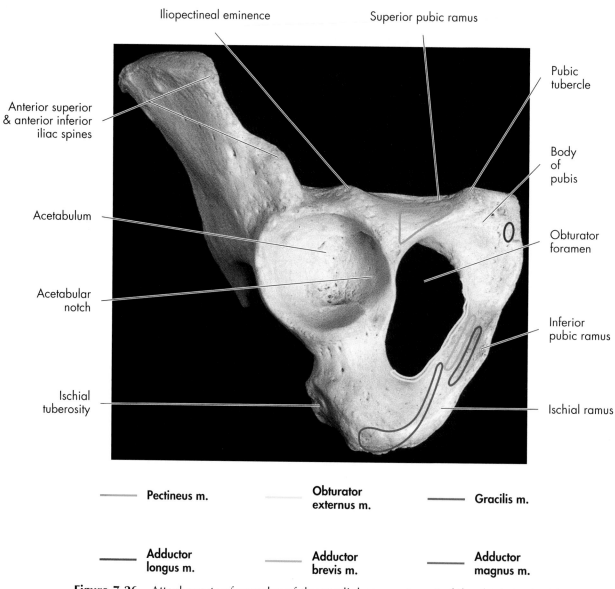

Iliopectineal eminence

Superior pubic ramus

Pubic tubercle

Anterior superior & anterior inferior iliac spines

Body of pubis

Acetabulum

Obturator foramen

Acetabular notch

Inferior pubic ramus

Ischial tuberosity

Ischial ramus

——— Pectineus m.

Obturator externus m.

——— Gracilis m.

——— Adductor longus m.

Adductor brevis m.

——— Adductor magnus m.

Figure 7-26   Attachments of muscles of the medial compartment of the thigh to the hip bone.

See PRINCIPLES, FIG. 7-23

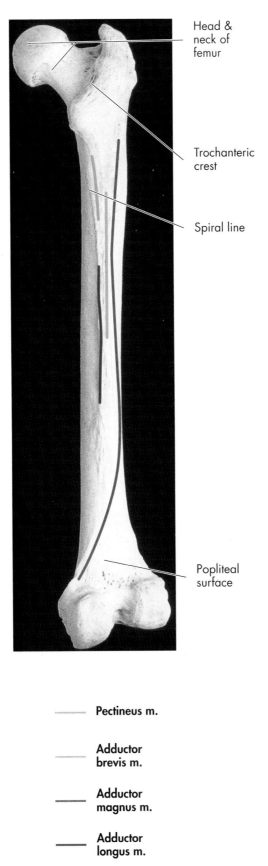

Head & neck of femur

Trochanteric crest

Spiral line

Popliteal surface

Pectineus m.

Adductor brevis m.

Adductor magnus m.

Adductor longus m.

Figure 7-27 Femoral attachments of the muscles of the medial compartment of the thigh.

See **DISSECTIONS**, Section 6,
pp. 2 and 3; Section 7, p. 5

See **PRINCIPLES**, Fig. 7-28

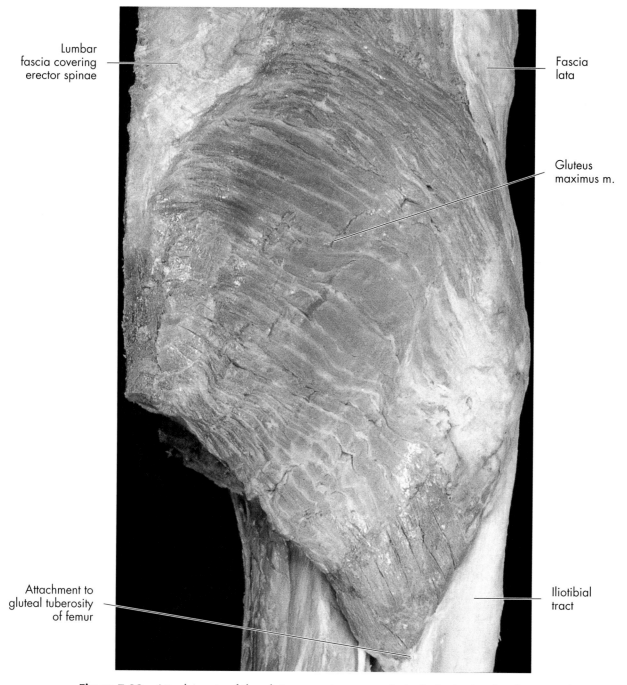

Lumbar
fascia covering
erector spinae

Fascia
lata

Gluteus
maximus m.

Attachment to
gluteal tuberosity
of femur

Iliotibial
tract

Figure 7-28   Attachments of the gluteus maximus muscle include the lumbar fascia and
the iliotibial tract.

See **DISSECTIONS, SECTION 6,**
P. 3; **SECTION 7, P. 5**

See **PRINCIPLES, FIG. 7-29**

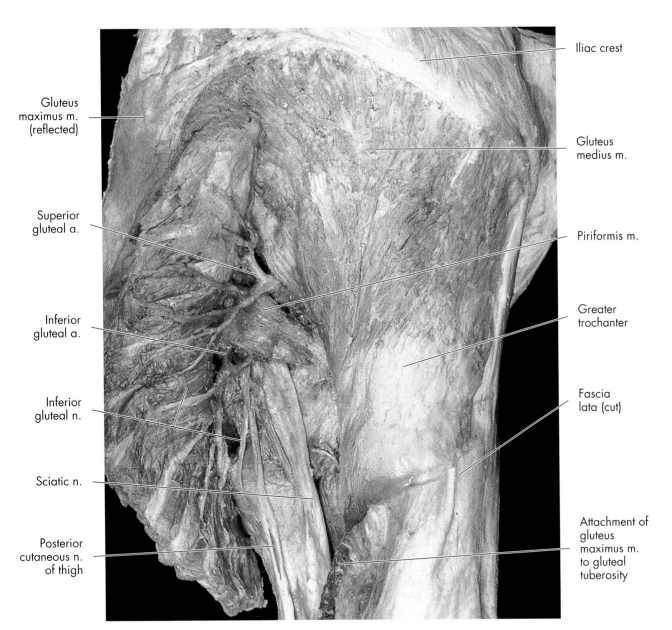

Figure 7-29   Reflection of gluteus maximus muscle exposing the gluteus medius and the neurovascular structures. *Intramuscular injections are frequently administered into the gluteal region (buttocks). Such injections are made superolaterally into the gluteal muscle to avoid injury to the sciatic nerve, which lies inferomedial to the injection site.*

See DISSECTIONS, Section 7, p. 5
See PRINCIPLES, Figs. 7-13, 7-36

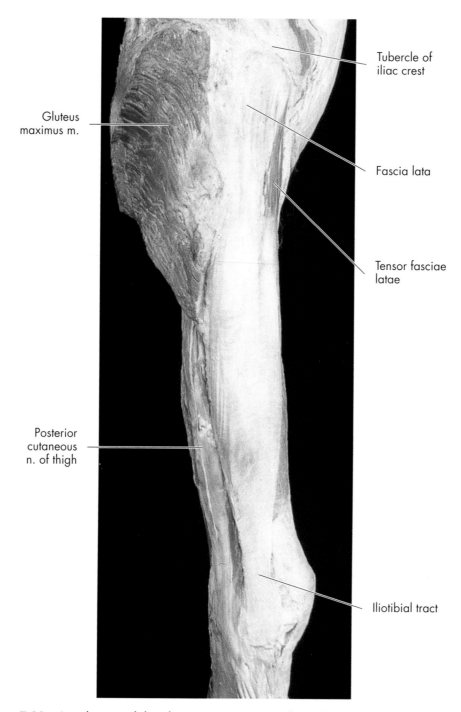

Tubercle of
iliac crest

Gluteus
maximus m.

Fascia lata

Tensor fasciae
latae

Posterior
cutaneous
n. of thigh

Iliotibial tract

Figure 7-30   Attachment of the gluteus maximus muscle and the tensor fasciae latae to the iliotibial tract.

See PRINCIPLES, Fig. 7-30

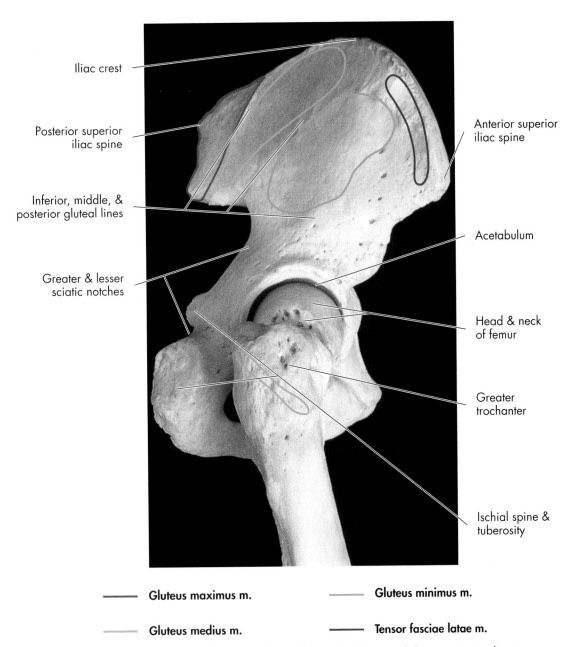

Iliac crest

Posterior superior
iliac spine

Inferior, middle, &
posterior gluteal lines

Greater & lesser
sciatic notches

Anterior superior
iliac spine

Acetabulum

Head & neck
of femur

Greater
trochanter

Ischial spine &
tuberosity

―――― Gluteus maximus m.   ―――― Gluteus minimus m.

―――― Gluteus medius m.   ―――― Tensor fasciae latae m.

Figure 7-31   Attachments of the gluteal muscles to the ilium and the greater trochanter.

SEE **DISSECTIONS**, SECTION 6,
PP. 3 AND 4; SECTION 7, P. 5

SEE **PRINCIPLES**, FIG. 7-33

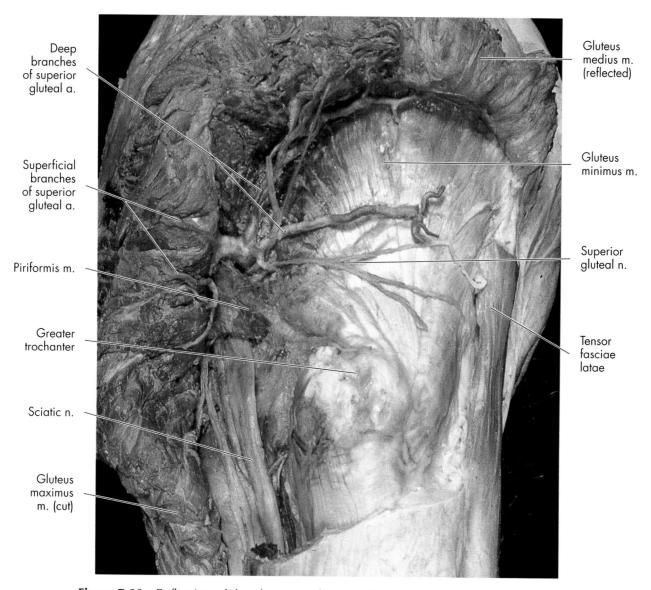

Deep
branches
of superior
gluteal a.

Superficial
branches
of superior
gluteal a.

Piriformis m.

Greater
trochanter

Sciatic n.

Gluteus
maximus
m. (cut)

Gluteus
medius m.
(reflected)

Gluteus
minimus m.

Superior
gluteal n.

Tensor
fasciae
latae

Figure 7-32   Reflection of the gluteus medius muscle reveals the gluteus minimus and the superior gluteal artery and nerve entering the buttock above the piriformis.

See **DISSECTIONS, Section 6,**
pp. 3 and 4; **Section 7, p. 6**

See **PRINCIPLES, Fig. 7-34**

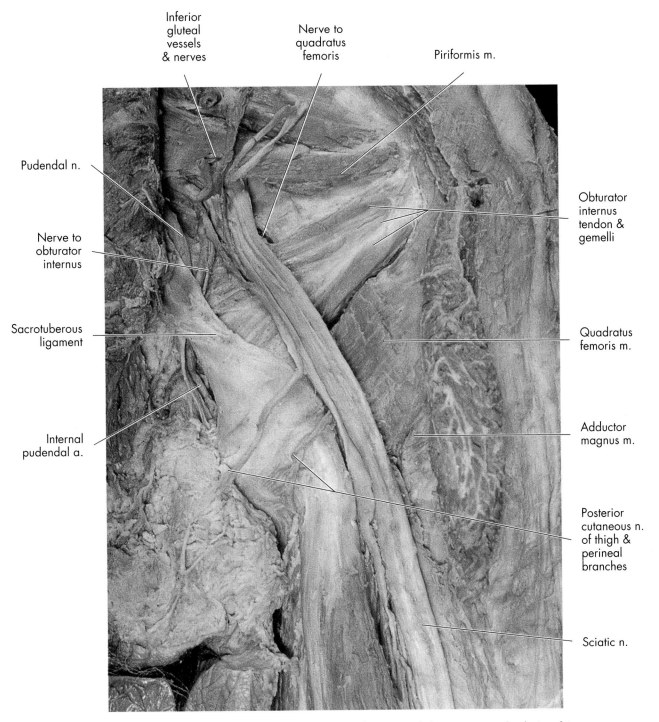

Inferior gluteal vessels & nerves

Nerve to quadratus femoris

Piriformis m.

Pudendal n.

Nerve to obturator internus

Sacrotuberous ligament

Internal pudendal a.

Obturator internus tendon & gemelli

Quadratus femoris m.

Adductor magnus m.

Posterior cutaneous n. of thigh & perineal branches

Sciatic n.

Figure 7-33 Structures emerging below the piriformis and the course and relationships of the sciatic nerve.

SEE **DISSECTIONS**, SECTION 7, P. 5

SEE **PRINCIPLES**, FIG. 7-32

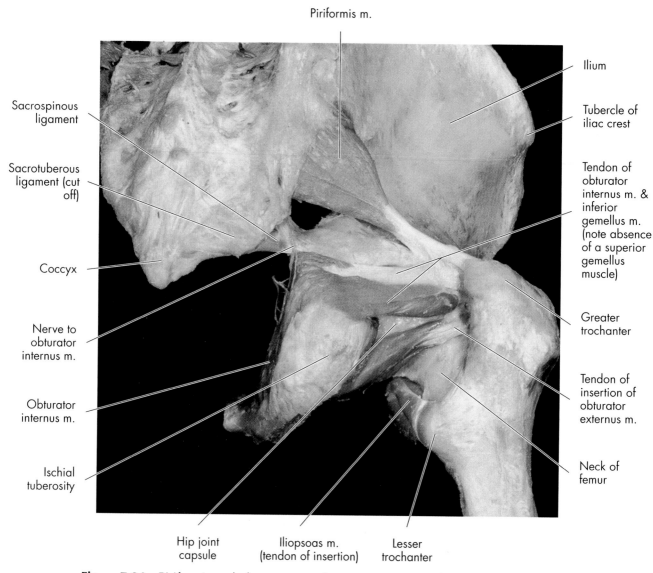

Piriformis m.

Ilium

Tubercle of iliac crest

Sacrospinous ligament

Tendon of obturator internus m. & inferior gemellus m. (note absence of a superior gemellus muscle)

Sacrotuberous ligament (cut off)

Coccyx

Greater trochanter

Nerve to obturator internus m.

Tendon of insertion of obturator externus m.

Obturator internus m.

Ischial tuberosity

Neck of femur

Hip joint capsule

Iliopsoas m. (tendon of insertion)

Lesser trochanter

Figure 7-34   Piriformis and obturator muscles, posterior view of the right side. This dissection illustrates the relationships of the piriformis and the obturator internus and externus muscles to the capsule of the hip joint and to the bony pelvis and femur.

See DISSECTIONS, Section 7, p. 6
See PRINCIPLES, Fig. 7-1

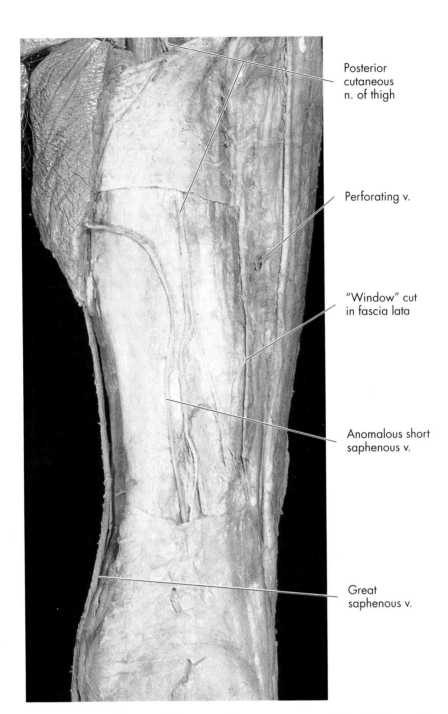

Posterior
cutaneous
n. of thigh

Perforating v.

"Window" cut
in fascia lata

Anomalous short
saphenous v.

Great
saphenous v.

Figure 7-35   Nerves and veins of the posterior compartment of the thigh seen through a "window" cut in the fascia lata. The short saphenous vein continues proximally to terminate in the great saphenous vein.

SEE DISSECTIONS, SECTION 7, P. 6
SEE PRINCIPLES, FIGS. 7-37, 7-38

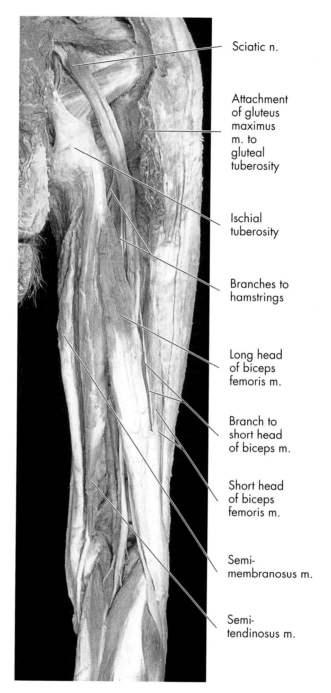

Sciatic n.

Attachment
of gluteus
maximus
m. to
gluteal
tuberosity

Ischial
tuberosity

Branches to
hamstrings

Long head
of biceps
femoris m.

Branch to
short head
of biceps m.

Short head
of biceps
femoris m.

Semi-
membranosus m.

Semi-
tendinosus m.

Figure 7-36   Principal contents of the posterior compartment of the thigh seen after removal of deep fascia.

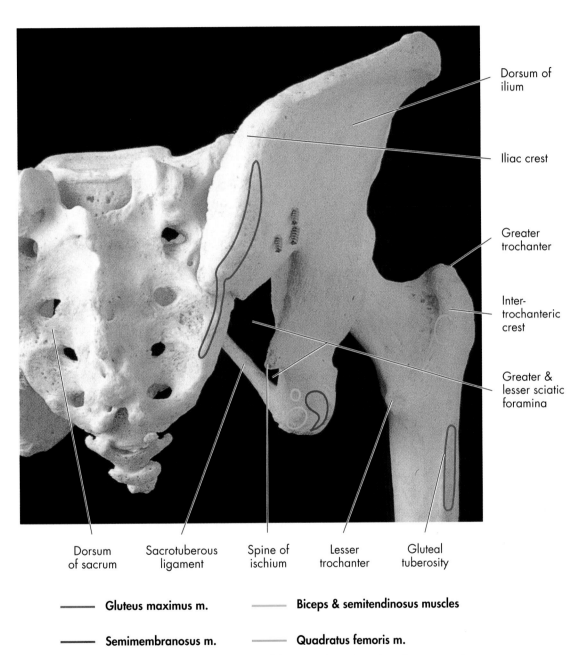

Dorsum of ilium

Iliac crest

Greater trochanter

Inter-trochanteric crest

Greater & lesser sciatic foramina

Dorsum of sacrum   Sacrotuberous ligament   Spine of ischium   Lesser trochanter   Gluteal tuberosity

—— Gluteus maximus m.   —— Biceps & semitendinosus muscles

—— Semimembranosus m.   —— Quadratus femoris m.

Figure 7-37 Posterior view of the sacrum and bony pelvis showing the sacrotuberous ligament with the greater and lesser sciatic foramina. The spine of the ischium is visible, but the sacrospinous ligament has been removed. Its course from the ischial spine to the sacrum makes the lesser sciatic notch into a foramen.

See PRINCIPLES, FIG. 7-17

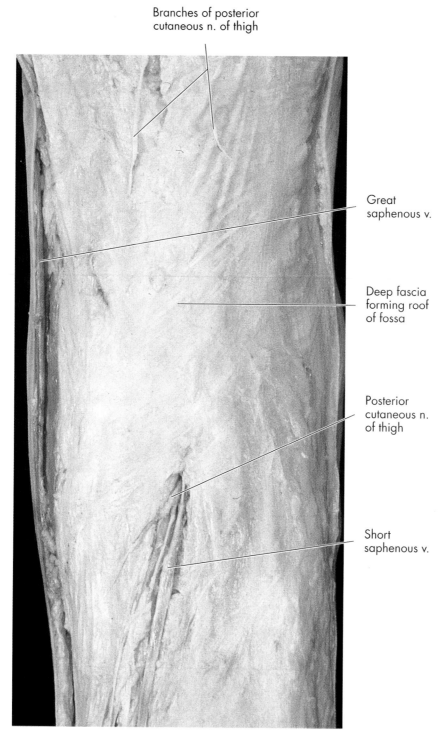

Branches of posterior
cutaneous n. of thigh

Great
saphenous v.

Deep fascia
forming roof
of fossa

Posterior
cutaneous n.
of thigh

Short
saphenous v.

Figure 7-38   Removal of skin and superficial fascia revealing the cutaneous nerves. The
short saphenous vein and accompanying nerve pierce the roof of the popliteal fossa.

See **DISSECTIONS,** Section 7, p. 12
See **PRINCIPLES,** Fig. 7-37

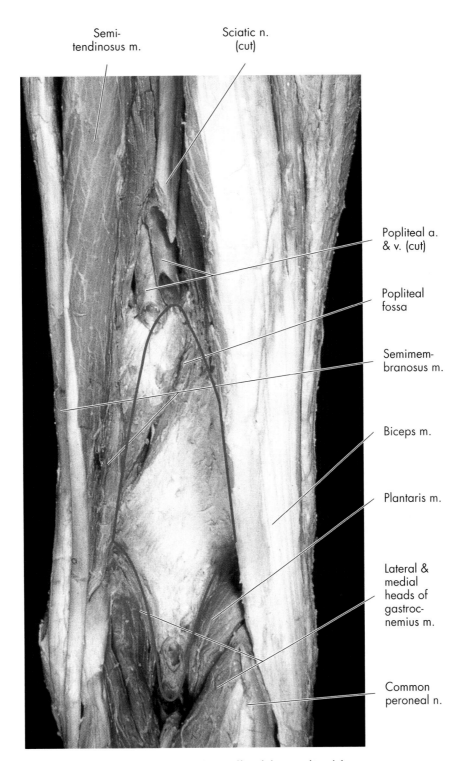

Semi-
tendinosus m.

Sciatic n.
(cut)

Popliteal a.
& v. (cut)

Popliteal
fossa

Semimem-
branosus m.

Biceps m.

Plantaris m.

Lateral &
medial
heads of
gastroc-
nemius m.

Common
peroneal n.

Figure 7-39 Muscles forming the walls of the popliteal fossa.

See DISSECTIONS, Section 7, p. 12
See PRINCIPLES, Fig. 7-55

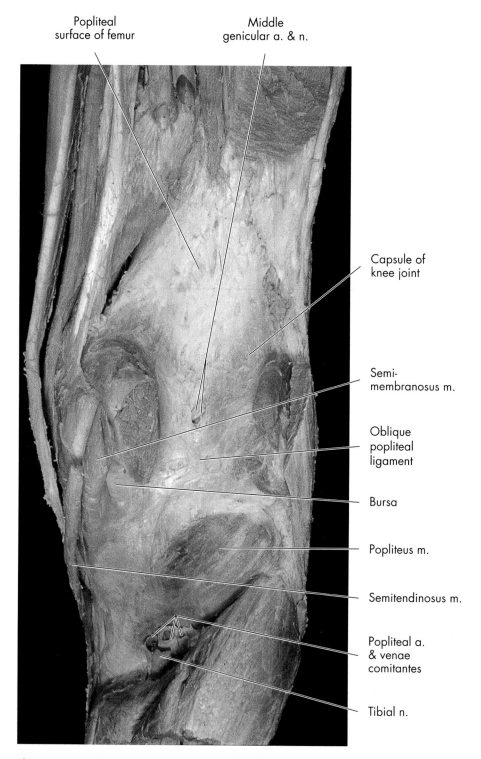

Popliteal surface of femur

Middle genicular a. & n.

Capsule of knee joint

Semi-membranosus m.

Oblique popliteal ligament

Bursa

Popliteus m.

Semitendinosus m.

Popliteal a. & venae comitantes

Tibial n.

Figure 7-40   Floor seen after removal of walls and contents of the fossa.

See **DISSECTIONS**, Section 7, p. 12
See **PRINCIPLES**, Figs. 7-47, 7-57, 7-58

Popliteal v. traversing opening
in adductor magnus m.

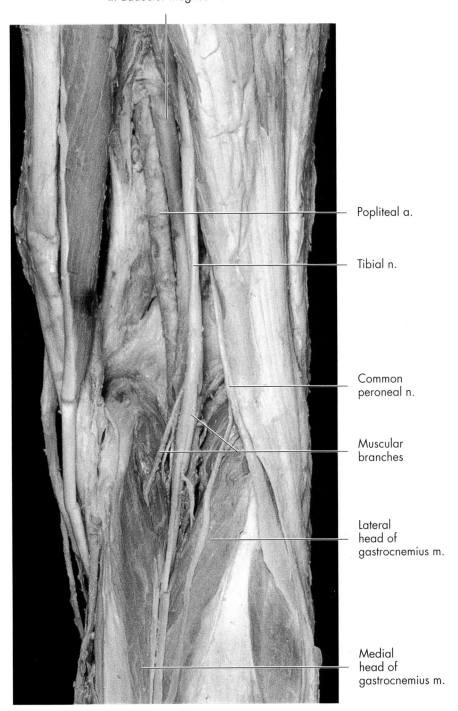

Popliteal a.

Tibial n.

Common
peroneal n.

Muscular
branches

Lateral
head of
gastrocnemius m.

Medial
head of
gastrocnemius m.

Figure 7-41 Principal vessels and nerves of the popliteal fossa revealed by removal of
fat.

See PRINCIPLES, Figs. 7-53, 7-54

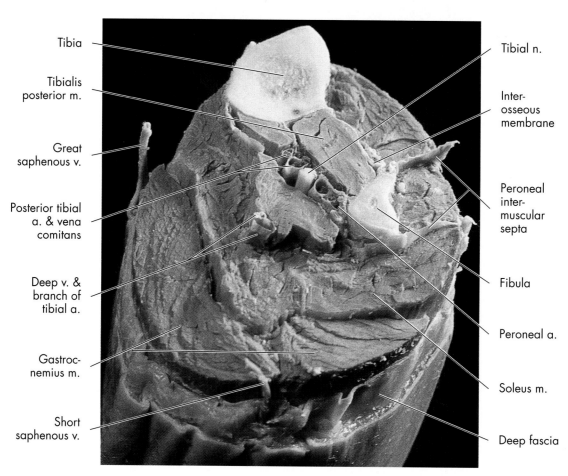

Tibia

Tibialis posterior m.

Great saphenous v.

Posterior tibial a. & vena comitans

Deep v. & branch of tibial a.

Gastrocnemius m.

Short saphenous v.

Tibial n.

Interosseous membrane

Peroneal intermuscular septa

Fibula

Peroneal a.

Soleus m.

Deep fascia

Figure 7-42   "Step" dissection showing the muscle layers in the upper third of the right leg and the location of principal nerves and vessels.

See **DISSECTIONS**, Section 7, p. 12
See **PRINCIPLES**, Fig. 7-17

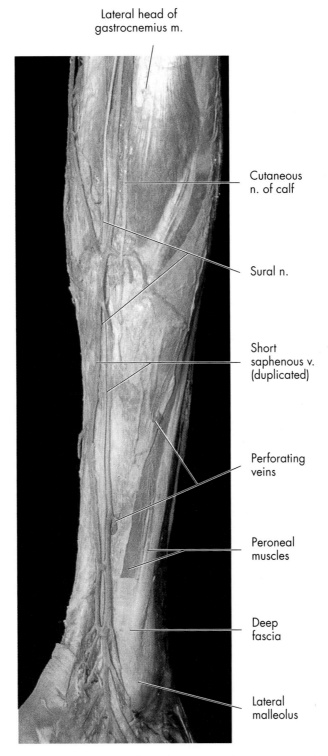

Lateral head of
gastrocnemius m.

Cutaneous
n. of calf

Sural n.

Short
saphenous v.
(duplicated)

Perforating
veins

Peroneal
muscles

Deep
fascia

Lateral
malleolus

Figure 7-43   Short saphenous vein and sural nerve. Perforating veins pierce the deep fascia to connect with deep veins in the calf muscles.

See DISSECTIONS, Section 7, p. 12
See PRINCIPLES, Fig. 7-50

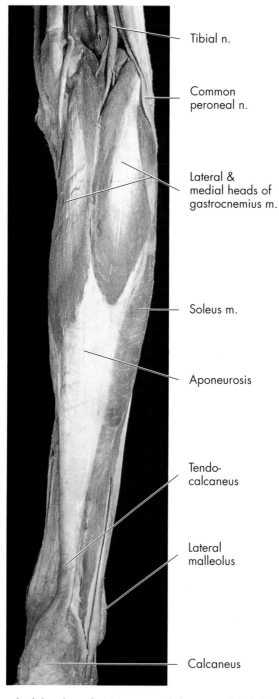

Tibial n.

Common
peroneal n.

Lateral &
medial heads of
gastrocnemius m.

Soleus m.

Aponeurosis

Tendo-
calcaneus

Lateral
malleolus

Calcaneus

Figure 7-44 Removal of the deep fascia to reveal the superficial flexor muscles, the gastrocnemius, and the soleus.

SEE PRINCIPLES, FIG. 7-51

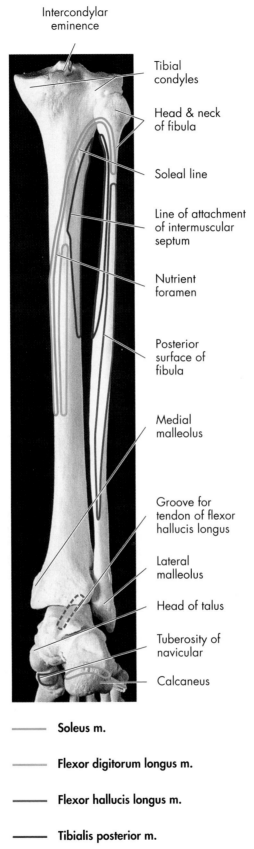

Intercondylar eminence

Tibial condyles

Head & neck of fibula

Soleal line

Line of attachment of intermuscular septum

Nutrient foramen

Posterior surface of fibula

Medial malleolus

Groove for tendon of flexor hallucis longus

Lateral malleolus

Head of talus

Tuberosity of navicular

Calcaneus

—— Soleus m.

—— Flexor digitorum longus m.

—— Flexor hallucis longus m.

—— Tibialis posterior m.

Figure 7-45 Posterior view of the bones of the leg and foot. The diagram shows attachments of muscles of the posterior compartment.

SEE DISSECTIONS, SECTION 7, P. 12
SEE PRINCIPLES, FIG. 7-55

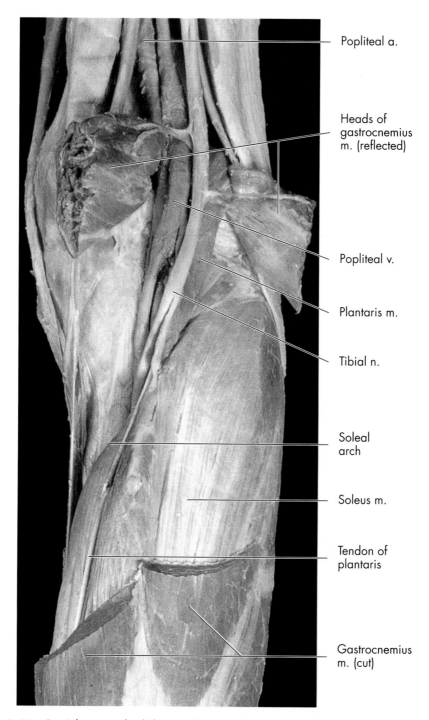

Popliteal a.

Heads of
gastrocnemius
m. (reflected)

Popliteal v.

Plantaris m.

Tibial n.

Soleal
arch

Soleus m.

Tendon of
plantaris

Gastrocnemius
m. (cut)

Figure 7-46 Partial removal of the two heads of the gastrocnemius reveals the soleus and the neurovascular bundle passing beneath the soleal arch to enter the calf.

SEE DISSECTIONS, SECTION 7, PP. 12 AND 13

SEE PRINCIPLES, FIGS. 7-57, 7-58

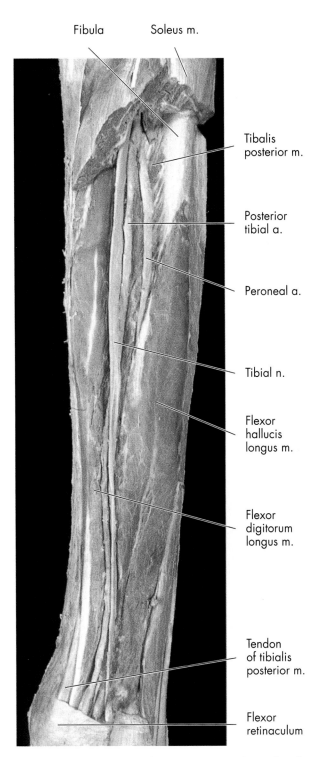

Fibula

Soleus m.

Tibalis posterior m.

Posterior tibial a.

Peroneal a.

Tibial n.

Flexor hallucis longus m.

Flexor digitorum longus m.

Tendon of tibialis posterior m.

Flexor retinaculum

Figure 7-47   Removal of the superficial flexor group to show the deep muscles of the compartment and the main neurovascular bundle.

See **DISSECTIONS**, Section 7, p. 14

See **PRINCIPLES**, Fig. 7-70

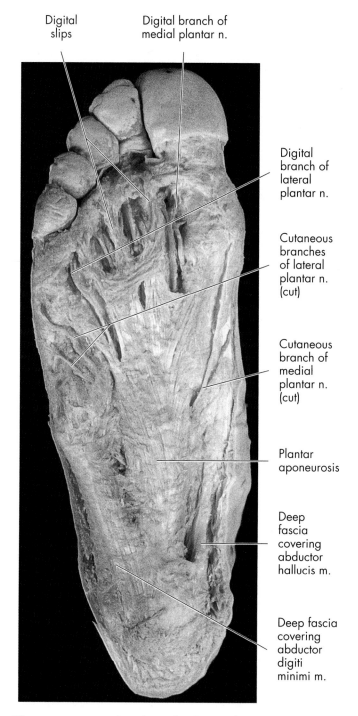

Digital
slips

Digital branch of
medial plantar n.

Digital
branch of
lateral
plantar n.

Cutaneous
branches
of lateral
plantar n.
(cut)

Cutaneous
branch of
medial
plantar n.
(cut)

Plantar
aponeurosis

Deep
fascia
covering
abductor
hallucis m.

Deep fascia
covering
abductor
digiti
minimi m.

Figure 7-48   Plantar aponeurosis, deep fascia, and cutaneous nerves revealed by removal of the skin of the sole.

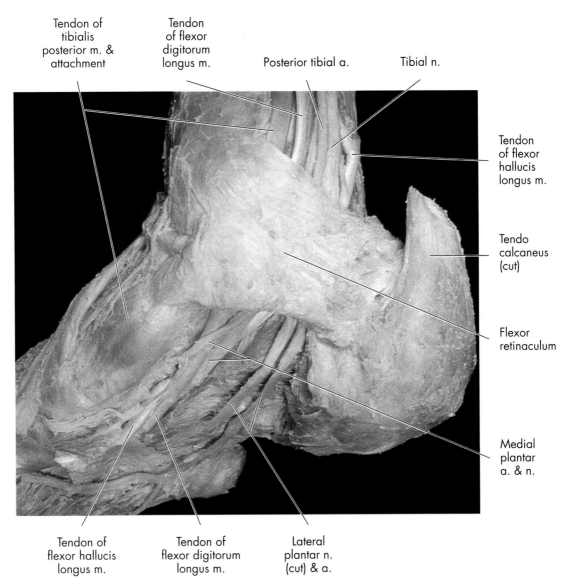

See **DISSECTIONS**, Section 7, p. 13
See **PRINCIPLES**, Figs. 7-63, 7-64

Tendon of
tibialis
posterior m. &
attachment

Tendon
of flexor
digitorum
longus m.

Posterior tibial a.

Tibial n.

Tendon
of flexor
hallucis
longus m.

Tendo
calcaneus
(cut)

Flexor
retinaculum

Medial
plantar
a. & n.

Tendon of
flexor hallucis
longus m.

Tendon of
flexor digitorum
longus m.

Lateral
plantar n.
(cut) & a.

Figure 7-49   Long tendons and the principal vessels and nerves from the posterior compartment of the leg passing deep to the flexor retinaculum to enter the sole of the foot.

See DISSECTIONS, Section 7, pp. 14 and 15

See PRINCIPLES, Fig. 7-79

Fibrous
flexor
sheaths

Tendon
of flexor
digitorum
brevis m.

Tendon
of flexor
digitorum
longus m.

Branches of
lateral plantar n.

Branches of
medial plantar n.

Abductor
digiti minimi m.

Flexor
digitorum
brevis m.

Abductor
hallucis m.

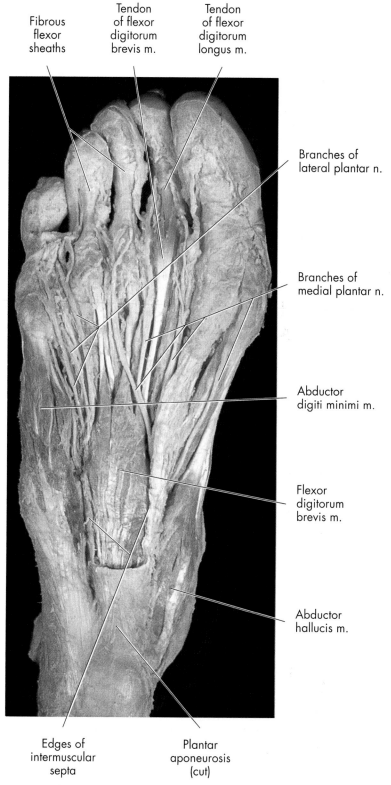

Edges of
intermuscular
septa

Plantar
aponeurosis
(cut)

Figure 7-50 Superficial intrinsic muscles and plantar nerves after removal of the deep fascia, part of the plantar aponeurosis, and the second fibrous tendon sheath. In this specimen, the flexor digitorum brevis muscle has only three tendons.

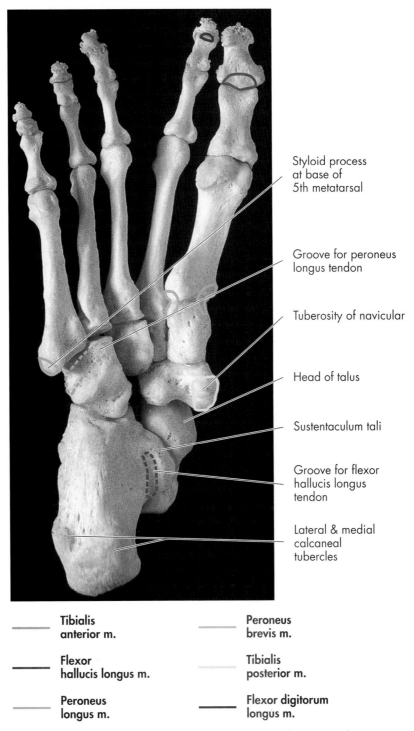

Styloid process
at base of
5th metatarsal

Groove for peroneus
longus tendon

Tuberosity of navicular

Head of talus

Sustentaculum tali

Groove for flexor
hallucis longus
tendon

Lateral & medial
calcaneal
tubercles

Tibialis anterior m.	Peroneus brevis m.
Flexor hallucis longus m.	Tibialis posterior m.
Peroneus longus m.	Flexor digitorum longus m.

Figure 7-51   Plantar view of bones of the foot showing attachments of some tendons.

See DISSECTIONS, Section 7, p. 15

See PRINCIPLES, Fig. 7-80

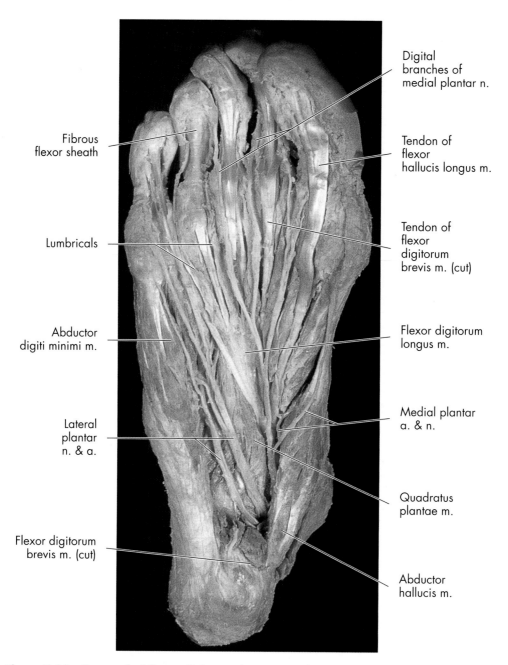

Digital branches of medial plantar n.

Tendon of flexor hallucis longus m.

Tendon of flexor digitorum brevis m. (cut)

Flexor digitorum longus m.

Medial plantar a. & n.

Quadratus plantae m.

Abductor hallucis m.

Fibrous flexor sheath

Lumbricals

Abductor digiti minimi m.

Lateral plantar n. & a.

Flexor digitorum brevis m. (cut)

Figure 7-52   Removal of flexor digitorum brevis muscle to reveal the plantar nerves and arteries, which enter the sole deep to the abductor hallucis.

SEE DISSECTIONS, SECTION 7, P. 15

SEE PRINCIPLES, FIG. 7-80

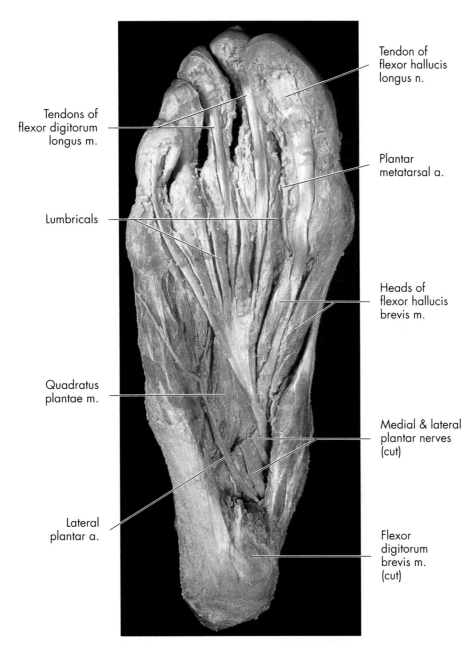

Tendon of
flexor hallucis
longus n.

Tendons of
flexor digitorum
longus m.

Plantar
metatarsal a.

Lumbricals

Heads of
flexor hallucis
brevis m.

Quadratus
plantae m.

Medial & lateral
plantar nerves
(cut)

Lateral
plantar a.

Flexor
digitorum
brevis m.
(cut)

Figure 7-53   Tendons of flexor digitorum longus, flexor hallucis longus, as well as quadratus plantae, and the lumbrical muscles after removal of medial and lateral plantar nerves and the tendons of the flexor digitorum brevis.

SEE DISSECTIONS, SECTION 7, P. 16

SEE PRINCIPLES, FIGS. 7-81, 7-83

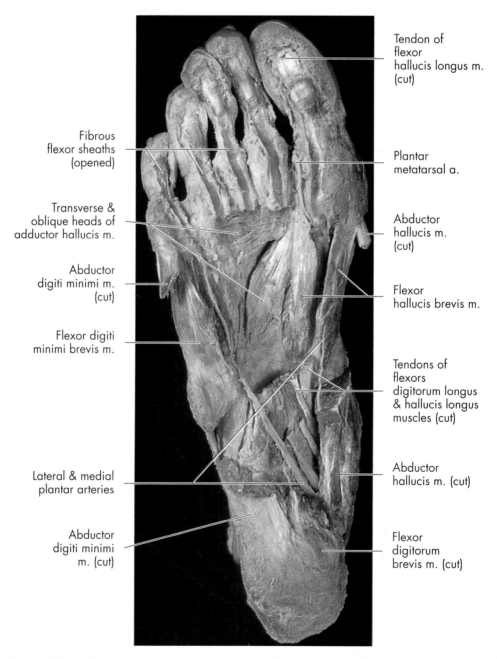

Tendon of flexor hallucis longus m. (cut)

Fibrous flexor sheaths (opened)

Plantar metatarsal a.

Transverse & oblique heads of adductor hallucis m.

Abductor hallucis m. (cut)

Abductor digiti minimi m. (cut)

Flexor hallucis brevis m.

Flexor digiti minimi brevis m.

Tendons of flexors digitorum longus & hallucis longus muscles (cut)

Lateral & medial plantar arteries

Abductor hallucis m. (cut)

Abductor digiti minimi m. (cut)

Flexor digitorum brevis m. (cut)

Figure 7-54   Deep intrinsic muscles revealed by removal of long flexor tendons and abductors of the great and little toes.

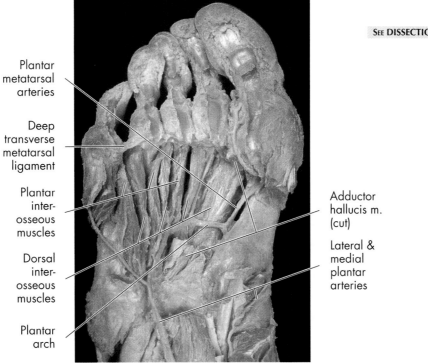

Plantar metatarsal arteries

Deep transverse metatarsal ligament

Plantar interosseous muscles

Dorsal interosseous muscles

Plantar arch

Adductor hallucis m. (cut)

Lateral & medial plantar arteries

Figure 7-55   Interosseous muscles and the plantar arterial arch exposed by removing the adductor hallucis.

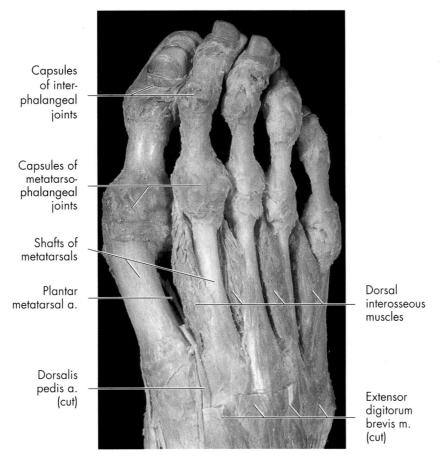

Capsules of interphalangeal joints

Capsules of metatarsophalangeal joints

Shafts of metatarsals

Plantar metatarsal a.

Dorsalis pedis a. (cut)

Dorsal interosseous muscles

Extensor digitorum brevis m. (cut)

Figure 7-56   Dorsal aspect of the foot showing the dorsal interosseous muscles after partial removal of the extensor digitorum brevis. Extensor expansions have been removed to show joint capsules.

See DISSECTIONS, Section 7, p. 16
See PRINCIPLES, Fig. 7-69, A

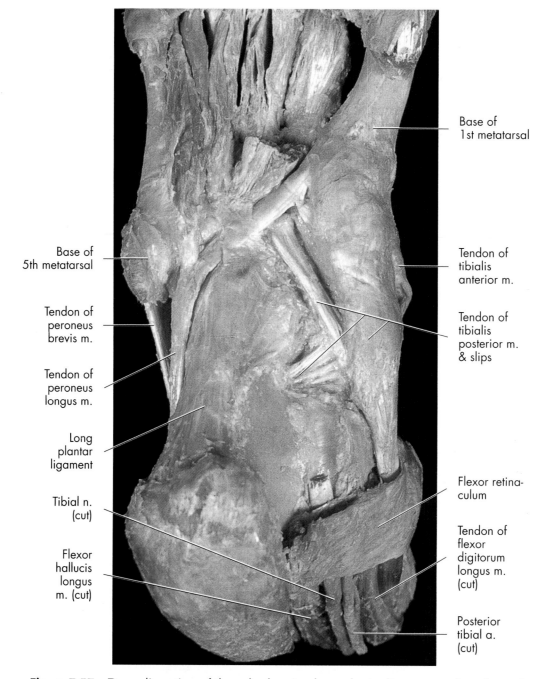

Base of
1st metatarsal

Base of
5th metatarsal

Tendon of
tibialis
anterior m.

Tendon of
peroneus
brevis m.

Tendon of
tibialis
posterior m.
& slips

Tendon of
peroneus
longus m.

Long
plantar
ligament

Tibial n.
(cut)

Flexor retina-
culum

Tendon of
flexor
digitorum
longus m.
(cut)

Flexor
hallucis
longus
m. (cut)

Posterior
tibial a.
(cut)

Figure 7-57   Deep dissection of the sole showing long plantar ligament and tendons of the peroneus longus and the tibialis posterior.

See **DISSECTIONS,** Section 7, p. 16
See **PRINCIPLES,** Fig. 7-69, *A*

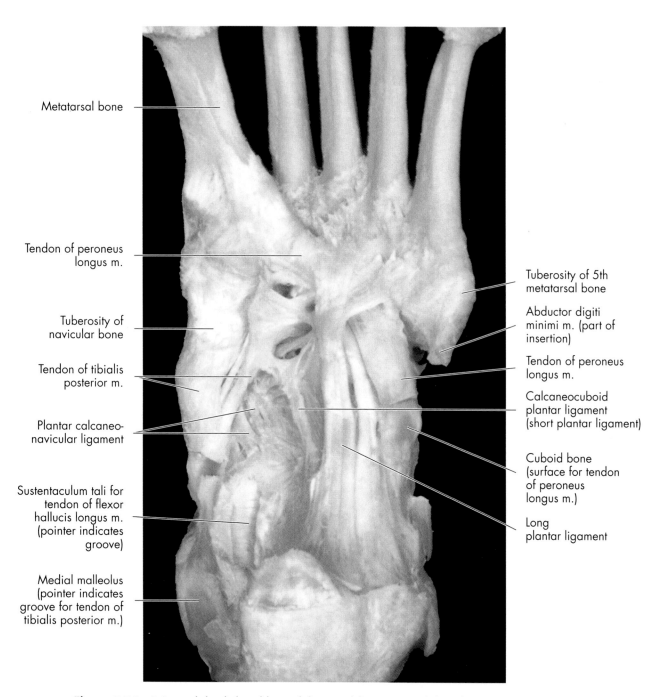

Metatarsal bone

Tendon of peroneus longus m.

Tuberosity of navicular bone

Tendon of tibialis posterior m.

Plantar calcaneo-navicular ligament

Sustentaculum tali for tendon of flexor hallucis longus m. (pointer indicates groove)

Medial malleolus (pointer indicates groove for tendon of tibialis posterior m.)

Tuberosity of 5th metatarsal bone

Abductor digiti minimi m. (part of insertion)

Tendon of peroneus longus m.

Calcaneocuboid plantar ligament (short plantar ligament)

Cuboid bone (surface for tendon of peroneus longus m.)

Long plantar ligament

Figure 7-58 Joints of the left ankle and foot and ligaments of the plantar aspect of the foot.

See DISSECTIONS, Section 7, p. 16

See PRINCIPLES, Fig. 7-69, A

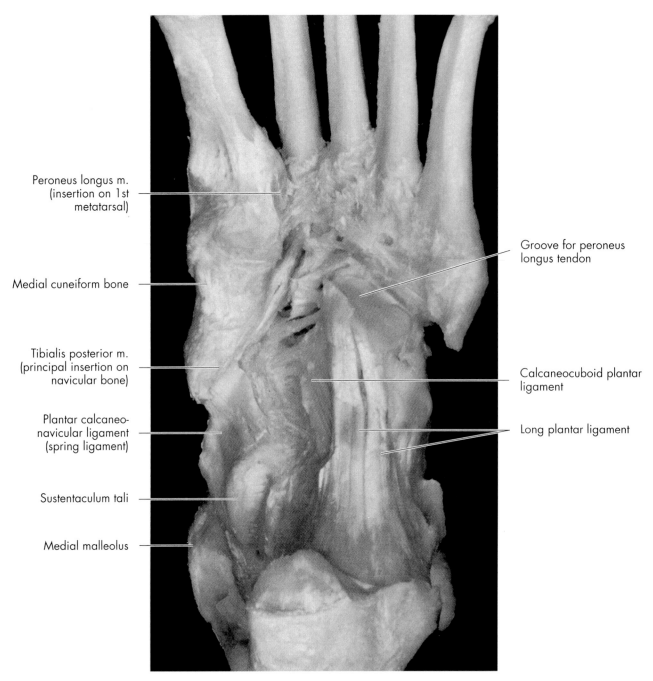

Peroneus longus m.
(insertion on 1st
metatarsal)

Medial cuneiform bone

Tibialis posterior m.
(principal insertion on
navicular bone)

Plantar calcaneo-
navicular ligament
(spring ligament)

Sustentaculum tali

Medial malleolus

Groove for peroneus
longus tendon

Calcaneocuboid plantar
ligament

Long plantar ligament

Figure 7-59   Joints of the left ankle and foot showing the deep layer of ligaments of the plantar aspect of the foot.

See PRINCIPLES, Figs. 7-53, 7-54

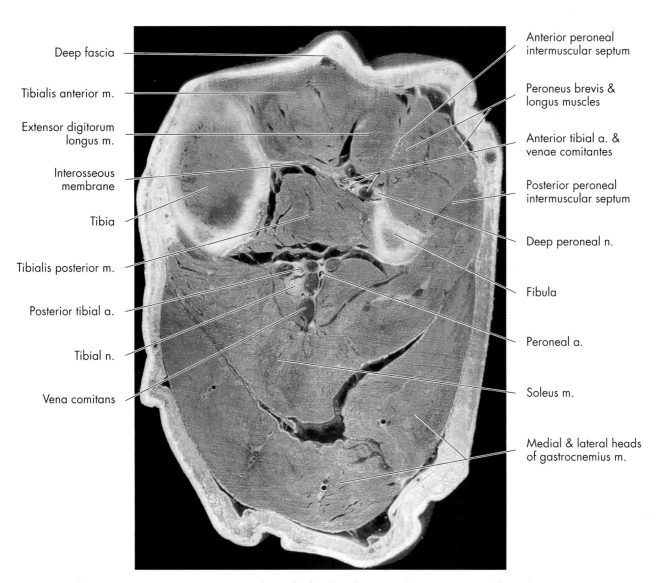

Deep fascia

Tibialis anterior m.

Extensor digitorum longus m.

Interosseous membrane

Tibia

Tibialis posterior m.

Posterior tibial a.

Tibial n.

Vena comitans

Anterior peroneal intermuscular septum

Peroneus brevis & longus muscles

Anterior tibial a. & venae comitantes

Posterior peroneal intermuscular septum

Deep peroneal n.

Fibula

Peroneal a.

Soleus m.

Medial & lateral heads of gastrocnemius m.

Figure 7-60   Transverse section through the leg showing the anterior and lateral compartments and their contents.

See **DISSECTIONS**, Section 7, pp. 9 and 17

See **PRINCIPLES**, Fig. 7-78

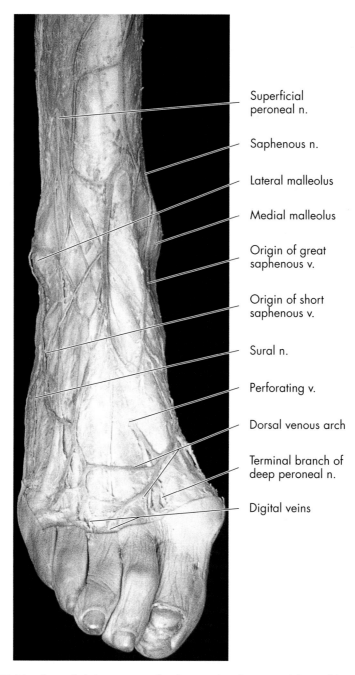

Figure 7-61   Superficial nerves and veins on the dorsum of the ankle and foot.

See **DISSECTIONS**, Section 7, p. 9

See **PRINCIPLES**, Fig. 7-17

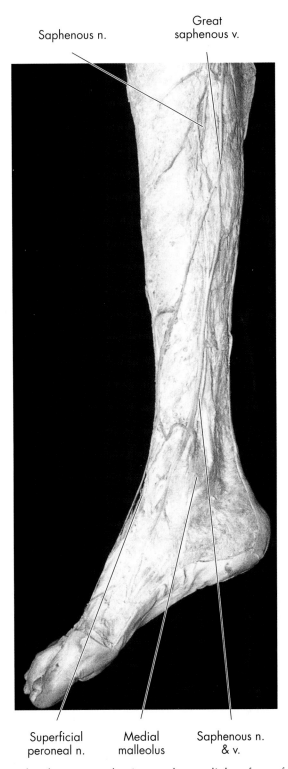

Saphenous n.

Great
saphenous v.

Superficial
peroneal n.

Medial
malleolus

Saphenous n.
& v.

Figure 7-62 Superficial nerves and veins on the medial surface of the leg and foot.

SEE **DISSECTIONS**, SECTION 7, PP. 9 AND 11

SEE **PRINCIPLES**, FIG. 7-59

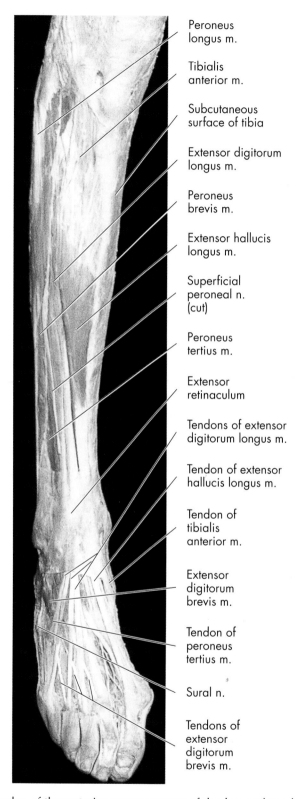

Peroneus
longus m.

Tibialis
anterior m.

Subcutaneous
surface of tibia

Extensor digitorum
longus m.

Peroneus
brevis m.

Extensor hallucis
longus m.

Superficial
peroneal n.
(cut)

Peroneus
tertius m.

Extensor
retinaculum

Tendons of extensor
digitorum longus m.

Tendon of extensor
hallucis longus m.

Tendon of
tibialis
anterior m.

Extensor
digitorum
brevis m.

Tendon of
peroneus
tertius m.

Sural n.

Tendons of
extensor
digitorum
brevis m.

Figure 7-63   Muscles of the anterior compartment of the leg and tendons on the dorsum of the foot seen after removal of the deep fascia. The extensor retinaculum has been retained.

SEE **DISSECTIONS,** SECTION 7, P. 10
SEE **PRINCIPLES,** FIG. 7-76

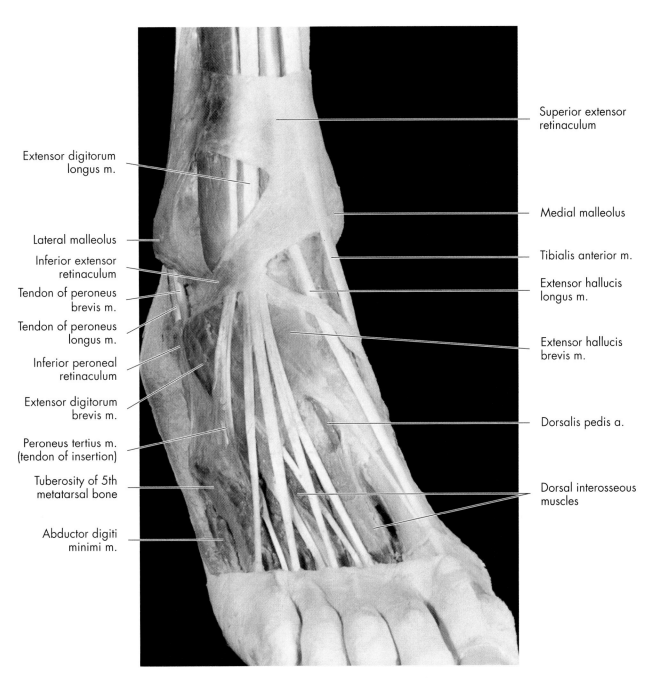

Extensor digitorum longus m.

Lateral malleolus

Inferior extensor retinaculum

Tendon of peroneus brevis m.

Tendon of peroneus longus m.

Inferior peroneal retinaculum

Extensor digitorum brevis m.

Peroneus tertius m. (tendon of insertion)

Tuberosity of 5th metatarsal bone

Abductor digiti minimi m.

Superior extensor retinaculum

Medial malleolus

Tibialis anterior m.

Extensor hallucis longus m.

Extensor hallucis brevis m.

Dorsalis pedis a.

Dorsal interosseous muscles

Figure 7-64   Dissection of the dorsolateral aspect of the left foot and ankle. The tendons, muscles, and retinacula of the dorsum of the foot are viewed anteriorly. Nerves, blood vessels, and fascia of the leg and foot have been removed.

SEE **PRINCIPLES**, FIG. 7-51

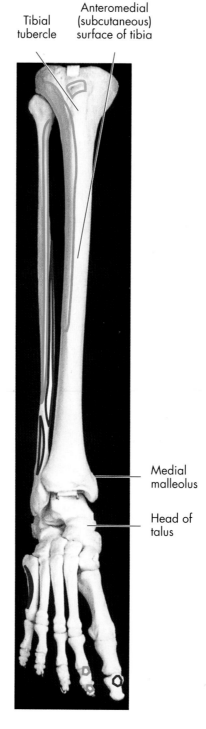

Tibial
tubercle

Anteromedial
(subcutaneous)
surface of tibia

Medial
malleolus

Head of
talus

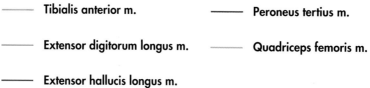

——— Tibialis anterior m.   ——— Peroneus tertius m.

——— Extensor digitorum longus m.   ——— Quadriceps femoris m.

——— Extensor hallucis longus m.

Figure 7-65   Anterior view of bones of the leg and foot showing attachments of muscles of the anterior compartment.

See DISSECTIONS, Section 7, p. 10

See PRINCIPLES, Fig. 7-76

Anterior tibial a. &
venae comitantes

Great saphe-
nous v.

Medial
malleolus

Tibialis anterior m.

Extensor hallucis
longus m.

Extensor digitorum
brevis m.

Tendons of extensor
digitorum longus m.

Deep peroneal n.

Tendon of
peroneus
tertius m.

Tendon of extensor
hallucis brevis m.

Dorsalis pedis a.

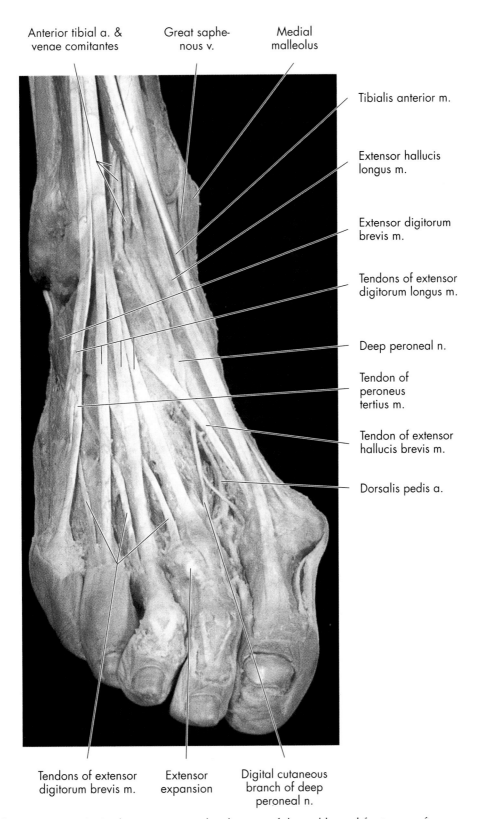

Tendons of extensor
digitorum brevis m.

Extensor
expansion

Digital cutaneous
branch of deep
peroneal n.

Figure 7-66   Principal structures on the dorsum of the ankle and foot seen after removal
of the extensor retinaculum.

See DISSECTIONS, Section 7, p. 11

See PRINCIPLES, Fig. 7-60

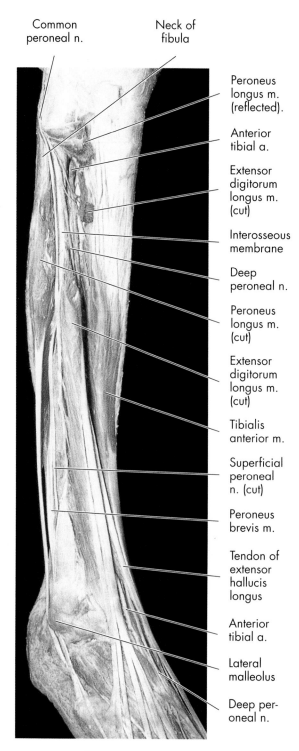

Common
peroneal n.

Neck of
fibula

Peroneus
longus m.
(reflected).

Anterior
tibial a.

Extensor
digitorum
longus m.
(cut)

Interosseous
membrane

Deep
peroneal n.

Peroneus
longus m.
(cut)

Extensor
digitorum
longus m.
(cut)

Tibialis
anterior m.

Superficial
peroneal
n. (cut)

Peroneus
brevis m.

Tendon of
extensor
hallucis
longus

Anterior
tibial a.

Lateral
malleolus

Deep per-
oneal n.

Figure 7-67   Common peroneal nerve and its branches and the anterior tibial artery
seen after deep dissection of both compartments.

See **DISSECTIONS**, Section 7, p. 11
See **PRINCIPLES**, Fig. 7-60

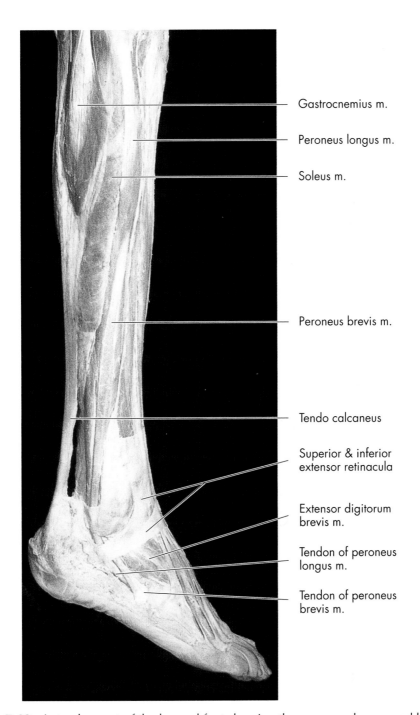

Gastrocnemius m.

Peroneus longus m.

Soleus m.

Peroneus brevis m.

Tendo calcaneus

Superior & inferior extensor retinacula

Extensor digitorum brevis m.

Tendon of peroneus longus m.

Tendon of peroneus brevis m.

Figure 7-68 Lateral aspect of the leg and foot showing the peroneus longus and brevis.

SEE PRINCIPLES, FIG. 7-51

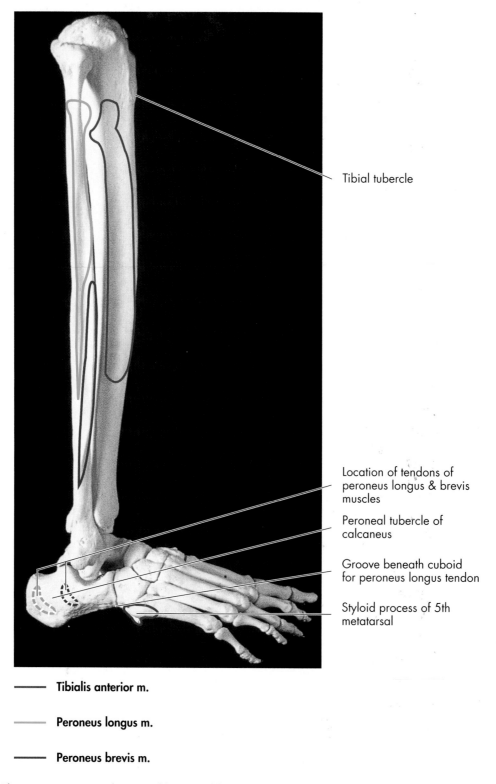

Tibial tubercle

Location of tendons of
peroneus longus & brevis
muscles

Peroneal tubercle of
calcaneus

Groove beneath cuboid
for peroneus longus tendon

Styloid process of 5th
metatarsal

—— Tibialis anterior m.

—— Peroneus longus m.

—— Peroneus brevis m.

Figure 7-69   Lateral view of bones of leg and foot showing attachments of the muscles
of the lateral and anterior compartments.

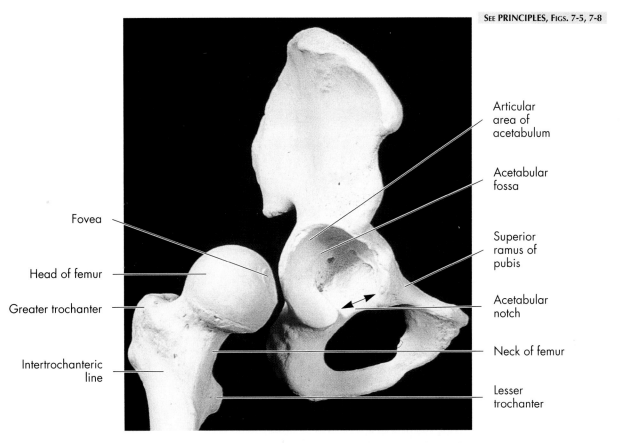

Figure 7-70 Articular surfaces of the hip joint comprise the acetabulum of the hip bone and the head of the femur.

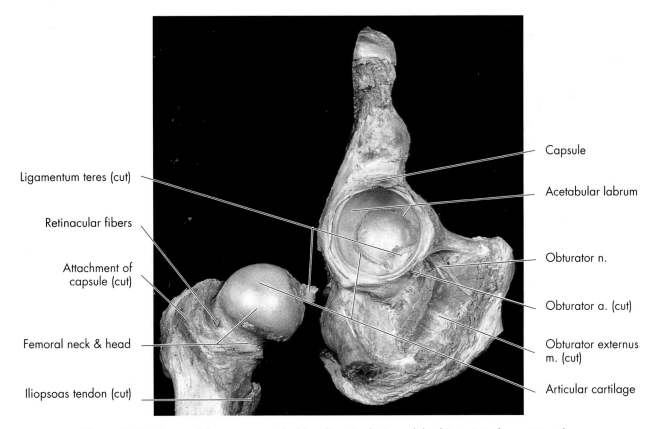

Figure 7-71 Internal features revealed by disarticulation of the hip joint after cutting the ligaments and joint capsule.

See **DISSECTIONS**, Section 7, p. 7

See **PRINCIPLES**, Fig. 7-7

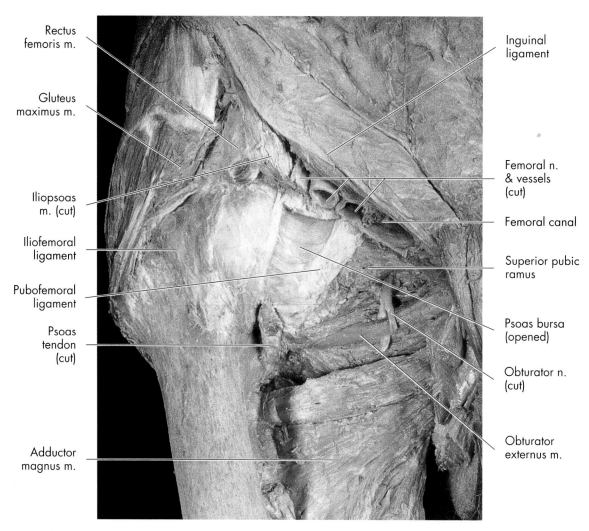

Rectus
femoris m.

Gluteus
maximus m.

Iliopsoas
m. (cut)

Iliofemoral
ligament

Pubofemoral
ligament

Psoas
tendon
(cut)

Adductor
magnus m.

Inguinal
ligament

Femoral n.
& vessels
(cut)

Femoral canal

Superior pubic
ramus

Psoas bursa
(opened)

Obturator n.
(cut)

Obturator
externus m.

Figure 7-72   Anterior surface of the joint capsule and its associated ligaments and immediate relations.

See DISSECTIONS, Section 7, p. 7

See PRINCIPLES, Fig. 7-9

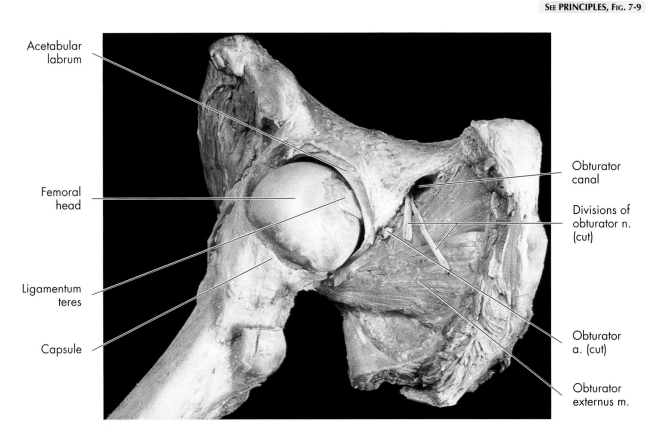

Acetabular labrum

Femoral head

Ligamentum teres

Capsule

Obturator canal

Divisions of obturator n. (cut)

Obturator a. (cut)

Obturator externus m.

Figure 7-73 Joint capsule opened anteriorly to show the interior of the joint. The femur has been abducted and externally rotated.

Ligament of femoral head (pointer near attachment of ligament to fovea of head of femur)

Synovial membrane covering fat pad within acetabular fossa

Acetabular margin

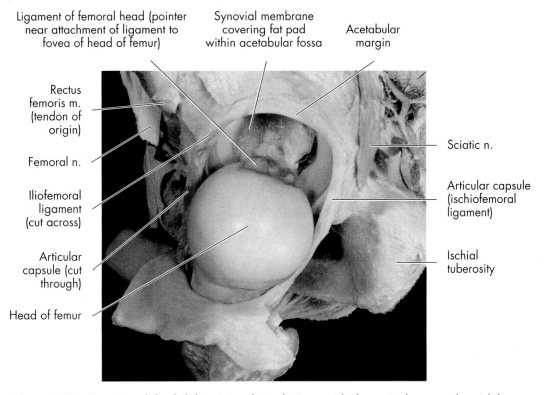

Rectus femoris m. (tendon of origin)

Femoral n.

Iliofemoral ligament (cut across)

Articular capsule (cut through)

Head of femur

Sciatic n.

Articular capsule (ischiofemoral ligament)

Ischial tuberosity

Figure 7-74 Interior of the left hip joint, lateral view, with the articular capsule widely opened. The femur has been partially dislocated from the acetabulum and adducted to show the ligamentum teres of the femoral head and the acetabular labrum.

See DISSECTIONS, Section 7, p. 7
See PRINCIPLES, Fig. 7-7

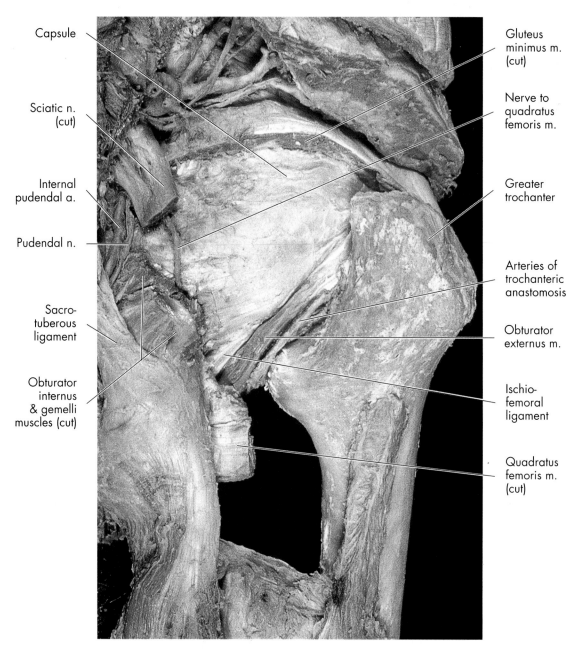

Capsule

Sciatic n. (cut)

Internal pudendal a.

Pudendal n.

Sacro-tuberous ligament

Obturator internus & gemelli muscles (cut)

Gluteus minimus m. (cut)

Nerve to quadratus femoris m.

Greater trochanter

Arteries of trochanteric anastomosis

Obturator externus m.

Ischio-femoral ligament

Quadratus femoris m. (cut)

Figure 7-75   Posterior surface of the joint capsule, the ischiofemoral ligament, and close relationships.

Symphysis pubis   Pectineus m.   Femoral v., a., & n.   Ilipsoas m.   Sartorius m.

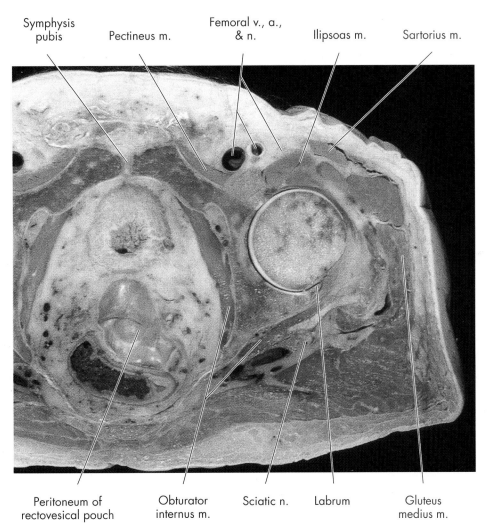

Peritoneum of rectovesical pouch   Obturator internus m.   Sciatic n.   Labrum   Gluteus medius m.

Figure 7-76   Transverse section through the hip joint showing its relationships.

See PRINCIPLES, Fig. 7-5

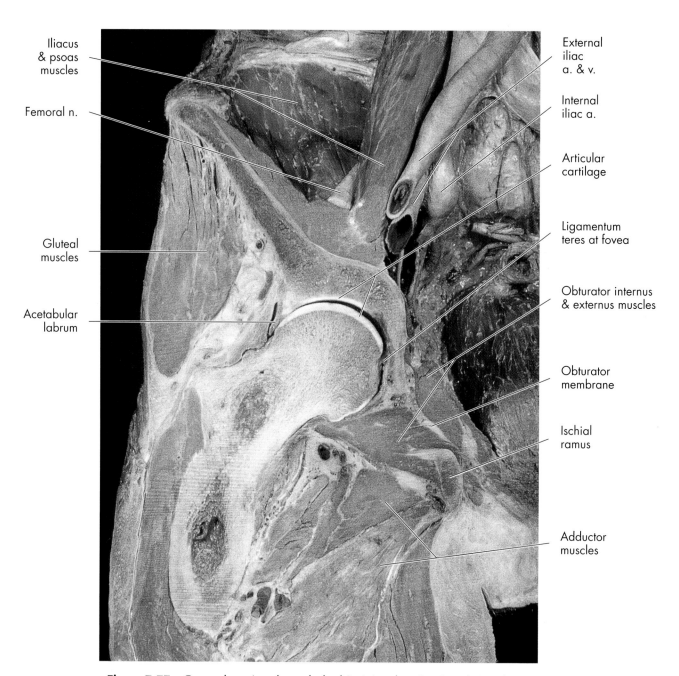

Iliacus & psoas muscles

Femoral n.

Gluteal muscles

Acetabular labrum

External iliac a. & v.

Internal iliac a.

Articular cartilage

Ligamentum teres at fovea

Obturator internus & externus muscles

Obturator membrane

Ischial ramus

Adductor muscles

Figure 7-77   Coronal section through the hip joint showing its relationships.

SEE PRINCIPLES, FIG. 7-41

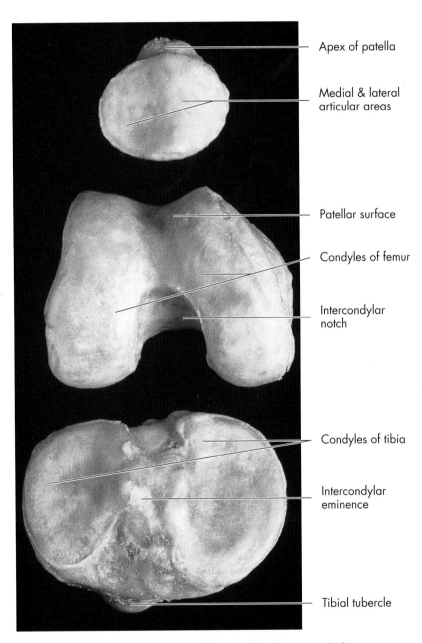

Apex of patella

Medial & lateral articular areas

Patellar surface

Condyles of femur

Intercondylar notch

Condyles of tibia

Intercondylar eminence

Tibial tubercle

Figure 7-78   Articular surfaces of the patella, femur, and tibia.

SEE PRINCIPLES, FIG. 7-43

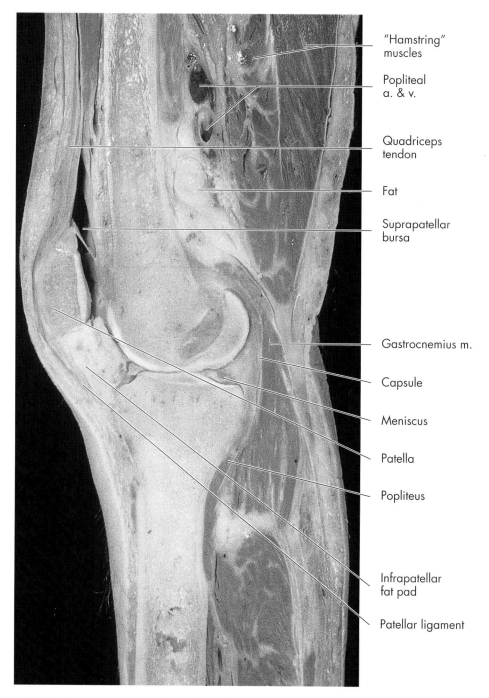

"Hamstring" muscles

Popliteal a. & v.

Quadriceps tendon

Fat

Suprapatellar bursa

Gastrocnemius m.

Capsule

Meniscus

Patella

Popliteus

Infrapatellar fat pad

Patellar ligament

Figure 7-79   Sagittal section through the knee joint showing the articular surfaces and their relationships.

See DISSECTIONS, SECTION 7, p. 8
See PRINCIPLES, FIG. 7-41

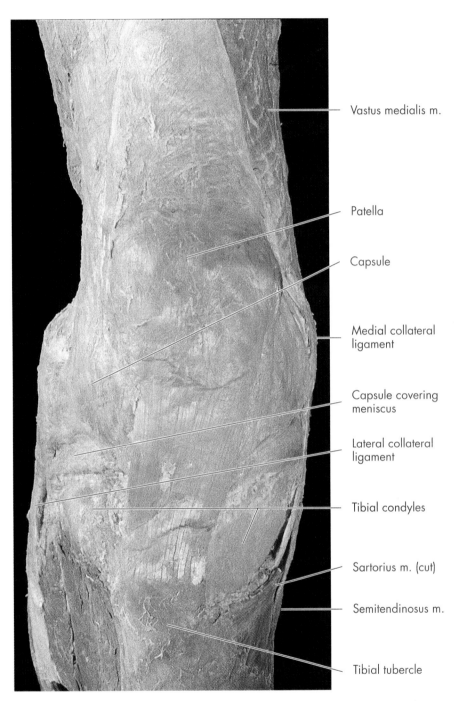

Vastus medialis m.

Patella

Capsule

Medial collateral
ligament

Capsule covering
meniscus

Lateral collateral
ligament

Tibial condyles

Sartorius m. (cut)

Semitendinosus m.

Tibial tubercle

Figure 7-80   Superficial dissection of the knee joint from the anterior aspect showing the
ligamentum patellae, capsule, and collateral ligaments.

SEE **DISSECTIONS**, SECTION 7, P. 12

SEE **PRINCIPLES**, FIG. 7-55

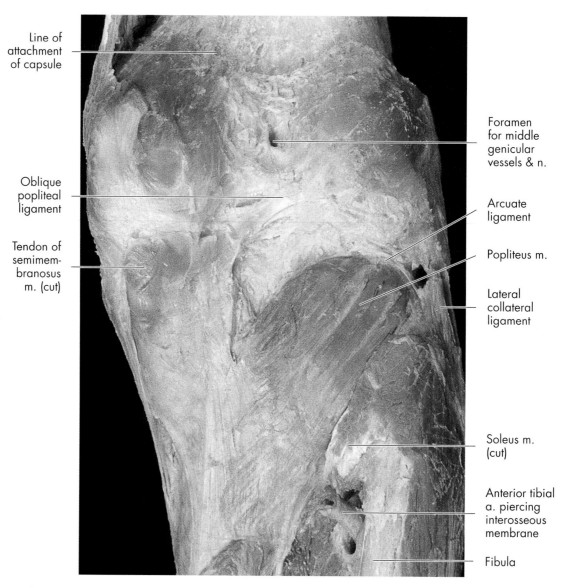

Line of attachment of capsule

Oblique popliteal ligament

Tendon of semimembranosus m. (cut)

Foramen for middle genicular vessels & n.

Arcuate ligament

Popliteus m.

Lateral collateral ligament

Soleus m. (cut)

Anterior tibial a. piercing interosseous membrane

Fibula

Figure 7-81   Posterior aspect of the knee joint showing the capsule, popliteus, and semimembranosus insertion.

See DISSECTIONS, Section 7, p. 12
See PRINCIPLES, Fig. 7-40

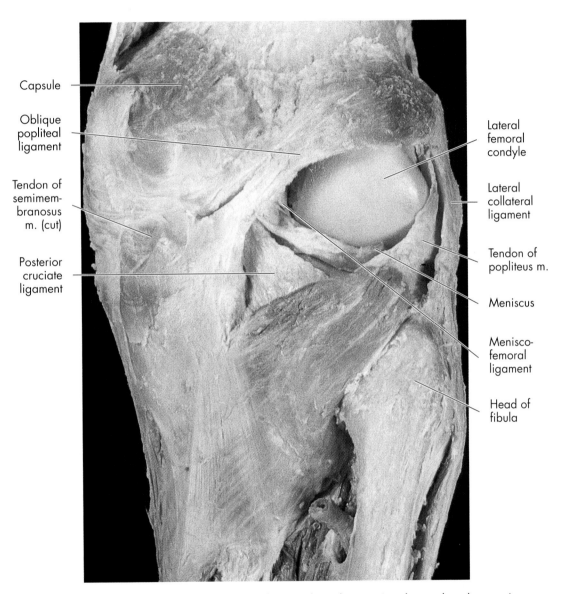

Figure 7-82 Partial removal of the capsule revealing the meniscofemoral and posterior cruciate ligaments and the tendon of the popliteus.

See DISSECTIONS, Section 7, p. 8

See PRINCIPLES, Fig. 7-40

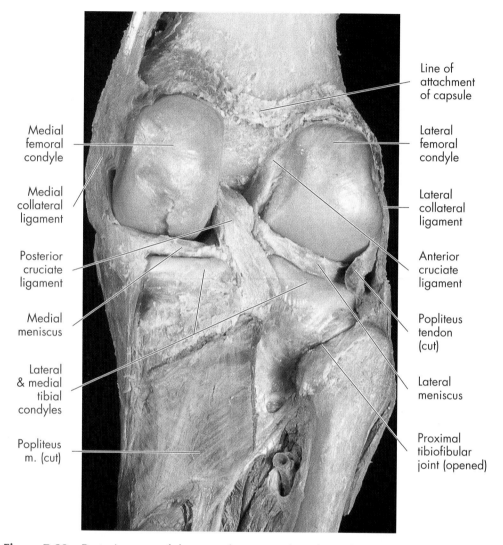

Medial femoral condyle

Medial collateral ligament

Posterior cruciate ligament

Medial meniscus

Lateral & medial tibial condyles

Popliteus m. (cut)

Line of attachment of capsule

Lateral femoral condyle

Lateral collateral ligament

Anterior cruciate ligament

Popliteus tendon (cut)

Lateral meniscus

Proximal tibiofibular joint (opened)

Figure 7-83   Posterior part of the capsule removed to show the cruciate ligaments and menisci. *Stability of the knee joint largely depends on the muscles and tough ligaments that cross the joint. The collateral ligaments are subject to rupture in blunt injury to the lateral or medial side of the joint. The lateral stability of the joint is assessed, immediately after injury, by passively stressing the joint and noting its lateral and medial range as compared with the normal contralateral joint (uninjured knee). Cruciate ligament tears are common in football players and skiers who are subject to injuries from pressure behind the knee (as in "clipping" or stress from a fall that may occur with skiing). Testing for anterior cruciate rupture is undertaken by flexing the knee and pulling the tibia forward on the thigh. If the leg slips forward at the knee (bureau drawer sign), the anterior cruciate ligament is ruptured. If the tibia moves backward unduly when the leg is pushed backward, the posterior cruciate is torn.*

SEE **DISSECTIONS, SECTION 7, P. 8**
SEE **PRINCIPLES, FIG. 7-39**

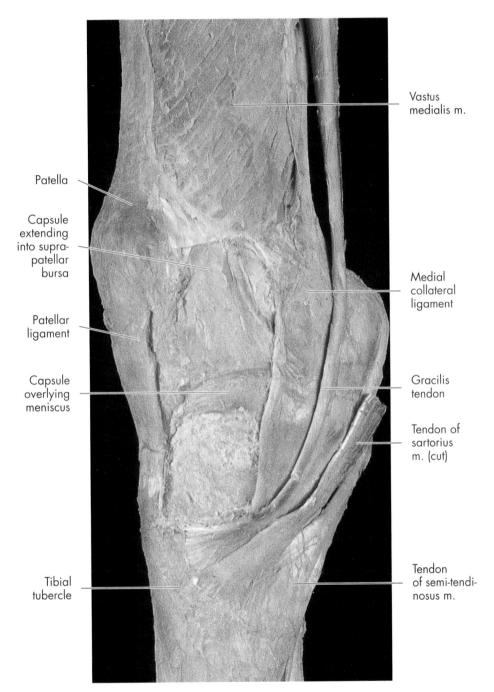

Figure 7-84   Superficial dissection of the knee joint from the medial aspect showing the medial collateral ligament, capsule, and insertions of the sartorius, gracilis, and semi-tendinosus muscles.

See DISSECTIONS, Section 7, p. 8
See PRINCIPLES, Figs. 7-40 and 7-46

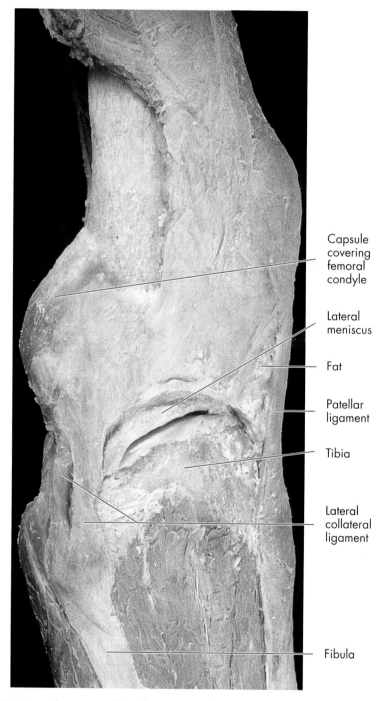

Capsule
covering
femoral
condyle

Lateral
meniscus

Fat

Patellar
ligament

Tibia

Lateral
collateral
ligament

Fibula

Figure 7-85   Lateral aspect of the knee joint showing the collateral ligament and the meniscus revealed by removing part of the capsule.

See **DISSECTIONS**, Section 7, p. 8
See **PRINCIPLES**, Fig. 7-40

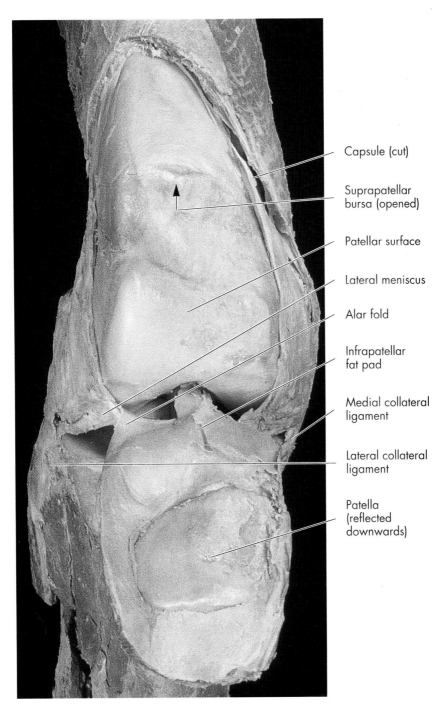

Capsule (cut)

Suprapatellar
bursa (opened)

Patellar surface

Lateral meniscus

Alar fold

Infrapatellar
fat pad

Medial collateral
ligament

Lateral collateral
ligament

Patella
(reflected
downwards)

Figure 7-86   Interior of the joint revealed by opening the capsule anteriorly and reflecting the patella downwards.

See **DISSECTIONS**, Section 7, p. 8

See **PRINCIPLES**, Fig. 7-44

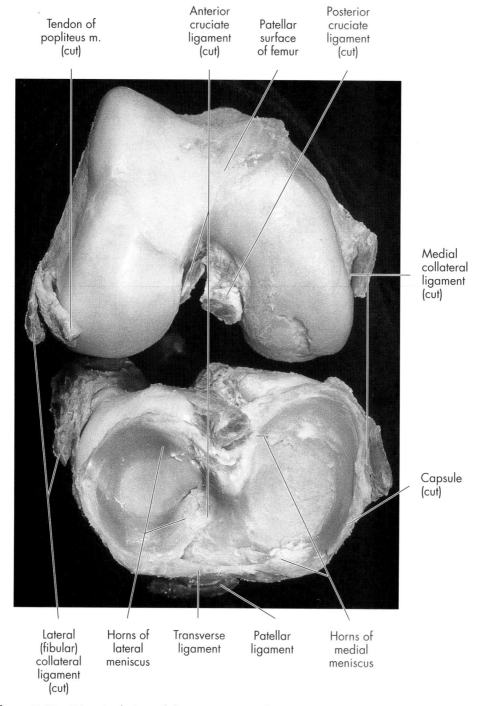

Tendon of popliteus m. (cut)

Anterior cruciate ligament (cut)

Patellar surface of femur

Posterior cruciate ligament (cut)

Medial collateral ligament (cut)

Capsule (cut)

Lateral (fibular) collateral ligament (cut)

Horns of lateral meniscus

Transverse ligament

Patellar ligament

Horns of medial meniscus

Figure 7-87   Disarticulation of the joint to reveal menisci and attachments of the cruciate ligaments.

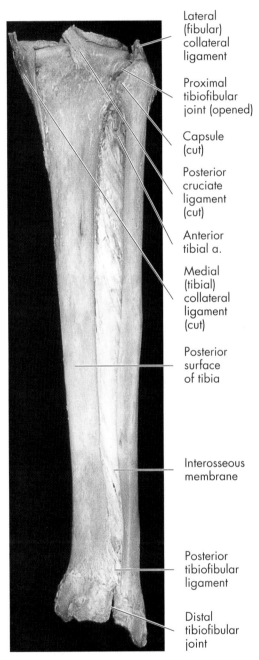

Lateral
(fibular)
collateral
ligament

Proximal
tibiofibular
joint (opened)

Capsule
(cut)

Posterior
cruciate
ligament
(cut)

Anterior
tibial a.

Medial
(tibial)
collateral
ligament
(cut)

Posterior
surface
of tibia

Interosseous
membrane

Posterior
tibiofibular
ligament

Distal
tibiofibular
joint

Figure 7-88   Posterior view of the tibia and fibula showing the tibiofibular joints and the interosseous membrane. The lower part of the tibiofibular ligament has been removed.

See PRINCIPLES, Fig. 7-74

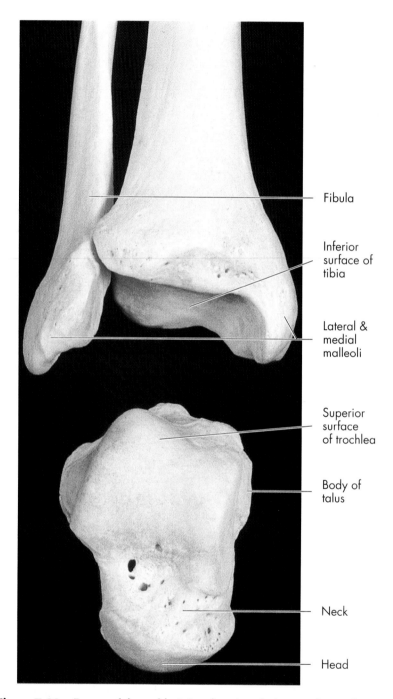

Fibula

Inferior
surface of
tibia

Lateral &
medial
malleoli

Superior
surface
of trochlea

Body of
talus

Neck

Head

Figure 7-89   Bones of the ankle joint showing their articular surfaces.

See PRINCIPLES, Fig. 7-74

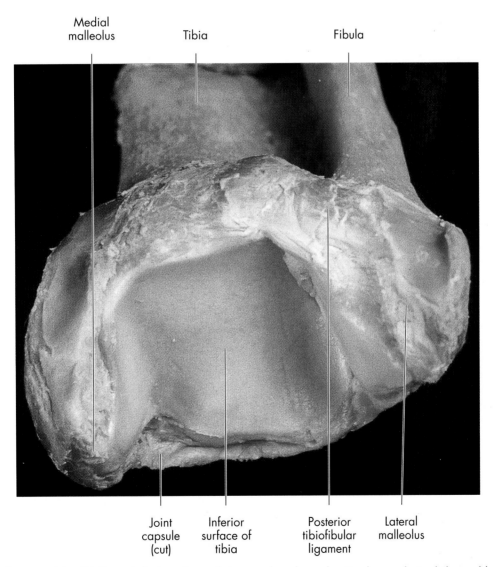

Medial malleolus Tibia Fibula

Joint capsule (cut) Inferior surface of tibia Posterior tibiofibular ligament Lateral malleolus

Figure 7-90 Oblique inferior view of the wedge-shaped articular socket of the ankle joint.

SEE PRINCIPLES, FIG. 7-74

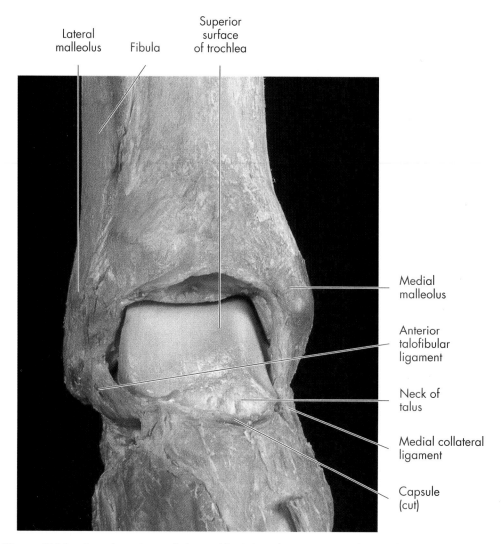

Lateral
malleolus   Fibula

Superior
surface
of trochlea

Medial
malleolus

Anterior
talofibular
ligament

Neck of
talus

Medial collateral
ligament

Capsule
(cut)

Figure 7-91   Anterior view of the ankle joint showing articular surfaces revealed by removal of the capsule.

See PRINCIPLES, Fig. 7-74

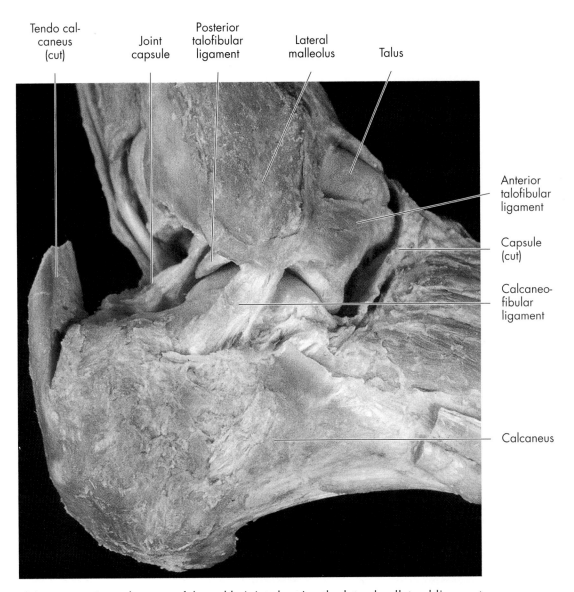

Tendo cal-
caneus
(cut)

Joint
capsule

Posterior
talofibular
ligament

Lateral
malleolus

Talus

Anterior
talofibular
ligament

Capsule
(cut)

Calcaneo-
fibular
ligament

Calcaneus

Figure 7-92   Lateral aspect of the ankle joint showing the lateral collateral ligament, which consists of the anterior and posterior talofibular ligaments and the calcaneofibular ligament.

See PRINCIPLES, FIGS. 7-74, 7-66, 7-67

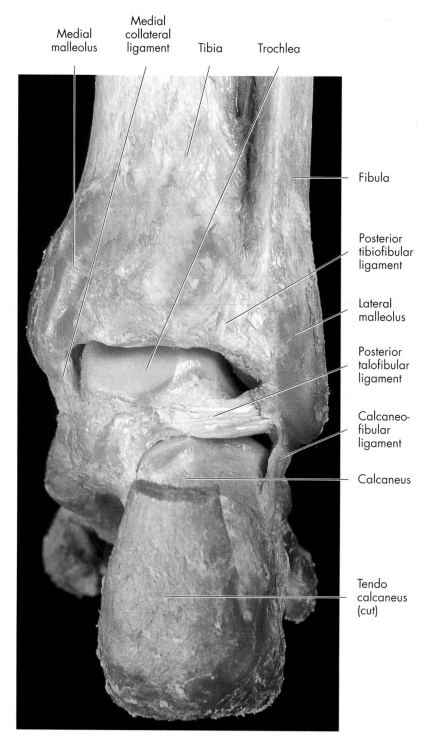

Medial
malleolus

Medial
collateral
ligament

Tibia

Trochlea

Fibula

Posterior
tibiofibular
ligament

Lateral
malleolus

Posterior
talofibular
ligament

Calcaneo-
fibular
ligament

Calcaneus

Tendo
calcaneus
(cut)

Figure 7-93   Posterior view of the ankle joint showing the articular surface of the talus after removal of the capsule.

See **PRINCIPLES**, Figs. 7-63, 7-74

Tendon of tibialis anterior (cut)

Sustentaculum tali

Trochlea

Tendo calcaneus (cut)

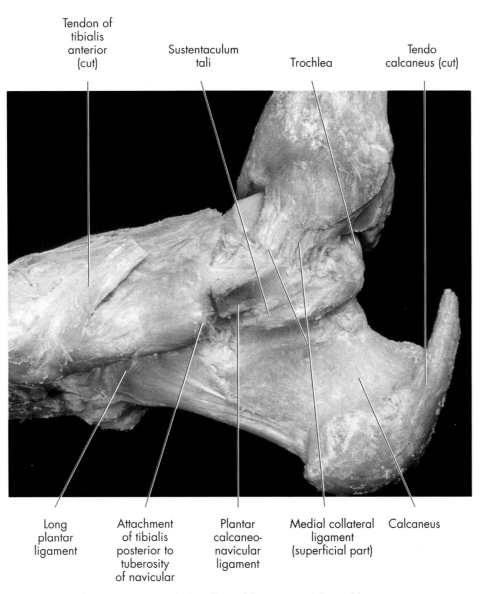

Long plantar ligament

Attachment of tibialis posterior to tuberosity of navicular

Plantar calcaneo-navicular ligament

Medial collateral ligament (superficial part)

Calcaneus

Figure 7-94   Medial collateral ligament of the ankle joint.

See PRINCIPLES, FIG. 7-74

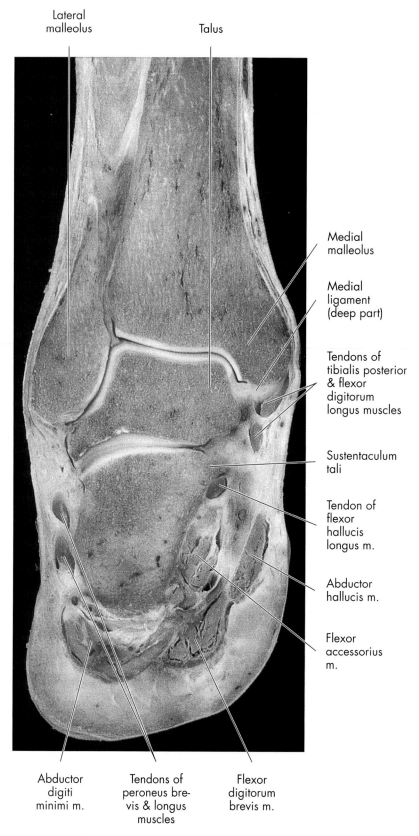

Figure 7-95   Coronal section through the ankle and talocalcaneal joints showing their relationships.

SEE **PRINCIPLES**, FIG. 7-64

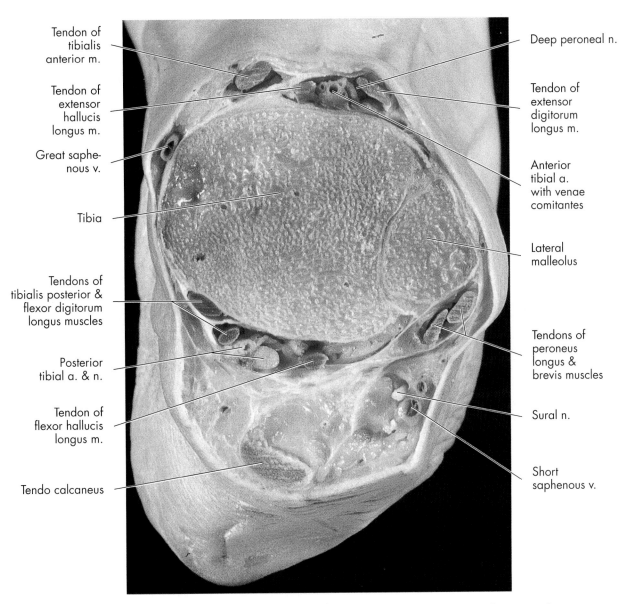

Tendon of
tibialis
anterior m.

Tendon of
extensor
hallucis
longus m.

Great saphe-
nous v.

Tibia

Tendons of
tibialis posterior &
flexor digitorum
longus muscles

Posterior
tibial a. & n.

Tendon of
flexor hallucis
longus m.

Tendo calcaneus

Deep peroneal n.

Tendon of
extensor
digitorum
longus m.

Anterior
tibial a.
with venae
comitantes

Lateral
malleolus

Tendons of
peroneus
longus &
brevis muscles

Sural n.

Short
saphenous v.

Figure 7-96   Transverse section immediately above the ankle joint cavity showing relationships of structures at this level.

SEE PRINCIPLES, FIG. 7-67, *A*

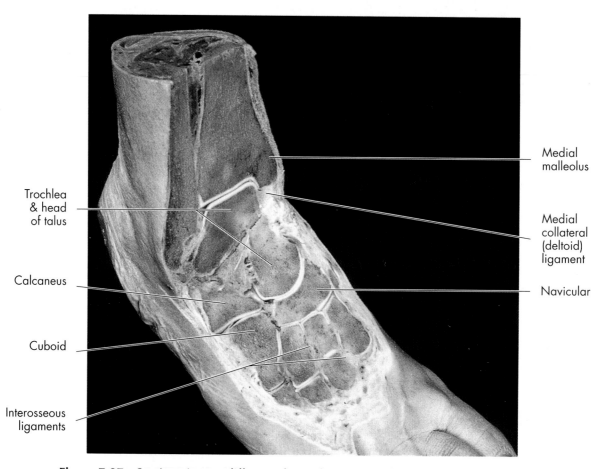

Medial
malleolus

Trochlea
& head
of talus

Medial
collateral
(deltoid)
ligament

Calcaneus

Navicular

Cuboid

Interosseous
ligaments

Figure 7-97   Sections in two different planes through the ankle and foot to show ankle and tarsal joints.

See **DISSECTIONS**, Section 7, p. 17

See **PRINCIPLES**, Fig. 7-69

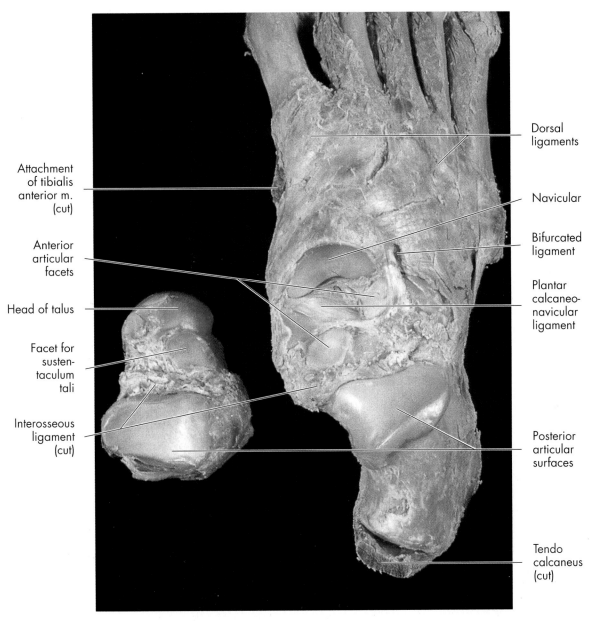

Dorsal
ligaments

Navicular

Bifurcated
ligament

Plantar
calcaneo-
navicular
ligament

Posterior
articular
surfaces

Tendo
calcaneus
(cut)

Attachment
of tibialis
anterior m.
(cut)

Anterior
articular
facets

Head of talus

Facet for
susten-
taculum
tali

Interosseous
ligament
(cut)

Figure 7-98 Talocalcaneal and talonavicular joints. The talus has been disarticulated and turned over.

See **PRINCIPLES, FIG. 7-68**

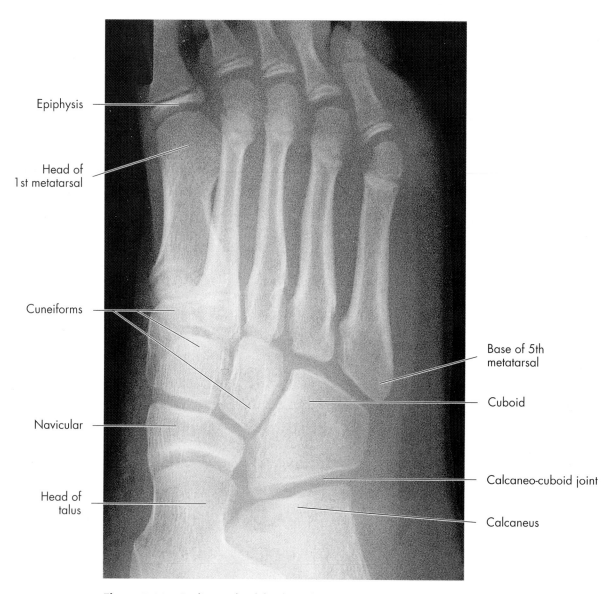

Epiphysis

Head of
1st metatarsal

Cuneiforms

Navicular

Head of
talus

Base of 5th
metatarsal

Cuboid

Calcaneo-cuboid joint

Calcaneus

Figure 7-99   Radiograph of the foot showing the tarsal bones and joints.

See PRINCIPLES, FIG. 7-71

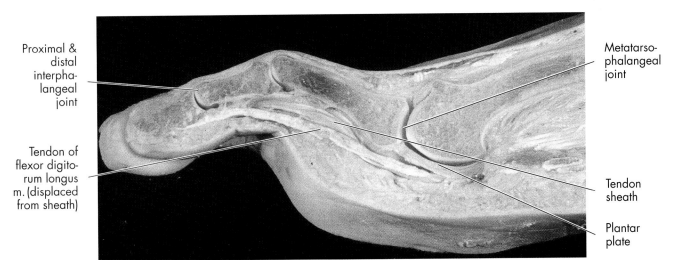

Proximal & distal interphalangeal joint

Tendon of flexor digitorum longus m. (displaced from sheath)

Metatarsophalangeal joint

Tendon sheath

Plantar plate

Figure 7-100 Sagittal section through the third toe showing the metatarsophalangeal and interphalangeal joints.

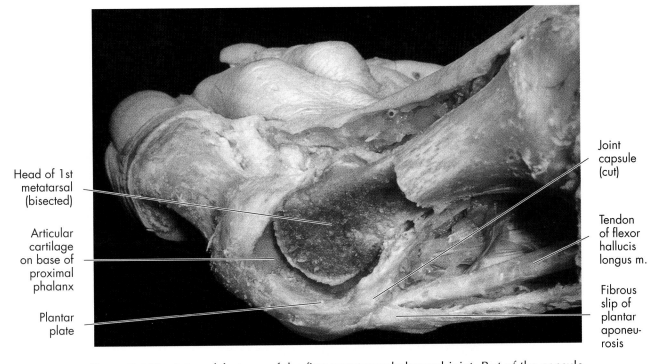

Head of 1st metatarsal (bisected)

Articular cartilage on base of proximal phalanx

Plantar plate

Joint capsule (cut)

Tendon of flexor hallucis longus m.

Fibrous slip of plantar aponeurosis

Figure 7-101 Internal features of the first metatarsophalangeal joint. Part of the capsule and the distal part of the metatarsal bone have been removed.

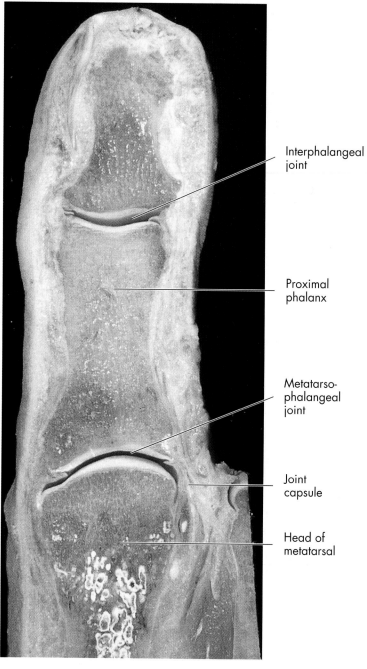

Interphalangeal joint

Proximal phalanx

Metatarso-phalangeal joint

Joint capsule

Head of metatarsal

Figure 7-102   Longitudinal section through the great toe showing its joints.

SEE **PRINCIPLES**, FIG. 7-73

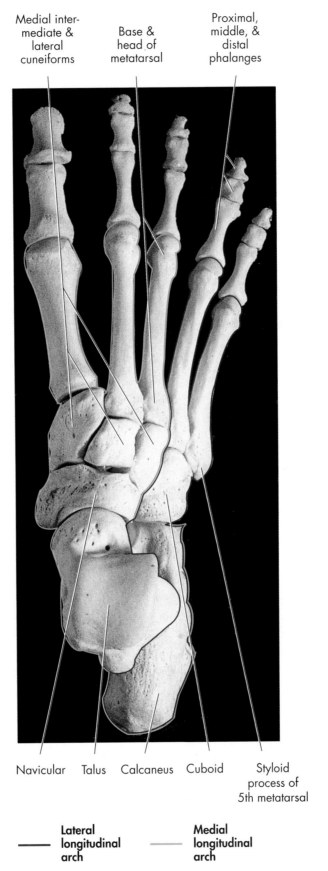

Medial inter-
mediate &
lateral
cuneiforms

Base &
head of
metatarsal

Proximal,
middle, &
distal
phalanges

Navicular   Talus   Calcaneus   Cuboid   Styloid
process of
5th metatarsal

—— Lateral
longitudinal
arch

—— Medial
longitudinal
arch

Figure 7-103 Dorsal aspect of the bones of the foot showing the medial and lateral longitudinal arches.

SEE **PRINCIPLES**, FIG. 7-61

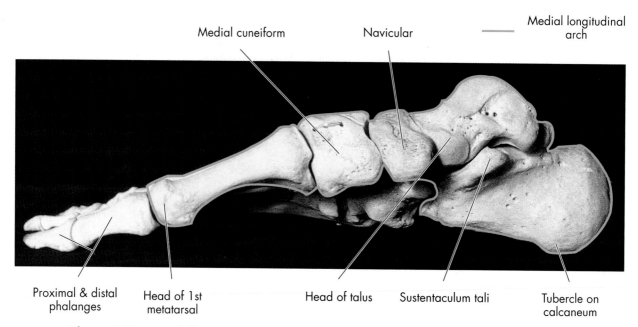

Medial cuneiform   Navicular   ——— Medial longitudinal arch

Proximal & distal phalanges   Head of 1st metatarsal   Head of talus   Sustentaculum tali   Tubercle on calcaneum

Figure 7-104 Medial aspect of the bones of the foot showing the medial longitudinal arch.

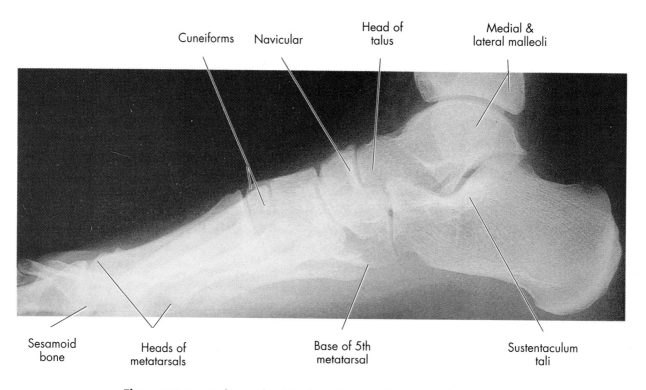

Cuneiforms   Navicular   Head of talus   Medial & lateral malleoli

Sesamoid bone   Heads of metatarsals   Base of 5th metatarsal   Sustentaculum tali

Figure 7-105 Radiograph of the foot showing the longitudinal arches.

See PRINCIPLES, Fig. 7-72

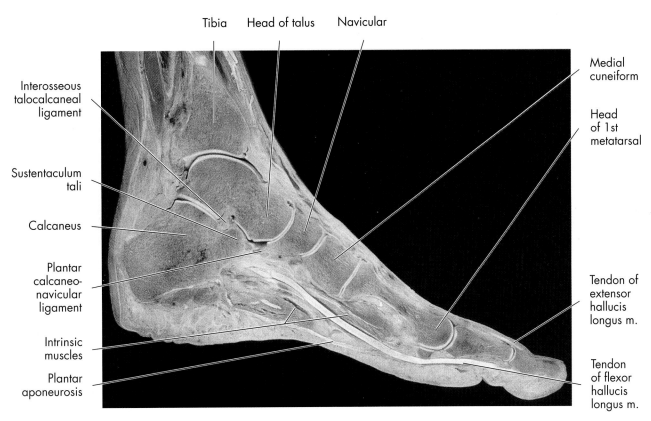

Tibia   Head of talus   Navicular

Interosseous
talocalcaneal
ligament

Medial
cuneiform

Head
of 1st
metatarsal

Sustentaculum
tali

Calcaneus

Plantar
calcaneo-
navicular
ligament

Tendon of
extensor
hallucis
longus m.

Intrinsic
muscles

Plantar
aponeurosis

Tendon
of flexor
hallucis
longus m.

Figure 7-106   Sagittal section of the foot showing the medial longitudinal arch.

Glossary

This glossary provides the *Nomina Anatomica (NA)* equivalents for many of the English terms used in the text. Items that differ only by the adjectives in the list to the right are often given in stem form only. Thus, 'nervus gluteus' is included but not 'nervus gluteus inferior' or 'nervus gluteus superior'.

right/left: dexter/sinister
medial/lateral: medialis/lateralis
anterior/posterior: anterior/posterior
superior/inferior: superior/inferior
external/internal: externus/internus
superficial/deep: superficialis/profundus

ENGLISH	NOMINA ANATOMICA	ENGLISH	NOMINA ANATOMICA
A		arachnoid mater	–arachnoid mater
abdomen	–abdomen	granulations	–granulationes arachnoideales
acetabulum	–acetabulum	arch	–arcus
Achilles tendon	–tendo calcaneus	aortic	–arcus aortae
acromion	–acromion	anterior, of atlas	–arcus anterior atlantis
adenoid	–tonsilla pharyngealis	of azygos vein	–arcus venae azygos
ala of sacrum	–ala sacralis	dorsal venous, of foot	–arcus venosus dorsalis pedis
ampulla		dorsal venous, of hand	–rete venosus dorsalis manus
of rectum	–ampulla recti	neural	–arcus vertebrae
of uterine tube	–ampulla tubae uterinae	palmar, arterial, of hand	–arcus palmaris
of vas deferens	–ampulla ductus deferentis	planter	–arcus plantaris
of Vater	–ampulla hepatopancreatica	posterior, of atlas	–arcus posterior atlantis
anastomosis	–vas anastomoticum	tendinous, of levator ani	–arcus tendineus, m. levator ani
angle, subcostal	–angulus infrasternalis	vertebral (neural)	–arcus vertebralis
annulus fibrosus	–annulus fibrosus	area, bare of liver	–area nuda
ansa cervicalis	–ansa cervicalis	arm	–brachium
subclavia	–ansa subclavia	arteriole	–arteriola
antrum	–antrum	artery	–arteria
maxillary	–sinus maxillarius	auricular, posterior	–a. auricularis posterior
of stomach	–antrum pyloricum	axillary	–a. axillaris
anus	–anus	basilar	–a. basilaris
aorta	–aorta	brachial	–a. brachialis
abdominal	–aorta abdominalis	cecal	–a. caecalis
arch	–arcus aortae	celiac	–truncus coeliacus
bifurcation	–bifurcatio aortae	carotid	
sinus	–sinus aortae	common	–a. carotis communis
thoracic		external	–a. carotis externa
ascending	–pars ascendens aortae	internal	–a. carotis interna
descending	–pars descendens aortae	cerebral, middle	–a. cerebri media
apex	–apex	cervical	
aponeurosis	–aponeurosis	deep	–a. cervicalis profunda
bicipital	–aponeurosis musculi bicipitis brachii	transverse	–a. transversa cervicis
epicranial	–galea aponeurotica	circumflex branch of right coronary	–ramus circumflexus
palatine	–aponeurosis palatina	femoral	–a. circumflexa femoris
palmar	–aponeurosis palmaris	humeral	–a. circumflexa humeri
plantar	–aponeurosis plantaris	scapular	–a. circumflexa scapulae
apparatus, lacrimal	–apparatus lacrimalis	colic	
appendage, atrial	–auricula	left	–a. colica sinistra
appendix	–appendix vermiformis	middle	–a. colica media
epiploicae	–appendices epiploicae	right	–a. colica dextra
vermiform	–appendix vermiformis	collateral	–a. collateralis

Reprinted from Gosling JA, Harris PF, Humpherson JR, Whitmore I, Willan PLT: *Human anatomy: text and colour atlas,* London, 1990, Gower.

ENGLISH	NOMINA ANATOMICA
artery (*cont.*)	
communicating	–a. communicans
coronary	–a. coronaria
cystic	–a. cystica
deep	
of clitoris	–a. profunda clitoridis
of penis	–a. profunda penis
digital	–aa. digitales
dorsal	
of clitoris	–a. dorsalis clitoridis
of penis	–a. dorsalis penis
dorsalis pedis	–a. dorsalis pedis
epigastric	–a. epigastrica
facial	–a. facialis
femoral	–a. femoralis
gastric	–a. gastrica
gastroduodenal	–a. gastroduodenalis
gastroepiploic	–a. gastro-omentalis
gluteal	–a. glutealis
hepatic	–a. hepatica communis
ileal	–aa. ileales
ileocolic	–a. ileocolica
iliac	
common	–a. iliaca communis
external	–a. iliaca externa
internal	–a. iliaca interna
intercostal	–aa. intercostales
anterior	–rami intercostales anteriores
posterior	–aa. intercostales posteriores
interosseous, common	–a. interossea communis
interventricular	
anterior	–ramus interventricularis anterior
inferior	–ramus interventricularis posterior
jejunal	–aa. jejunales
lingual	–a. lingualis
lumbar	–aa. lumbales
marginal, of heart	–ramus marginalis dexter
maxillary	–a. maxillaris
meningeal, middle	–a. meningea media
mesenteric	–a. mesenterica
metacarpal	–aa. metacarpales
metatarsal	–aa. metatarsales
musculophrenic	–a. musculophrenica
nutrient	–a. nutricia
obturator	–a. obturatoria
abnormal obturator	–a. obturatoria accessoria
occipital	–a. occipitalis
ophthalmic	–a. ophthalmica
ovarian	–a. ovarica
pancreaticoduodenal	–a. pancreaticoduodenalis
peroneal	–a. fibularis
pharyngeal, ascending	–a. pharyngea ascendens
phrenic, inferior	–a. phrenica inferior
plantar	–a. plantaris
popliteal	–a. poplitea
profunda	
brachii	–a. profunda brachii
femoris	–a. profunda femoris
pudenal	
external	–aa. pudendae externae
internal	–a. pudenda interna
pulmonary	–a. pulmonalis
radial	–a. radialis
rectal	–a. rectalis
renal	–a. renalis
retinal, central	–a. centralis retinae
sacral, median	–a. sacralis mediana
sigmoid	–aa. sigmoideae
splenic	–a. splenica
subclavian	–a. subclavia
subscapular	–rami subscapulares
suprarenal	–a. suprarenalis
suprascapular	–a. suprascapularis

ENGLISH	NOMINA ANATOMICA
temporal, superficial	–a. temporalis superficialis
testicular	–a. testicularis
thoracic	
internal	–a. thoracica interna
lateral	–a. thoracica lateralis
superior	–a. thoracica superior
thoracoacromial	–a. thoracoacromialis
thyrocervical	–a. thyrocervicalis
thyroid	–a. thyroidea
tibial	–a. tibialis
ulnar	–a. ulnaris
umbilical, obliterated	–a. umbilicalis, pars occlusa
uterine	–a. uterina
vertebral	–a. vertebralis
vesical	–a. vesicalis
articulation (joint)	–articulatio
atlas vertebra	–atlas
atrial appendage	–auricula
atrioventricular	
bundle	–fasciculus atrioventricularis
groove	–sulcus coronarius
orifice	–ostium atrioventriculare
atrium of heart	–atrium cordis
autonomic nervous system	–systema nervosum autonomicum
axilla	–axilla
axis vertebra	–axis
axon	–axon

B

ENGLISH	NOMINA ANATOMICA
base	–basis
of cranium	–basis cranii
of heart	–basis cordis
of lung	–basis pulmonis
bifurcation	–bifurcatio
bladder	–vesica
gall	–vesica biliaris
urinary	–vesica urinaria
blood vessels	
body	–corpus
border	–margo
branch	–ramus
breast	–mamma
areola	–areola mammae
glandular elements	–glandula mammaria
lactiferous duct	–ductus lactiferi
nipple	–papilla mammaria
bronchopulmonary segments	–segmenta bronchopulmonalia
bronchus	–bronchus
main, principal	–bronchus principalis
bulb	
of penis	–bulbus penis
of vestibule	–bulbus vestibuli
bundle of His (atrioventricular)	–fasciculus atrioventricularis
bundle branch	–crus
bursa	–bursa synovialis
infrapatellar	–bursa infrapatellaris
olecranon	–bursa subcutanea olecrani
omental	–bursa omentalis
prepatellar	–bursa subcutanea prepatellaris
semimembranosus	–bursa musculi semimembranosi
subacromial	–bursa subacromialis
subscapular	–bursa subtendinea musculi subscapularis
suprapatellar	–bursa suprapatellaris
buttock	–regio glutealis

C

ENGLISH	NOMINA ANATOMICA
calcaneum	–calcaneus
calf	–sura
calices	–calices renales
canal	

ENGLISH	NOMINA ANATOMICA
canal (*cont.*)	
anal	–canalis analis
carotid	–canalis caroticus
carpal	–canalis carpi
cervical	–canalis cervicis uteri
femoral	–canalis femoralis
hypoglossal	–canalis hypoglossi
inguinal	–canalis inguinalis
nasolacrimal	–canalis nasolacrimalis
obturator	–canalis obturatorius
optic	–canalis opticus
pudendal	–canalis pudendalis
pyloric	–canalis pyloricus
subsartorial	–canalis adductorius
vertebral	–canalis vertebralis
capillaries	–vasa capillare
capitate bone	–os capitatum
capsule, articular	–capsula articularis
carina	–carina tracheae
carpal bones	–ossa carpi
carpus	–carpus
cartilage	
articular	–cartilago articularis
arytenoid	–cartilago arytenoidea
costal	–cartilago costalis
cricoid	–cartilago cricoidea
elastic	–cartilago elastica
fibrocartilage	–cartilago fibrosa
hyaline	–cartilago hyalina
thyroid	–cartilago thyroidea
tracheal	–cartilagines trachealis
cauda equina	–cauda equina
cavity	
abdominal	–cavitas abdominale
nasal	–cavitas nasi
pelvis	–cavitas pelvis
pericardial	–cavitas pericardialis
peritoneal	–cavitas peritonealis
pleural	–cavitas pleuralis
thorax	–cavitas thoracis
uterine	–cavitas uteri
cecum	–caecum
cerebellum	–cerebellum
cerebrospinal fluid	–liquor cerebrospinalis
cerebrum	–cerebrum
cervix, uterine	–cervix uteri
chordae tendineae	–chordae tendineae
circle of Willis	–circulus arteriosus cerebri
cisterna chyli	–cisterna chyli
clavicle	–clavicula
clitoris	–clitoris
clivus	–clivus
coccyx	–os coccygis
colliculus, seminal	–colliculus seminalis
colon	–colon
ascending	–colon ascendens
descending	–colon descendens
sigmoid	–colon sigmoideum
transverse	–colon transversum
column	
anal	–columna anales
vertebral	–columna vertebrales
cervical	–vertebrae cervicales
coccygeal	–vertebrae coccygeae
lumbar	–vertebrae lumbales
sacral	–vertebrae sacrales (os sacrum)
thoracic	–vertebrae thoracicae
colliculus, seminal	–colliculus seminalis
concha, nasal	–concha nasalis
conducting system of heart	–systema conducens cordis
condyle	
femoral	–condylus femoris
tibial	–condylus tibiae

ENGLISH	NOMINA ANATOMICA
conjunctiva	–tunica conjunctiva
connective tissue	–textus connectivus
cord	
of brachial plexus	–plexus brachialis
lateral	–fasciculus lateralis
medial	–fasciculus medialis
posterior	–fasciculus posterior
spermatic	–funiculus spermaticus
spinal	–medulla spinalis
cornea	–cornea
corpus	
cavernosum	–corpus cavernosum
spongiosum	–corpus spongiosum
cranium	–cranium
crest	
sacral	–crista sacralis
urethral	–crista urethralis
crista	–crista
galli	–crista galli
terminalis	–crista terminalis
crus	
of clitoris	–crus clitoridis
of diaphragm	–crus partis lumbalis diaphragmatis
of penis	–crus penis
cuboid bone	–os cuboideum
cuneiform bone	–os cuneiforme
curve, curvature	–curvatura gastrica
cusp	–cuspis
of aortic valve	–valvula semilunares
of mitral valve	–cuspis valvula mitrealis
of pulmonary	–valvula semilunaris
of tricuspid valve	–cuspis valvula tricuspidalis

D

ENGLISH	NOMINA ANATOMICA
dens	–dens axis
dermatomes	–dermatomi
diaphragm	–diaphragma (thoraco-abdominale)
pelvic	–diaphragma pelvis
urogential	–diaphragma urogenitale
diaphragma sellae	–diaphragma sellae
digits	
of hand (fingers)	–digiti manus
of foot (toes)	–digiti pedis
disk	
articular cartilage	–discus articularis
intervertebral	–discus intervertebralis
diverticulum, ileal (Meckel's)	–diverticulum ilei
dorsum	
of foot	–dorsum pedis
of hand	–dorsum manus
duct	
bile	–ductus choledochus
cystic	–ductus cysticus
efferent of testis	–ductuli efferentes testis
ejaculatory	–ductus ejaculatorius
hepatic	–ductus hepaticus
nasolacrimal	–ductus nasolacrimalis
pancreatic	–ductus pancreaticus
accessory	–ductus pancreaticus accessorius
thoracic	–ductus thoracicus
ductus	
arteriosus	–ductus arteriosus
deferens	–ductus deferens
duodenum	–duodenum
papilla	–papilla duodeni
dura mater	–dura mater

E

ENGLISH	NOMINA ANATOMICA
ear	–auris
external	–auris externa
eminence	

ENGLISH	NOMINA ANATOMICA	ENGLISH	NOMINA ANATOMICA
eminence —*cont'd*		fold	
hypothenar	–eminentia hypothenar	aryepiglottic	–plica aryepiglottica
iliopectineal	–eminentia iliopubica	horizontal, of rectum	–plicae transversae recti
intercondylar	–eminentia intercondylaris	peritoneal	–plica peritonealis
thenar	–eminentia thenar	vestibular	–plica vestibularis
enlargement		vocal	–plica vocalis
cervical	–intumescentia cervicalis	foot	–pes
lumbosacral	–intumescentia lumbosacralis	dorsal surface	–dorsum pedis
epicondyle	–epicondylus	sole	–planta pedis
epidermis	–epidermis	foramen	
epididymis	–epididymis	epiploic	–foramen omentale
epiglottis	–epiglottis	intervertebral	–foramen intervertebrale
epiphysis	–epiphysis	jugular	–foramen jugulare
esophagus	–oesophagus	lacerum	–foramen lacerum
ethmoid bone	–os ethmoidale	magnum	–foramen magnum
eyeball	–bulbus oculi	nutrient	–foramen nutriens
eyelashes	–cilia	obturator	–foramen obturatum
eyelid	–palpebra	ovale	–foramen ovale
		rotundum	–foramen rotundum
		sacral	–foramina sacralia
F		sciatic	–foramen ischiadicum
		spinosum	–foramen spinosum
face	–facies	transversarium	–foramen transversarium
muscles	–mm. faciales	forearm	–antebrachium
nerve	–n. facialis	fornix, vaginal	–fornix vaginae
falx cerebri	–falx cerebri	fossa	
fascia	–fascia	acetabular	–fossa acetabuli
bulbi	–vagina bulbi	cranial	–fossa cranii
cremasteric	–fascia cremasterica	cubital	–fossa cubitalis
deep	–fascia profunda	glenoid	–cavitas glenoidalis
dorsum of foot	–fascia dorsalis pedis	infraspinous	–fossa infraspinatus
leg	–fascia cruris	infratemporal	–fossa infratemporalis
iliac	–fascia iliaca	intersigmoid	–recessus intersigmoideus
investing	–fascia cervicalis: lamina superficialis	ischiorectal	–fossa ischioanalis
lata	–fascia lata	lacrimal	–fossa sacci lacrimalis
lumbar	–fascia thoracolumbalis	navicular	–fossa navicularis urethrae
neck	–fascia cervicalis	ovalis	–fossa ovalis
obturator	–fascia obturatoria	ovarian	–fossa ovarica
pelvic	–fascia pelvis	paraduodenal	–recessus duodenalis
penile	–fascia penis	peritoneal	–fossae peritonealis
pharyngobasilar	–fascia pharyngobasilaris	popliteal	–fossa poplitea
pretracheal	–fascia cervicalis: lamina pretrachealis	pterygopalatine	–fossa pterygopalatina
prevertebral	–fascia cervicalis: lamina prevertebralis	retrocecal	–recessus retrocaecalis
renal	–fascia renalis	subscapular	–fossa subscapularis
spermatic	–fascia spermatica	supraspinous	–fossa supraspinatis
superficial	–fascia superficialis	temporal	–fossa temporalis
thoracolumbar (lumbar)	–fascia thoracolumbalis	of temporal bone	–fossa mandibularis
transversalis	–fascia transversalis	fourchette	–commissura labiorum posterior
fat		frenulum	–frenulum
perinephric	–corpus adiposum pararenale	frontal bone	–os frontale
femur	–femur	fundus	–fundus
fiber	–fibra		
fibrocartilage	–cartilago fibrosa		
filum terminale	–filum terminale	**G**	
fimbriae	–fimbriae tubae		
fingers	–digiti manus	gallbladder	–vesica bilaris
index	–index	ganglion	
little	–digitus minimus	ciliary	–ganglion ciliae
middle	–digitus medius	otic	–ganglion oticum
ring	–digitus annularis	parasympathetic	–ganglion parasympathicum
fissure	–fissura	pterygopalatine	–ganglion pterygopalatinum
of liver		stellate	–ganglion cervicothoracicum
for ligamentum teres	–fissura ligamenti teretis	submandibular	–ganglion submandibulare
for ligamentum venosum	–fissura ligamenti venosi	sympathetic	–ganglion sympathicum
of lung		thoracic	–ganglia thoracica
horizontal	–fissura horizontalis	genitalia, external	–organa genitalia externa
oblique	–fissura obliqua	female	–organa genitalia feminina externa
orbital	–fissura orbitalis	male	–organa genitalia masculina externa
palpebral	–rima palpebrarum	girdle	
flexure		pectoral	–cingulum pectorale
duodenojejunal	–flexura duodenojejunalis	pelvic	–cingulum membri inferioris
colic	–flexura coli	gland	–glandula
floor		bulbourethral	–glandula bulbourethralis
pelvic	–diaphragma pelvis	greater vestibular	–glandula vestibularis major

ENGLISH	NOMINA ANATOMICA	ENGLISH	NOMINA ANATOMICA
gland (*cont.*)		hip	–articulatio coxae
lacrimal	–glandula lacrimalis	intercarpal	–articulationes intercarpales
parathyroid	–glandula parathyroidea	intermetacarpal	–articulationes intermetacarpales
parotid	–glandula parotidea	intermetatarsal	–articulationes intermetatarsales
prostate	–prostata	interphalangeal	–articulationes interphalangeales
sublingual	–glandula sublingualis	knee	–articulatio genus
submandibular	–glandula submandibularis	lumbosacral	–articulo lumbosacralis
suprarenal	–glandula suprarenalis	manubriosternal	–symphysis manubriosternalis
thyroid	–glandula thyroidea	metacarpophalangeal	–articulationes metacarpophalangeales
glans		metatarsophalangeal	–articulationes metatarsophalangeales
of clitoris	–glans clitoridis	midcarpal	–articulatio mediocarpalis
of penis	–glans penis	radiocarpal	–articulatio radiocarpalis
groove		radioulnar	–articulatio radioulnaris
atrioventricular	–sulcus coronarius	sacrococcygeal	–articulatio sacrococcygea
in liver for inferior vena cava	–sulcus venae cavae	sacroiliac	–articulatio sacroiliaca
subcostal	–sulcus costae	shoulder (glenohumeral)	–articulatio humeri
gutters		sternoclavicular	–articulatio sternoclavicularis
paracolic	–sulci paracolici	subtalar	–articulatio subtalaris
		synovial	–articulationes synoviales
		talocalcaneal	–articulatio subtalaris
H		talocalcaneonavicular	–articulatio talocalcaneonavicularis
hamate bone	–os hamatum	tarsal	–articulatio tarsi
hamulus		tarsometatarsal	–articulationes tarsometatarsales
of hamate	–hamulus ossis hamati	temporomandibular	–articulatio temporomandibularis
of pterygoid	–hamulus pterygoideus	wrist	–articulatio radiocarpalis
hand	–manus		
dorsal surface	–dorsum manus		
palm of	–palma manus	**K**	
haustrations	–haustra	kidney	–ren
head	–caput		
of rib	–caput costae		
heart	–cor	**L**	
conducting system	–systema conducens cordis	labia	
hemisphere, cerebral	–hemispherium cerebralis	majora	–labia majora pudendi
hiatus semilunaris	–hiatus semilunaris	minora	–labia minora pudendi
hilum	–hilum	labrum	
hindbrain	–rhombencephalon	acetabular	–labrum acetabulare
hip bone	–os coxae	glenoid	–labrum glenoidale
humerus	–humerus	lacunae (venous) of	
hyoid bone	–os hyoideum	superior sagittal sinus	–lacunae laterales
		lamina, vertebral	–lamina arcus vertebrae
		laryngopharynx	–pars laryngea pharyngis
I		larynx	–larynx
ileum	–ileum	leg	–crus
ilium	–os ilii	ligament	–ligamentum
impression		annular, of radius	–ligamentum annulare radii
cardiac, of left lung	–impressio cardiaca	arcuate	
incisura angularis	–incisura angularis	of diaphragm	–ligamentum arcuatum diaphragmatis
infundibulum		of knee	–ligamentum popliteum arcuatum
of right ventricle	–conus arteriosus	arteriosum	–ligamentum arteriosum
inlet		atlantooccipital	–ligamentum altantooccipitale
thoracic	–apertura thoracica superior	broad, of uterus	–ligamentum latum uteri
pelvic	–apertura pelvis superior	calcaneofibular	–ligamentum calcaneofibulare
intestine		calcaneonavicular, 'spring'	–ligamentum calcaneonaviculare
large	–intestinum crassum	plantare	
small	–intestinum tenue	capsular	–ligamenta capsularia
ischium	–os ischii	collateral	–ligamentum collaterale
		coracoacromial	–ligamentum coracoacromial
		coracoclavicular	–ligamentum coracoclaviculare
J		coronary	–ligamentum coronarium
jejunum	–jejunum	costoclavicular	–ligamentum costoclaviculare
joint		cricothyroid	–ligamentum cricothyroideum medianum
acromioclavicular	–articulatio acromioclavicularis		
ankle	–articulatio talocruris	cruciate of atlas	–ligamentum cruciforme atlantis
atlantoaxial	–articulatio atlantoaxialis	deltoid of ankle	–ligamentum mediale
atlantooccipital	–articulatio atlantooccipitalis	denticulate	–ligamentum denticulatum
calcaneocuboid	–articulatio calcaneocuboidea	extracapsular	–ligamenta extracapsularia
carpometacarpal	–articulationes carpometacarpales	falciform	–ligamentum falciforme hepatis
cartilaginous	–articulationes cartilaginea	gastrosplenic	–ligamentum gastrosplenicum
elbow	–articulatio cubiti	glenohumeral	–ligamenta glenohumeralia
fibrous	–articulationes fibrosae	iliofemoral	–ligamentum iliofemorale
foot	–articulationes pedis	iliolumbar	–ligamentum iliolumbale
hand	–articulationes manus	inguinal	–ligamentum inguinale

ENGLISH	NOMINA ANATOMICA	ENGLISH	NOMINA ANATOMICA
ligament (*cont.*)		urethral	–ostium urethrae
intercarpal	–ligamenta intercarpalia	Meckel's diverticulum	–diverticulum ilei
interosseous, sacroiliac	–ligamenta sacroiliaca interossea	mediastinum	–mediastinum
intracapsular	–ligamenta intracapsularia	medulla oblongata	–medulla oblongata
ischiofemoral	–ligamentum ischiofemorale	membrane	
lacunar	–ligamentum lacunare	aryepiglottic	–membrana quadrangularis
lienorenal	–ligamentum splenorenale	atlantooccipital	–membranum atlantooccipitale
longitudinal	–ligamentum longitudinale	cricovocal (cricothyroid)	–conus elasticus
meniscofemoral	–ligamentum meniscofemorale	intercostal	
metatarsal, deep transverse	–ligamentum metatarsale transversum profundum	anterior	–membrana intercostalis externa
		posterior	–membrana intercostalis interna
nuchae	–ligamentum nuchae	interosseous	
oblique popliteal	–ligamentum popliteum obliquum	radioulnar	–membrana interossea antebrachii
palpebral	–ligamentum palpebrale	tibiofibular	–membrana interossea cruris
patellar	–ligamentum patellae	perineal	–membrana perinei
pisohamate	–ligamentum pisohamatum	suprapleural	–membrana suprapleuralis
pisometacarpal	–ligamentum pisometacarpale	synovial	–membrana synovialis
plantar	–ligamenta tarsi plantaria	thyrohyoid	–membrana thyrohyoidea
pubofemoral	–ligamentum pubofemorale	meninges	–meninges
puboprostatic	–ligamentum puboprostaticum	meniscus	–meniscus
pulmonary	–ligamentum pulmonale	mesentery	–mesenterium
round		mesoappendix	–mesoappendix
of liver	–ligamentum teres hepatis	mesocolon	
of ovary	–ligamentum ovarii proprium	sigmoid	–mesocolon sigmoideum
of uterus	–ligamentum teres uteri	transverse	–mesocolon transversum
sacroiliac	–ligamenta sacroilaca	mesovarium	–mesovarium
sacrospinous	–ligamentum sacrospinale	metacarpal bones	–ossa metacarpi
sacrotuberous	–ligamentum sacrotuberale	metacarpus	–metacarpus
scapular, transverse	–ligamentum transversum scapulae	metatarsal bones	–ossa metatarsi
'spring'	–ligamentum calcaneonaviculare	moderator band	–trabecula septomarginalis
plantare		mons pubis	–mons pubis
stylohyoid	–ligamentum stylohyoideum	mouth	–cavitas oris
talofibular	–ligamentum talofibulare	muscle	–musculus
teres		abductor	
of hip joint	–ligamentum capitis femoris	digiti minimi	–m. abductor digiti minimi
of liver	–ligamentum teres hepatis	hallucis	–m. abductor hallucis
tibiofibular	–ligamentum tibiofibulare	pollicis brevis	–m. abductor pollicis brevis
triangular	–ligamentum triangulare	pollicis longus	–m. abductor pollicis longus
venosum	–ligamentum venosum	adductor	
limb, lower	–membrum inferius	brevis	–m. adductor brevis
foot	–pes	hallucis	–m. adductor hallucis
dorsum	–dorsum pedis	longus	–m. adductor longus
sole	–planta pedis	magnus	–m. adductor magnus
leg	–crus	pollicis	–m. adductor pollicis
thigh	–femur	anconeus	–m. anconeus
limb, upper	–membrum superius	auricular	–mm. auriculares
line, arcuate	–linea arcuata	biceps brachii	–m. biceps brachii
linea		biceps femoris	–m. biceps femoris
alba	–linea alba	bipennate	–m. bipennatus
semilunaris	–linea semilunaris	brachialis	–m. brachialis
lingula, of left lung	–lingula pulmonis sinistri	brachioradialis	–m. brachioradialis
liver	–hepar	buccinator	–m. buccinator
lobe	–lobus	bulbospongiosus	–m. bulbospongiosus
caudate	–lobus caudatus	cardiac	–m. cardiacus striatus
quadrate	–lobus quadratus	ciliary	–m. ciliaris
lunate bone	–os lunatum	coccygeus	–m. coccygeus
lung	–pulmo	compressor nares	–m. nasalis: pars transversum
lymphatic vessel	–vasa lymphatica	constrictor of pharynx	–m. constrictor pharyngis
		coracobrachialis	–m. coracobrachialis
M		cremaster	–m. cremaster
malleolus	–malleolus	cricoarytenoid	–m. cricoarytenoideus
mandible	–mandibula	cricothyroid	–m. cricothyroideus
manubrium	–manubrium sterni	dartos	–m. dartos
margin, costal	–arcus costalis	deltoid	–m. deltoideus
mater		depressor anguli oris	–m. depressor angulioris
arachnoid	–arachnoid mater	depressor labii inferioris	–m. depressor labii inferioris
dura	–dura mater	detrusor	–m. detrusor vesicae
pia	–pia mater	digastric	–m. digastricus
maxilla	–maxilla	dilator nares	–m. nasalis: pars alaris
meatus		dilator pupillae	–m. dilator pupillae
acoustic	–meatus acusticus	erector spinae	–m. erector spine
nasal	–meatus nasi	extensor	
		carpi radialis brevis	–m. extensor carpi radialis brevis

ENGLISH	NOMINA ANATOMICA
muscle (*cont.*)	
carpi radialis longus	–m. extensor carpi radialis longus
carpi ulnaris	–m. extensor carpi ulnaris
digiti minimi	–m. extensor digiti minimi
digitorum	–m. extensor extensor digitorum
brevis	–m. extensor digitorum brevis
longus	–m. extensor digitorum longus
hallucis brevis	–m. extensor hallucis brevis
hallucis longus	–m. extensor hallucis longus
indicis	–m. extensor indicis
pollicis brevis	–m. extensor pollicis brevis
pollicis longus	–m. extensor pollicis longus
extraocular	–mm. bulbi oculi
of facial expression	–mm. faciales
flexor	
accessorius	–m. quadratus plantae
carpi radialis	–m. flexor carpi radialis
carpi ulnaris	–m. flexor carpi ulnaris
digiti minimi	–m. flexor digiti minimi
digiti minimi brevis	–m. flexor digiti minimi brevis
digitorum	
brevis	–m. flexor digitorum brevis
longus	–m. flexor digitorum longus
profundus	–m. flexor digitorum profundus
superficialis	–m. flexor digitorum superficialis
hallucis brevis	–m. flexor hallucis brevis
hallucis longus	–m. flexor hallucis longus
pollicis brevis	–m. flexor pollicis brevis
pollicis longus	–m. flexor pollicis longus
gastrocnemius	–m. gastrocnemius
gemelli	–mm. gemelli
genioglossus	–m. genioglossus
geniohyoid	–m. geniohyoideus
gluteus	
maximus	–m. gluteus maximus
medius	–m. gluteus medius
minimus	–m. gluteus minimus
gracilis	–m. gracilis
hyoglossus	–m. hyoglossus
iliacus	–m. iliacus
iliococcygeus	–m. iliococcygeus
iliopsoas	–m. iliopsoas
infrahyoid	–mm. infrahyoidei
infraspinatus	–m. infraspinatus
interarytenoid	–m. arytenoideus
intercostal	
external	–mm. intercostales externi
innermost	–mm. intercostales intimi
internal	–mm. intercostales interni
interosseous	–mm. interossei dorsales
dorsal	–mm. interossei plantares
plantar	–mm. interossei palmares
palmar	–m. ischiocavernosus
ischiocavernosus	–mm. laryngis
laryngeal, intrinsic	–m. latissimus dorsi
latissimus dorsi	
levator	–m. levator ani
ani	–m. levator veli palatini
palati	–m. levator palpebrae superioris
palpebrae superioris	–m. levator scapulae
scapulae	–mm. lumbricales
lumbrical	–m. masseter
masseter	–m. mentalis
mentalis	–m. multipennatus
multipennate	–m. mylohyoideus
mylohyoid	
oblique	
external	–m. obliquus externus abdominis
inferior	–m. obliquus inferior
internal	–m. obliquus internus abdominis
superior	–m. obliquus superior
obturator externus	–m. obturator externus
obturator internus	–m. obturator externus
occipitofrontalis	–m. occipitofrontalis
omohyoid	–m. omohyoideus
opponens digiti minimi	–m. opponens digiti minimi
opponens pollicis	–m. opponens pollicis
orbicularis oculi	–m. orbicularis oculi
orbicularis oris	–m. orbicularis oris
palatoglossus	–m. palatoglossus
palatopharyngeus	–m. palatopharyngeus
palmaris brevis	–m. palmaris brevis
palmaris longus	–m. palmaris longus
papillary	–mm. papillares
pectinati	–mm. pectinati
pectineus	–m. pectineus
pectoralis major	–m. pectoralis major
pectoralis minor	–m. pectoralis minor
peroneus	
brevis	–m. peroneus brevis
longus	–m. peroneus longus
tertius	–m. peroneus tertius
pharyngeal	–tunica muscularis pharyngis
piriformis	–m. piriformis
plantaris	–m. plantaris
platysma	–m. platysma
popliteus	–m. popliteus
pronator quadratus	–m. pronator quadratus
pronator teres	–m. pronator teres
psoas major	–m. psoas major
psoas minor	–m. psoas minor
pterygoid	–m. pterygoideus
pubococcygeus	–m. pubococcygeus
pyramidalis	–m. pyramidalis
quadratus femoris	–m. quadratus femoris
quadratus lumborum	–m. quadratus lumborum
quadriceps femoris	–m. quadriceps femoris
rectus	
abdominis	–m. rectus abdominis
of eye	–mm. recti bulbi
femoris	–m. rectus femoris
rhomboid major	–m. rhomboideus major
rhomboid minor	–m. rhomboideus minor
salpingopharyngeus	–m. salpingopharyngeus
sartorius	–m. sartorius
scalenus	
anterior	–m. scalenus anterior
medius	–m. scalenus medius
posterior	–m. scalenus posterior
semimembranosus	–m. semimembranosus
semitendinosus	–m. semitendinosus
serratus	
anterior	–m. serratus anterior
posterior	
inferior	–m. serratus posterior inferior
superior	–m. serratus posterior superior
skeletal	–textus muscularis striatus skeletalis
smooth	–textus muscularis nonstriatus
soleus	–m. soleus
sphincter	
anal	
external	–m. sphincter ani externus
deep part	–pars profunda
subcutaneous part	–pars subcutanea
superficial part	–pars superficialis
internal	–m. sphincter ani internus
pupillae	–m. sphincter pupillae
urethral	–m. sphincter urethrae
splenius capitis	–m. splenius capitis
splenius cervicis	–m. splenius cervicis
sternohyoid	–m. sternohyoideus
sternomastoid	–m. sternocleidomastoideus
sternothyroid	–m. sternothyroideus
styloglossus	–m. styloglossus
stylohyoid	–m. stylohyoideus
stylopharyngeus	–m. stylopharyngeus

ENGLISH	NOMINA ANATOMICA
muscle (*cont.*)	
subscapularis	–m. subscapularis
supinator	–m. supinator
supraspinatus	–m. supraspinatus
temporalis	–m. temporalis
tensor fasciae latae	–m. tensor fasciae latae
tensor palati	–m. tensor veli palatini
teres major	–m. teres major
teres minor	–m. teres minor
thyroarytenoid	–m. thyroarytenoideus
thyrohyoid	–m. thyrohyoideus
tibialis anterior	–m. tibialis anterior
tibialis posterior	–m. tibialis posterior
transversospinal	–mm. transversospinales
transversus abdominis	–m. transversus abdominis
transversus thoracis	–m. transversus thoracis
trapezius	–m. trapezius
triceps brachii	–m. triceps brachii
unipennate	–m. unipennatus
uvular	–m. uvulae
vastus	
intermedius	–m. vastus intermedius
lateralis	–m. vastus lateralis
medialis	–m. vastus medialis
voluntary striated	–textus muscularis striatus skeletalis
zygomaticus major	–m. zygomaticus major
zygomaticus minor	–m. zygomaticus minor
myocardium	–m. myocardium

N

ENGLISH	NOMINA ANATOMICA
nasopharynx	–pars nasalis pharyngis
neck	–cervix, collum
of femur	–collum femoris
of humerus	
anatomic	–collum anatomicum
surgical	–collum chirurgicum
of radius	–collum radii
of uterus	–cervix uteri
nerve	–nervus
abducens (VI)	–n. abducens
accessory (XI)	–n. accessorius
alveolar	–n. alveolaris
auricular, great	–n. auricularis magnus
auriculotemporal	–n. auriculotemporalis
autonomic	–systema nervosum autonomicum
axillary	–n. axillaris
buccal	–n. buccalis
cervical, transverse	–n. transversus colli
chorda tympani	–chorda tympani
ciliary	–nn. ciliares
coccygeal	–n. coccygeus
cranial	–nn. craniales
cutaneous	
of thigh	–n. cutaneous femoris
antebrachial	–n. cutaneous antebrachial
brachial	–n. cutaneous brachii
digital	–nn. digitales
dorsal	
of clitoris	–n. dorsalis clitoridis
of penis	–n. dorsalis penis
scapular	–n. dorsalis scapulae
facial (VII)	–n. facialis
in parotid gland	–plexus intraparotideus
femoral	–n. femoralis
frontal	–n. frontalis
genitofemoral	–n. genitofemoralis
glossopharyngeal (IX)	–n. glossopharyngeus
gluteal	–n. gluteus
hypoglossal (XII)	–n. hypoglossus
iliohypogastric	–n. iliohypogastricus
ilioinguinal	–n. ilioinguinalis
intercostal	–nn. intercostales

ENGLISH	NOMINA ANATOMICA
interosseus	–n. interosseus
lacrimal	–n. lacrimalis
laryngeal	
recurrent	–n. laryngeus recurrens
superior	–n. laryngeus superior
lingual	–n. lingualis
long thoracic (serratus anterior)	–n. thoracicus longus
lumbar	–nn. lumbales
mandibular (V3)	–n. mandibularis
masseteric	–n. massetericus
maxillary (V2)	–n. maxillaris
median	–n. medianus
musculocutaneous	–n. musculocutaneus
mylohyoid	–n. mylohyoideus
nasociliary	–n. nasociliaris
nasopalatine	–n. nasopalatini
obturator	–n. obturatorius
occipital	
greater	–n. occipitalis major
lesser	–n. occipitalis minor
oculomotor (III)	–n. oculomotorius
olfactory (I)	–nn. olfactorii
opthalmic (V1)	–n. ophthalmicus
optic (II)	–n. opticus
palatine	
greater	–n. palatinus major
lesser	–nn. palatini minores
pectoral	–n. pectoralis
perineal	–nn. perineales
peroneal	
common	–n. fibularis communis
deep	–n. fibularis profundus
superficial	–n. fibularis superficialis
phrenic	–n. phrenicus
plantar	–n. plantaris
of pterygoid canal	–n. canalis pterygoidei
pudenal	–n. pudendus
to quadratus femoris	–n. musculi quadrati femoris
radial	–n. radialis
rectal inferior	–nn. rectales inferiores
sacral	–nn. sacrales
saphenous	–n. saphenus
sciatic	–n. ischiadicus
spinal	–nn. spinales
anterior rami	–rami anteriores
posterior rami	–rami posteriores
splanchnic	–n. splanchnicus
pelvic	–nn. pelvici splanchnici
subcostal	–n. subcostalis
subscapular	–nn. subcostalis
supraclavicular	–nn. supraclaviculares
supraorbital	–n. supraorbitalis
suprascapular	–n. suprascapularis
supratrochlear	–n. supratrochlearis
sural	–n. suralis
temporal, deep	–nn. temporales profundi
thoracic, long	–n. thoracicus longus
thoracodorsal	–n. thoracodorsalis
tibial	–n. tibialis
trigeminal (V)	–n. trigeminus
mandibular division (V3)	–n. mandibularis
maxillary division (V2)	–n. maxillaris
ophthalmic division (V1)	–n. ophthalmicus
trochlear (IV)	–n. trochlearis
ulnar	–n. ulnaris
vagus (X)	–n. vagus
vestibulocochlear (VIII)	–n. vestibulocochlearis
zygomatic	–n. zygomaticus
zygomaticofacial	–ramus zygomaticofacialis
zygomaticotemporal	–ramus zygomaticotemporalis
nervi erigentes	–nn. pelvici splanchnici
nervous system	–system nervosa
autonomic	–pars autonomica

ENGLISH	NOMINA ANATOMICA
nervous system (*cont.*)	
parasympathetic	–pars parasympathetica
sympathetic	–pars sympathetica
central	–pars centralis
peripheral	–pars peripherica
neuron	–neuron
nipple	–papilla mammaria
lactiferous duct	–ductus lactiferi
node	
atrioventricular	–nodus atrioventricularis
lymph	–nodus lymphaticus
aortic	–nodi lymphatici aortici
axillary	–nodi lymphatici axillares
cervical	–nodi lymphatici cervicales
iliac	–nodi lymphatici iliaci
inguinal	–nodi lymphatici inguinales
popliteal	–nodi lymphatici popliteales
supraclavicular	–nodi lymphatici supraclaviculares
sinoatrial	–nodus sinuatrialis
nose	–regio nasalis
nostrils	–nares
notch, cardiac of left lung	–incisura cardiaca
nucleus pulposus	–nucleus pulposus

O

ENGLISH	NOMINA ANATOMICA
occipital bone	–os occipitale
olecranon process	–olecranon
omentum	–omentum
bursa	–bursa omentalis
greater	–omentum majus
lesser	–omentum minus
opening	
of diaphragm	
aortic	–hiatus aorticus
caval	–foramen venae cavae
esophageal	–hiatus oesophageus
saphenous	–hiatus saphenus
vaginal	–ostium vaginae
oral cavity	–cavitas oris
orbit	–orbita
eyelids	–palpebrae
lacrimal apparatus	–apparatus lacrimalis
septum	–septum orbitale
orifice	–ostium
of stomach	
cardiac	–ostium cardiacum
pyloric	–ostium pyloricum
ureteric	–ostium ureteris
oropharynx	–pars oralis pharyngis
os, external	–ostium uteri
ovary	–ovarium

P

ENGLISH	NOMINA ANATOMICA
palate	
hard	–palatum durum
soft	–palatum molle
palatine bone	–os palatinum
palm	–palma manus
pancreas	–pancreas
papilla, duodenal	–papilla duodeni
parietal bone	–os parietale
part	–pars
patella	–patella
pedicle, vertebral	–pediculus arcus vertebrae
pelvis	–pelvis
floor (diaphragm)	–diaphragma pelvis
girdle	–cingulum membri inferioris
inlet	–apertura pelvis superior
renal	–pelvis renalis
of ureter	–pelvis renalis
penis	–penis

ENGLISH	NOMINA ANATOMICA
pericardium	–pericardium
fibrous	–pericardium fibrosum
serous	–pericardium serosum
perineum	–perineum
periosteum	–periosteum
peritoneum	–peritoneum
epiploic foramen	–foramen omentale
parietal	–peritoneum parietale
retroperitoneal organ	–organum extraperitoneale
visceral	–peritoneum viscerale
Peyer's patches	–folliculi lymphatici aggregati
phalanges	–ossa digitorum
pharynx	–pharynx
pia mater	–pia mater
pisiform bone	–os pisiforme
plate, cribriform	–lamina cribrosa
pleura	–pleura
cervical	–capula pleurae
mediastinal	–pleura mediastinalis
parietal	–pleura parietalis
visceral	–pleura visceralis
plexus	
nervous	–plexus nervosus
aortic	–plexus aorticus
brachial	–plexus brachialis
cardiac	–plexus cardiacus
celiac	–plexus coeliacus
cervical	–plexus cervicalis
esophageal	–plexus oesophagealis
hypogastric	–plexus hypogastricus
lumbar	–plexus lumbalis
pelvic	–pars pelvica systematis autonomica
pharyngeal	–plexus pharyngeus
pulmonary	–plexus pulmonalis
sacral	–plexus sacralis
venous	–plexus venosus
pampiniform	–plexus pampiniformis
prostatic	–plexus venosus prostaticus
pterygoid	–plexus pterygoideus
uterine	–plexus venosus uterinus
vesical	–plexus venosus vesicalis
plicae circulares	–plicae circulares
pneumatized bone	–os pneumaticum
pole	–extremitas
pons	–pons
porta hepatis	–porta hepatis
pouch	
of Douglas	–excavatio rectouterina
perineal	–spatium perinei
rectouterine	–excavatio rectouterina
rectovesical	–excavatio rectovesicalis
vesicouterine	–excavatio vesicouterina
prepuce	–preputium
process	
articular	–processus articularis
clinoid	–processus clinoideus
coracoid	–processus coracoideus
coronoid	–processus coronoideus
mastoid	–processus mastoideus
odontoid	–dens axis
spinous	–processus spinosus
styloid	–processus styloideus
transverse	–processus transversus
uncinate	–processus uncinatus
xiphoid	–processus xiphoideus
promontory of sacrum	–promontorium basi ossis sacri
protruberance, occipital	–protruberantia occipitalis
pubic bone	–os pubis
pylorus	–pylorus

R

ENGLISH	NOMINA ANATOMICA
radius	–radius

ENGLISH	NOMINA ANATOMICA
raphe	–raphe
anococcygeal	–ligamentum anococcygeum
pterygomandibular	–raphe pterygomandibularis
recess	
costodiaphragmatic	–recessus costodiaphragmaticus
sphenoethmoidal	–recessus sphenoethmoidalis
rectum	–rectum
retinaculum	
extensor, ankle	–retinaculum musculorum extensorum
extensor, wrist	–retinaculum extensorum
flexor, ankle	–retinaculum musculorum flexorum
flexor, wrist	–retinaculum flexorum
peroneal	–retinaculum musculorum peroneorum
rib	–os costale
false	–costae spuriae
floating	–costae fluitantes
true	–costae verae
ridge	
palatoglossal	–arcus palatoglossus
palatopharyngeal	–arcus palatopharyngeus
ring	
femoral	–annulus femoralis
fibrotendinous	–annulus tendineus communis
inguinal	–annulus inguinalis
root	–radix
of lung	–radix pulmonis
of mesentery	–radix mesenterii
of penis	–radix penis
rugae	–rugae
of stomach	–plicae gastrici

S

sac, lesser peritoneal	–bursa omentalis
sacrum	–os sacrum
scaphoid bone	–os scaphoideum
scapula	–scapula
scrotum	–scrotum
segments, bronchopulmonary	–segmenta bronchopulmonalia
sella turcica	–sella turcica
septum	
interatrial	–septum interatriale
intermuscular	–septum intermusculare
interventricular	–septum interventriculare
nasal	–septum nasi
orbitale	–septum orbitale
rectovesical	–septum rectovesicale
sesamoid bones	–ossa sesamoidea
sheath	
axillary	–fascia axillaris
carotid	–vagina carotica
fibrous flexor	–vaginae fibrosae digitorum
rectus	–vaginae musculi recti abdominis
synovial	–vaginae synoviales
shoulder joint	–articulatio humeri
sinus	–sinus
aortic	–sinus aortae
cartoid	–sinus caroticus
paranasal	–sinus paranasales
ethmoidal	–sinus ethmoidales
frontal	–sinus frontalis
maxillary	–sinus maxillaris
sphenoidal	–sinus sphenoidalis
pericardial	
oblique	–sinus obliquus pericardii
transverse	–sinus transversus pericardii
prostatic	–sinus prostaticus
pulmonary	–sinus trunci pulmonalis
renal	–sinus renalis
venous	
coronary	–sinus coronarius
dural	–sinus durae matris
cavernous	–sinus cavernosus

ENGLISH	NOMINA ANATOMICA
petrosal	–sinus petrosus
sagittal	–sinus sagittalis
sigmoid	–sinus sigmoideus
straight	–sinus rectus
transverse	–sinus transversus
skeleton	–skeleton
skin	–cutis
skull	–cranium
small intestine	–intestinum tenue
space	
extradural	–spatium epidurale
intercostal	–spatium intercostale
subarachnoid	–spatium subarachnoideum
subhepatic	–recessus subhepatici
subphrenic	–recessus subphrenici
sphenoid bone	–os sphenoidale
sphincter	–musculus sphincter
anal	–m. sphincter ani
of Oddi	–m. sphincter ampullae hepato-pancreatica
pupillae	–m. sphincter pupillae
pyloric	–m. sphincter pyloricus
urethral, external	–m. sphincter urethrae
spine	–columna vertebralis
cervical	–vertebrae cervicales
ischial	–spina ischiadica
lumbar	–vertebrae lumbales
of scapula	–spina scapulae
thoracic	–vertebrae thoracicae
spleen	–splen
sternum	–sternum
stomach	–gaster
cardiac notch	–incisura cardiaca
greater curvature	–curvatura gastrica major
lesser curvature	–curvatura gastrica minor
rugae	–plicae gastricae
sulcus	
intertubercular	–sulcus intertubercularis
terminalis	–sulcus terminalis
sustentaculum tali	–sustentaculum tali
sutures	–sutura
symphysis, pubic	–symphysis pubica

T

taeniae coli	–taeniae coli
tail	–cauda
talus bone	–talus
tarsal bones	–ossa tarsi
temporal bone	–os temporali
tendinous intersections	–intersectiones tendineae
tendon	
calcaneus (Achilles)	–tendo calcaneus
central, of diaphragm	–centrum tendineum
conjoint	–falx inguinalis
tentorium cerebelli	–tentorium cerebelli
testis	–testis
thigh	–femur
thorax	–thorax
bones	–ossa thoracis
inlet	–apertura thoracis superior
outlet	–apertura thoracis inferior
thumb	–pollex
thymus	–thymus
tibia	–tibia
tissue, connective	–textus connectivus
toe	–digitus pedis
great	–hallux
tongue	–lingua
muscles	–musculi linguae
tonsil	–tonsilla
trabeculae carneae	–trabeculae carneae
trachea	–trachea

ENGLISH	NOMINA ANATOMICA	ENGLISH	NOMINA ANATOMICA
tract, iliotibial	–tractus iliotibialis	ileocecal	–valva ileocaecalis
trapezium bone	–os trapezium	vena cava, inferior	–valvula venae cavae inferioris
trapezoid bone	–os trapezoideum	venous	–valvula venosa
tree, bronchial	–arbor bronchialis	vas deferens	–ductus deferens
triangle		vein	–vena
anal	–regio analis	axillary	–v. axillaris
femoral	–trigonum femorale	azygos	–v. azygos
of neck, anterior	–regio cervicalis anterior	basilic	–v. basilica
of neck, posterior	–regio cervicalis lateralis	brachiocephalic	–v. brachiocephalica
urogenital	–regio urogenitalis	cardiac	–vv. cordis
trigone, bladder	–trigonum vesicae	cava	–v. cava
triquetral bone	–os triquetrum	cephalic	–v. cephalica
trochlea	–trochlea	comitantes	–vv. comitantes
trunk		cystic	–v. cystica
brachiocephalic	–truncus brachiocephalicus	deep dorsal of penis	–v. dorsalis profunda penis
costocervical	–truncus costocervicalis	diploic	–vv. diploicae
lumbosacral	–truncus lumbosacralis	epigastric	–v. epigastrica
pulmonary	–truncus pulmonalis	femoral	–v. femoralis
sympathetic	–truncus sympatheticus	gastric	–vv. gastricae
tube		gastroepiploic	–v. gastroomentalis
auditory (Eustachian)	–tuba auditiva	hemiazygos	–v. hemiazygos
uterine	–tuba uterina	accessory	–v. hemiazygos accessoria
intramural part	–pars uterina	hepatic	–vv. hepaticae
tubercle, tuberosity		ileocolic	–v. ileocolica
calcaneal	–tuberculum calcanei	iliac	–v. iliaca
deltoid	–tuberositas deltoidea	intercostal	–vv. intercostales
gluteal	–tuberositas glutealis	jugular	–v. jugularis
infraglenoid	–tuberculum infraglenoidale	median cubital	–v. media cubiti
ischial	–tuber ischiadicum	meningeal	–vv. meningeae
pubic	–tuberculum pubicum	mesenteric	–v. mesenterica
radial	–tuberositas radii	musculophrenic	–vv. musculophrenicae
of rib	–tuberculum costae	ophthalmic	–v. ophthalmica
scalene	–tuberculum musculi scaleni anterioris	popliteal	–v. poplitea
supraglenoid	–tuberculum supraglenoidale	portal	–v. portae hepatis
tibial	–tuberositas tibiae	pudendal, external	–vv. pudendae externae
of ulna	–tuberositas ulnae	pulmonary	–vv. pulmonales
tunica		renal	–v. renalis
albuginae	–tunica albuginea	retromandibular	–v. retromandibularis
vaginalis	–tunica vaginalis	sacral	–vv. sacrales
tunnel, carpal	–canalis carpi	saphenous, long	–v. saphena magna
		saphenous, short	–v. saphena parva
		splenic	–v. splenica
U		subclavian	–v. subclavia
ulna	–ulna	suprarenal	–v. suprarenalis
umbilicus	–umbilicus	thoracic, internal	–v. thoracica interna
urachus	–urachus or ligamentum umbilicae medianum	thyroid	–vv. thyroideae
ureter	–ureter	vertebral	–v. vertebralis
urethra	–urethra	ventricle of heart	–ventriculus cordis
female	–urethra feminina	vertebra	–vertebra
male	–urethra masculina	cervical	–vertebrae cervicales
crest	–crista urethralis	lumbar	–vertebrae lumbales
membranous	–pars membranacea	prominens	–vertebra prominens
prostatic	–pars prostatica	sacral	–vertebrae sacrales
spongy	–pars spongiosa	thoracic	–vertebrae thoracicae
uterus		vesicle, seminal	–vesicula seminalis
surfaces		vincula vasculosa	–vincula tendinum
posterosuperior	–facies intestinalis	vomer	–vomer
anteroinferior	–facies vesicalis		
utricle	–utriculus prostaticus		
uvula	–uvula	**W**	
		wrist	–carpus
V			
vagina	–vagina	**X**	
vaginal opening	–ostium vaginae	xiphisternum	–processus xiphoideus
valve			
of heart		**Z**	
aortic	–valva aortae	zygoma	–os zygomaticum
semilunar cusp	–valvula semilunaris		
mitral (bicuspid)	–valva atrioventricularis sinistra		
pulmonary	–valva trunci pulmonalis		
tricuspid	–valva atrioventricularis dextra		

Index